1992
YEAR BOOK OF
NEUROLOGY AND
NEUROSURGERY®

The 1992 Year Book® Series

Year Book of Anesthesia and Pain Management: Drs. Miller, Kirby, Ostheimer, Roizen, and Stoelting

Year Book of Cardiology®: Drs. Schlant, Collins, Engle, Frye, Kaplan, and O'Rourke

Year Book of Critical Care Medicine®: Drs. Rogers and Parrillo

Year Book of Dentistry®: Drs. Meskin, Currier, Kennedy, Leinfelder, Matukas, and Rovin

Year Book of Dermatologic Surgery: Drs. Swanson, Salasche, and Glogau

Year Book of Dermatology®: Drs. Sober and Fitzpatrick

Year Book of Diagnostic Radiology®: Drs. Federle, Clark, Gross, Madewell, Maynard, Sackett, and Young

Year Book of Digestive Diseases®: Drs. Greenberger and Moody

Year Book of Drug Therapy®: Drs. Lasagna and Weintraub

Year Book of Emergency Medicine®: Drs. Wagner, Burdick, Davidson, Roberts, and Spivey

Year Book of Endocrinology®: Drs. Bagdade, Braverman, Horton, Kannan, Landsberg, Molitch, Morley, Odell, Rogol, Ryan, and Sherwin

Year Book of Family Practice®: Drs. Berg, Bowman, Davidson, Dietrich, and Scherger

Year Book of Geriatrics and Gerontology®: Drs. Beck, Abrass, Burton, Cummings, Makinodan, and Small

Year Book of Hand Surgery®: Drs. Amadio and Hentz

Year Book of Health Care Management: Drs. Heyssel, Brock, King, and Steinberg, Ms. Avakian, and Messrs. Berman, Kues, and Rosenberg

Year Book of Hematology®: Drs. Spivak, Bell, Ness, Quesenberry, and Wiernik

Year Book of Infectious Diseases®: Drs. Wolff, Barza, Keusch, Klempner, and Snydman

Year Book of Infertility: Drs. Mishell, Paulsen, and Lobo

Year Book of Medicine®: Drs. Rogers, Bone, Cline, Braunwald, Greenberger, Utiger, Epstein, and Malawista

Year Book of Neonatal and Perinatal Medicine®: Drs. Klaus and Fanaroff

Year Book of Nephrology®: Drs. Coe, Favus, Henderson, Kashgarian, Luke, Myers, and Strom

Year Book of Neurology and Neurosurgery®: Drs. Currier and Crowell

Year Book of Neuroradiology: Drs. Osborn, Harnsberger, Halbach, and Grossman

Year Book of Nuclear Medicine®: Drs. Hoffer, Gore, Gottschalk, Sostman, Zaret, and Zubal

Year Book of Obstetrics and Gynecology®: Drs. Mishell, Kirschbaum, and Morrow

Year Book of Occupational and Environmental Medicine: Drs. Emmett, Brooks, Harris, and Schenker

Year Book of Oncology: Drs. Young, Longo, Ozols, Simone, Steele, and Weichselbaum

Year Book of Ophthalmology®: Drs. Laibson, Adams, Augsberger, Benson, Cohen, Eagle, Flanagan, Nelson, Reinecke, Sergott, and Wilson

Year Book of Orthopedics®: Drs. Sledge, Poss, Cofield, Frymoyer, Griffin, Hansen, Johnson, Simmons, and Springfield

Year Book of Otolaryngology–Head and Neck Surgery®: Drs. Bailey and Paparella

Year Book of Pathology and Clinical Pathology®: Drs. Gardner, Bennett, Cousar, Garvin, and Worsham

Year Book of Pediatrics®: Dr. Stockman

Year Book of Plastic, Reconstructive, and Aesthetic Surgery: Drs. Miller, Cohen, McKinney, Robson, Ruberg, and Whitaker

Year Book of Podiatric Medicine and Surgery®: Dr. La Porta

Year Book of Psychiatry and Applied Mental Health®: Drs. Talbott, Frances, Freedman, Meltzer, Perry, Schowalter, and Yudofsky

Year Book of Pulmonary Disease®: Drs. Bone and Petty

Year Book of Speech, Language, and Hearing: Drs. Bernthal, Hall, and Tomblin

Year Book of Sports Medicine®: Drs. Shephard, Eichner, Sutton, and Torg, Col. Anderson, and Mr. George

Year Book of Surgery®: Drs. Schwartz, Jonasson, Robson, Shires, Spencer, and Thompson

Year Book of Transplantation: Drs. Ascher, Hansen, and Strom

Year Book of Ultrasound: Drs. Merritt, Mittelstaedt, Carroll, and Nyberg

Year Book of Urology®: Drs. Gillenwater and Howards

Year Book of Vascular Surgery®: Dr. Bergan

Roundsmanship '92–'93: A Year Book® Guide to Clinical Medicine: Drs. Dan, Feigin, Quilligan, Schrock, Stein, and Talbot

1992

The Year Book of NEUROLOGY AND NEUROSURGERY®

"Published without interruption since 1902"

Neurology

Editor

Robert D. Currier, M.D.

McCarty Professor and Chairman Emeritus, Department of Neurology, University of Mississippi Medical Center, Jackson, Mississippi

Neurosurgery

Editor

Robert M. Crowell, M.D.

Director of Cerebrovascular Surgery, Massachusetts General Hospital and Harvard Medical School, Boston, Massachusetts

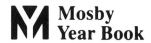
Mosby Year Book

St. Louis   Baltimore   Boston   Chicago   London   Philadelphia   Sydney   Toronto

Editor-in-Chief, Year Book Publishing: Kenneth H. Killion
Sponsoring Editor: Nancy G. Puckett
Manager, Medical Information Services: Edith M. Podrazik
Senior Medical Information Specialist: Terri Strorigl
Senior Medical Writer: David A. Cramer, M.D.
Assistant Director, Manuscript Services: Frances M. Perveiler
Associate Managing Editor, Year Book Editing Services: Elizabeth Fitch
Production Coordinator: Max F. Perez
Proofroom Manager: Barbara M. Kelly

Editorial Office:
Mosby-Year Book, Inc.
200 North LaSalle St.
Chicago, IL 60601

International Standard Serial Number: 0513-5117
International Standard Book Number: 0-8151-2141-5

Table of Contents

The material in this volume represents literature reviewed through March 1991.

Journals Represented

Mosby–Year Book subscribes to and surveys nearly 850 U.S. and foreign medical and allied health journals. From these journals, the Editors select the articles to be abstracted. Journals represented in this YEAR BOOK are listed below.

Acta Neurochirurgica
Acta Neurologica Scandinavica
Acta Orthopaedica Scandinavica
Acta Paediatrica Scandinavica
Alcohol and Alcoholism
Alzheimer's Disease and Associated Disorders
American Journal of Diseases of Children
American Journal of Neuroradiology
American Journal of Physiologic Imaging
American Journal of Psychiatry
American Journal of Roentgenology
American Surgeon
Anesthesia and Analgesia
Annals of Emergency Medicine
Annals of Internal Medicine
Annals of Neurology
Annals of Vascular Surgery
Aphasiology
Archives of Neurology
Archives of Otolaryngology–Head and Neck Surgery
Archives of Physical Medicine and Rehabilitation
Atherosclerosis
Brain and Cognition
Brain and Language
Brain–Journal of Neurology
British Journal of Cancer
British Journal of Psychiatry
British Medical Journal
Canadian Journal of Neurological Sciences
Cancer
Cancer Research
Cephalalgia
Clinica Chimica Acta
Cortex
Epilepsia
European Journal of Chiropractic
European Neurology
Headache
Hypertension
International Journal of Radiation, Oncology, Biology, and Physics
International Orthopaedics
Israel Journal of Medical Sciences
Journal de Radiologie
Journal of Bone and Joint Surgery (British Volume)
Journal of Clinical Investigation
Journal of Computer Assisted Tomography
Journal of Family Practice
Journal of Hypertension
Journal of Neurology, Neurosurgery and Psychiatry

Journal of Neuropathology and Experimental Neurology
Journal of Neurosurgery
Journal of Nuclear Medicine
Journal of Orthopaedic Research
Journal of Pediatrics
Journal of Reconstructive Microsurgery
Journal of Trauma
Journal of Vascular Surgery
Journal of the American Medical Association
Journal of the National Cancer Institute
Journal of the Neurological Sciences
Journal of the Royal Society of Medicine
Lancet
Life Sciences
Mayo Clinic Proceedings
Medical Journal of Australia
Movement Disorders
Muscle and Nerve
Nature
Neuro-Chirurgie
Neurobiology of Aging
Neurochirurgia
Neurology
Neuropsychologia
Neuroradiology
Neurosurgery
New England Journal of Medicine
Ophthalmology
PACE
Pain
Paraplegia
Pediatric Neurology
Pediatrics
Presse Medicale
Proceedings of the National Academy of Sciences
Psychological Medicine
ROFO: Fortschritte Auf Dem Gebiete Der Rontgenstrahlen Und Der
　　　Nuklearmedizin
Radiology
Science
Spine
Stroke
Surgical Neurology
Thorax
World Journal of Surgery

STANDARD ABBREVIATIONS

The following terms are abbreviated in this edition: acquired immunodeficiency syndrome (AIDS), central nervous system (CNS), cerebrospinal fluid (CSF), computed tomography (CT), electrocardiography (ECG), electroencephalogram (EEG), human immunodeficiency virus (HIV), and magnetic resonance (MR) imaging (MRI).

Publisher's Preface

The 1992 volume of the YEAR BOOK OF NEUROLOGY and NEUROSURGERY represents the tenth and final volume in which the Neurology section bears the stamp of Robert D. Currier, M.D. For the first seven of those volumes, he was co-editor of the section with the late Russell N. DeJong; since 1990, he has organized the section himself with invaluable collaboration from Drs. Appel, Evans, Galaburda, and Toole. Readers of this series no doubt have recognized Bob Currier's intellectual curiosity, enthusiasm, and clinical acumen throughout this decade of publishing.

Dr. Currier's successor beginning with the 1993 volume will be Walter G. Bradley, M.D., chairman of the Department of Neurology at University of Miami. Dr. Robert Crowell will continue to edit the Neurosurgery section.

The urge among those of us who have worked with Bob Currier these past several years is to fill the next few pages with emotional appreciation of his warmth and kindness, and with sincere admiration for his efficiency and resilience through many personal and professional challenges.

However, in the interest of brevity, suffice it to say that our work as publishers generally is a satisfying way to earn a living. Once in a while, when we work with someone like Bob Currier, our work transcends that, and it becomes a joyful way to live. For that transcendent experience, we are eternally grateful to Bob, and we wish him nothing but joy and satisfaction in all his future endeavors.

NEUROLOGY

ROBERT D. CURRIER, M.D.

Introduction

Although the YEAR BOOK series started in 1900, the first Neurology YEAR BOOK was published 2 years later in 1902—90 years ago. Volume 10 of that year's series was entitled, *Skin and Venereal Diseases, Nervous and Mental Diseases*. The editors were W.L. Baum and Hugh Patrick, with the collaboration of Charles Mix. Dr. Baum was professor of skin and venereal diseases at the Chicago Post-Graduate Medical School, and Dr. Patrick was clinical professor of nervous diseases at Northwestern University Medical School. The YEAR BOOKS in those days were intended for the general practitioner. There were 10 or 12 in the various specialty areas published each year. The physician would subscribe to them all and read them as they appeared throughout the year.

Hugh Patrick wrote a brief preface:

"In the preparation of the following pages, the Editor has kept constantly in mind the needs and wishes of the busy general practitioner, as he understands them. Consequently, in this brief indication of the year's literature, much of great interest has been omitted because of extreme technicality, multitudinous detail or inadaptability for immediate application in practice. For the same reason the Editor has felt in incumbent upon him to supplement the text with an occasional comment, adverse, commendatory or explanatory, which the reader will take for what he thinks it is worth. These comments are enclosed in brackets except when it is obvious that they emanate from the Editor."

It looks as though the editor in those days wrote the whole thing. Occasionally, an editorial note in brackets was inserted, but in general it was a summation of the literature of the previous year without comments. It could also be interpreted as being entirely comment. I like the part about taking it for what it is worth.

The journals reviewed were in three languages—English, French, and German. The only American journal devoted to the nervous system at that time was the *Journal of Nervous and Mental Diseases*. Reviewed was a most remarkable report by F.T. Stewart in the *Philadelphia Medical Journal* of June 7, 1902. A 26-year-old woman was shot with a 32-caliber revolver, ". . . the ball entering about one inch to the right of the 7th dorsal spine and passing directly into the spinal canal." There were "the ordinary symptoms of complete transverse lesion of the cord." At operation 3 hours later, the bullet was found in the spinal canal. The two ends of the spinal cord were separated by 3/4 of an inch, a finding that was verified by five physicians, all named, two assistants, the anesthetist, and an onlooker. The ends of the cord were approximated with catgut sutures after great difficulty, the cord tending to tear as the ends were pulled together. The dura could not be approximated. On the fifth day after operation the patient felt a sensation in her back when her calf was squeezed, and on the 42nd day a pin point was felt on each thigh. On the 60th day the patient could move her right toe readily, and at 16 months she flexed her toes, flexed and extended her legs, flexed and extended her thighs, and rotated her thighs; she was able to stand with either hand on the back of a chair, thus supporting much of the weight of her body, and had the sense of touch, temperature, and pain all over. The editor commented, ". . . with considerable diffidence, but a careful perusal of the paper leaves him with an unmistakable doubt that the spinal cord was completely severed." He believed that the rapidity of return of function precluded nerve regeneration. I wonder if those interested in spinal cord trauma and regeneration are aware of this paper?

By 1912 the YEAR BOOK had shed skin and venereal diseases and was entitled, *Nervous and Mental Diseases*. The editors were Hugh Patrick and Peter Bassoe of Rush Medical College. In it is recorded in four pages the only understandable explanation of psychoanalysis I have read, a review of an article by James J. Putnam (*Boston Med Surg J*, Jan 25, 1912). The review, and possibly the original, might be worth reading today. Patrick also commented on Charles H. Frazier's report of 63 surgically treated epileptic patients (*Therap Gaz*, March 1912). Frazier obtained "gratifying results" in 10% to 25% of his patients. In many cases, nothing was found at operation. Such were the beginnings of epilepsy surgery. In the same issue is a report by O. Foerster (*Berlin Clin Wochenschr*, May 20, 1912) on the beginnings of brain biopsy. Foerster had done 16 needle biopsies and had been able to diagnose paretic dementia, arteriosclerotic brain disease, and multiple sclerosis by this method. The editor commented that it was not likely to be adopted by anyone "outside the large clinics of continental Europe. Similar harpooning of the liver and spleen has also been practiced. . .but the method is not without danger." Wilson's description of progressive lenticular degeneration is given (*Brain* 34:295–509, 1912), 7 pages and several photographs. Twenty-four pages is given to poliomyelitis, the scourge of the day.

The 1922 YEAR BOOK OF NERVOUS AND MENTAL DISEASES, edited by Peter Bassoe alone, had much on syphilis, much on encephalitis lethargica in its myriad forms, and several comments on multiple sclerosis but nothing on amyotrophic lateral sclerosis or headache. The only mention of ischemic stroke was a note by H. Mella on cortical blindness secondary to bilateral calcarine softening.

The 1932 YEAR BOOK OF NEUROLOGY AND PSYCHIATRY, the Neurology portion still edited by Peter Bassoe, and the psychiatry portion by Franklin Ebaugh of Colorado, had much on migraine, which was listed as one of the neuroses, a listing that also included epilepsy and narcolepsy. A fine review article on migraine by Henry Alsop Riley (*Bull Neurol Inst, New York*, 2:429, 1932) was presented in some detail. No definite conclusion about either the cause or the treatment was reached. This is the first of these volumes that belonged to my father, and in it I find an old prescription blank on which his specialty is listed as neurology. That is a surprise. I had always thought that he considered himself a neuropsychiatrist. He had a back door to his office for the alienated gentry. Macdonald Critchley discussed a paper on the treatment of syphilis by David Lees (*Br J Vener Dis*, October, 1932). Critchley, a personal hero, is still in good form 60 years later. I sent him a copy of last year's YEAR BOOK. He replied with a lovely note: "Since I am now 91, I am, of course, retired, but I am still a victim of *cacoethes scribendi* (or scribbler's itch)," and included samples of his latest, all in good form. I have the same disease and hope that I can also scribble for eight decades.

The 1942 YEAR BOOK OF NEUROLOGY, PSYCHIATRY AND ENDOCRINOLOGY was edited by Hans Reese (Neurology), Nolan Lewis (Psychiatry), and E.L. Severinghaus (Endocrinology). Dr. Reese in his introduction comments that publications from the Axis-dominated areas reached the United States and YEAR BOOK only sporadically. He noted sadly the "upheavals and eruptions created by decivilized groups in a nation." This is the first of the modern era of YEAR BOOKS, which had by this time changed their focus from the general practitioner to the specialist. Again, ischemic strokes are given no notice, but cerebral hemorrhage, sinus thrombosis, sickle cell disease and its effect on the brain, Buerger's disease, and blast injury were. A long comment on a report from Albany College (*Arch Neurol Psychiatry* 47:645–661, 1942) on the improvement after thymectomy for thymoma experienced by a patient with myasthenia gravis was in the endocrinology, not the neurology, section. And, good grief, in the psychiatric section is reviewed an article by my mother's psychoanalyst brother, my uncle Ed (Edward D. Hoedemaker) (*Ann Intern Med* 17:486–495, 1942), on two patients who had chest sensations beginning in childhood that represented repressed anger against their fathers. In adult life coronary artery disease developed in both. I wonder how Uncle Ed got along with his father, my grandfather, whom I never knew. A little farther on is a comment on an article on war neuroses during the seige of Tobruk. Those Australians defending Tobruk are considered nowadays, 50 years later, as having been men of steel withstanding Rommel's Afrika Korps. But here's a report of 132 suffering from anxiety (*Med J Aust* 2:73–77, 1942)—of course, humans, just like the rest us.

The 1952 YEAR BOOK OF NEUROLOGY, PSYCHIATRY AND NEUROSURGERY (dropping Endocrinology and adding Neurosurgery), edited by Roland Mackay of Chicago, Nolan Lewis for psychiatry, and Percival Bailey for neurosurgery, finally accepted stroke as a neurologic disease. There are comments on Fisher's paper on the carotid artery syndrome—the eye on one side and the hemiplegia on the other, and an autopsy study of 100 stroke patients by Hicks and Warren—at autopsy, 60% had no thrombosis of any vessel that could be seen.

The 1962–1963 YEAR BOOK was edited by Mackay, Sam Wortis for Psychiatry, and Oscar Sugar for Neurosurgery. Mackay in the introduction noted the difficulty of selecting articles and commenting on the year's publications. "To make a relatively small but representative selection from the vast amount of each year's neurologic publications is an exercise of some daring; to summarize this selection in a few paragraphs designed to present the current visage of neurology is indeed presumptuous. To escape from one's personal myopia and bias, to judge between the significant and the trivial, and to assess relative importance requires a quixotic self-assurance that is quite artificial." He states in the introduction that, "vascular disorders of course still constitute a great bulk of the clinician's problems." He complained of the tendency to order studies rather than examine the patient, and gave vent to his feelings about the Wartenberg wheel in the sensory examination—"a thing of the devil." The 1972 YEAR BOOK OF NEUROLOGY AND NEUROSURGERY (Psychiatry was now omitted) was edited by Russell DeJong and Sugar and had much the same format as the present one. Dr. DeJong noted in the introduction that the publication time would be changed to the first of the year so it would be available to candidates in neurology and neurosurgery studying for their spring written examinations.

And, finally, 10 years ago I briefly reviewed peptides, muscle relaxants, stroke, parkinsonism, and multiple sclerosis. My introductory comments were the first in which I went afield from clinical neurology to consider things of general interest to neurologists such as the possible oversupply of neurologists, fees, and what should be included in the YEAR BOOK (actually, it now seems, an old theme). As you can see, the tendency to ramble has gotten worse, and the introduction you are reading may set a record for length of introductory remarks. My bias in selection of articles is now evident and for all to see. Not a single article on AIDS, the current scourge of the country and the world, has been included. My optimism last year that the disease might be peaking is gainsaid by a letter in the *New England Journal of Medicine* (Steel and Haverkos, *N Engl J Med* 325:65–66, 1991). It seems that the peak was a mirage, and the case numbers are still ascending. Why have we not selected an article about this disease, which more often than not affects the nervous system? The fact that most patients who have it are taken care of by internal medicine–infectious disease specialists is only an excuse. The truth is that I don't like the disease and have turned my back on it in the hopes that it will go away.

It's a good time to mention some names. During these 10 years there have been many at Year Book who have done most of the work. Rich Lampert, John Matusik, Nancy Gorham, Caroline Scoulas, Judy Plazyk, Carla White, and Nancy Puckett have been forever forgiving of my delays, memory lapses, and poor English. And those higher up in the Mosby–Year Book and Times Mirror organizations, most of whom I have never met, have kept the YEAR BOOK, which I remember on my Dad's cigar stand next to his pipe and dish of peanuts, alive and allowed the *KEY* concept to be born and nurtured; both should survive until the year 2002. Walter Bradley, do you hear?

Many neurologists have given depth to the YEAR BOOK and the KEY, two having become my friends in the process—Albert Galaburda and Stanley Appel. O.B. (Bev) Evans, Jim Toole, and Armin Haerer, already good friends, have with superb ability commented and brought together various topics for review. Robert Crowell in the traces with me these 10 years had not bucked or kicked once. Bill Anderson, Dan Darnley, Paul Richter, and Bob Joynt have kept me up with helpful feedback.

R.D. Currier, M.D.

1 Diagnostics and Imaging

Multiple Sclerosis: Specificity of MR for Diagnosis
Yetkin FZ, Haughton VM, Papke RA, Fischer ME, Rao SM (Med College of Wisconsin; Froedtert Mem Lutheran Hosp, Milwaukee)
Radiology 178:447–451, 1991   1–1

As many as 20% of control subjects have periventricular foci of high signal intensity on MR images. It is not clear how accurately radiologists are able to distinguish between these "bright objects" and plaques of multiple sclerosis.

The MR images from 92 patients with multiple sclerosis, 10 healthy controls, and 68 patients with hypertension or dementia were read by 2 experienced neuroradiologists in a blinded manner. Axial MR sections were acquired using a quadrature head coil.

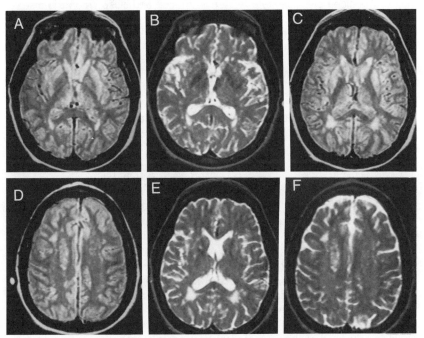

Fig 1–1.—A,C,E, proton density (2,000/20) and B,D,F, T2-weighted (2,000/70) MR images of a hypertensive control subject with nonspecific periventricular lesions. The images were read as negative for MS. (Courtesy of Yetkin FZ, Haughton VM, Papke RA, et al: *Radiology* 178:447–451, 1991.)

The specificity of an MR diagnosis of multiple sclerosis ranged from 95% to 99%, when considering true negative findings in relation to all non–multiple-sclerosis cases. The sensitivity of diagnosing multiple sclerosis ranged from 68%, when suspect cases were considered negative, to 80% when they were considered negative, to 80% when they were considered positive. Findings in a hypertensive control are shown in Figure 1–1. Agreement between the readers was excellent for all multiple sclerosis patients and controls. The MR diagnosis of multiple sclerosis is highly specific; nevertheless, up to 4% of healthy persons have periventricular changes that cannot be distinguished from multiple sclerosis on current criteria.

▶ These investigators found a 95% to 99% accuracy of MR in diagnosis of multiple sclerosis if the subjects' age and sex also were known. This article deals with patients with confirmed established multiple sclerosis. What we need now are tests that will have some predictive value in early multiple sclerosis. I suspect they will come, too. When they do arrive, we will know who is a candidate for treatment. It may be several years yet, however.

Harris et al. (1), in an interesting study of 6 patients with active multiple sclerosis, found that when MRI scanning was enhanced with gadolinium and done frequently, the lesions tended to come and go, usually lasted for less than a month, and were often not associated with clinical symptoms. This is confirmation of the blood brain barrier's tendency to open and close when the disease is active.— R.D. Currier, M.D.

Reference

1. Harris JO, et al: *Ann Neurol* 29:548, 1991.

Sydenham Chorea: MR Manifestations in Two Cases
Kienzle GD, Breger RK, Chun RWM, Zupanc ML, Sackett JF (Univ of Wisconsin Health Ctr, Madison)
AJNR 12:73–76, 1991   1–2

The acute onset of a unilateral choreiform movement disorder in a child who has recently had a febrile illness or streptococcal pharyngitis suggests Sydenham's chorea. The MR manifestations of Sydenham's chorea were described in 2 children.

Girl, 8 years, experienced bitemporal headaches accompanied by a mild fever, left arm and leg choreiform movements, facial weakness, drooling, and slurred speech. A throat culture demonstrated β-hemolytic streptococci. Within 44 days of symptom onset, MRI was done on 3 separate occasions. The initial study, done 3 days after symptom onset, showed signal intensity on T2-weighted images involving the head of the right caudate nucleus and contiguous part of the putamen and bridging striations. A mass effect on the adjacent frontal horn of the right lateral ventricle appeared on T1-weighted coronal images (Fig 1–2). Twelve

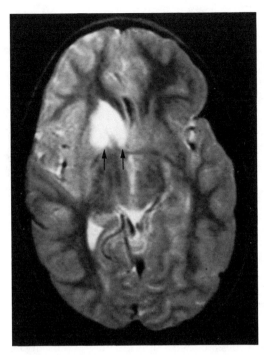

Fig 1–2.—Initial MR study in an 8-year-old girl obtained 3 days after onset of chorea. Axial T2-weighted (2,500/80/2) image shows increased signal intensity involving the head of the right caudate nucleus and contiguous anterior putamen *(arrows)*. (Courtesy of Kienzle GD, Breger RK, Chun RWM, et al: *AJNR* 12:73–76, 1991.)

days later axial T2-weighted images showed an interval reduction in the size of the right caudate and putaminal abnormalities. After gadopentetate dimeglumine administration, enhancement of the right caudate head and adjacent putamen was observed on T1-weighted images. Sydenham's chorea was diagnosed, and antibiotic therapy started.

In these 2 children, increased signal intensity in the corpus striatum contralateral to the symptomatic side was seen on T2-weighted images. Focal enhancement in the involved head of the caudate was demonstrated after gadopentetate dimeglumine administration. The MR findings correlated with anatomical areas thought to be susceptible to cross-reaction with IgG antibodies formed in association with streptococcal infection.

▶ There has been much discussion over the years of the site of pathology of Sydenham's chorea, and this may finally be the real thing. It's a fascinating finding and one that I would not have predicted. The head of the caudate and the putamen seem to be the preferred sites. These then are the lesions that cause chorea with no other manifestations. Klawans, in the same issue of *AJNR* (1), makes helpful remarks that aid our understanding of the syndrome, but why does this allergic phenomenon localize to the anterior basal ganglia region? The authors report that Husby et al. (2), examining patients with rheumatic fever, frequently found sera with IgG antibodies that demonstrated cross-reactivity and high affinity for antigens from the caudate and subthalamic nuclei.

Recently reported is a British study of the usefulness of the MRI scanner (3). These investigators found it was of help to the physician 73% of the time but did not improve the patient's quality of life measured over a 4-month period. I should think it beneficial to both physician and patient to know what was going on, and the quality-of-life benefit might well take longer than 4 months to be appreciated. To the neurologist, MRI is the eighth wonder of the world.— R.D. Currier, M.D.

References

1. Klawans HL: *AJNR* 12:77, 1991.
2. Husby G, et al: *J Exper Med* 144:1094, 1976.
3. Dixon AK, et al: *Br Med J* 302:79, 1991.
4.

Early Cerebral Infarction: Gadopentetate Dimeglumine Enhancement
Elster AD, Moody DM (Bowman Gray School of Medicine, Wake Forest Univ, Winston-Salem, NC)
Radiology 177:627–632, 1990   1–3

Preliminary studies have shown that gadopentetate dimeglumine enhances cerebral infarction in a manner similar to iodinated contrast agents used in CT. The early findings with dimeglumine enhancement were studied in 77 consecutive patients referred for cranial MRI within 2 weeks of the clinical onset of cerebral infarction.

Satisfactory images were acquired from 50 patients with subacute infarction. High-field-strength studies were carried out using spin-echo pulse sequencing. Gadopentetate dimeglumine was given intravenously in a dose of .1 mM/kg.

In 4 cases infarcts were seen only on unenhanced spin-density or T2-weighted images. Half of the patients had classic parenchymal enhance-

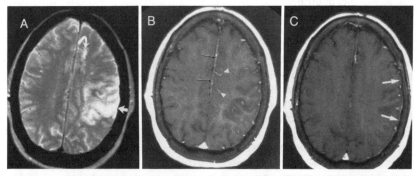

Fig 1–3.—Meningeal enhancement sign in a patient with a 2-day-old infarct of the right side of the posterior cerebral artery. **A,** T2-weighted image shows high signal intensity in the right occipital lobe consistent with an infarct. **B,C,** enhancement of the tentorium *(arrows)* is seen on axial (**B**) and coronal (**C**) images obtained after administration of gadopentetate dimeglumine. (Courtesy of Elster AD, Moody DM: *Radiology* 177:627–632, 1990.)

ment with gadopentetate dimeglumine, starting as early as 2–3 days after infarction. In many cases there was enhancement within vessels supplying the affected region. Contrast enhancement of the adjacent meninges (Fig 1–3) also was noted. A transitional phase of enhancement was seen in a few patients with infarcts 4–6 days old. The MR images showed either intravascular or meningeal enhancement as well as parenchymal enhancement in these cases, presumably reflecting vascular engorgement, sluggish blood flow, and early breakdown of the blood-brain barrier. Magnetic resonance imaging with gadopentetate dimeglumine demonstrates flow-related abnormalities before classic parenchymal enhancement develops in patients with early cerebral infarction.

▶ The enhanced MRI scan of stroke evolves from day 1, initially showing the vessels in the infarcted area, then the meninges over the infarct, and finally a combination of those appearances plus the infarction itself in the third stage. This explains some of those weird things we have been seeing on MRI scans.— R.D. Currier, M.D.

Cerebral Infarction: Early Detection by Means of Contrast-Enhanced Cerebral Arteries at MR Imaging
Sato A, Takahashi S, Soma Y, Ishii K, Kikuchi Y, Watanabe T, Sakamoto K
(Takeda Hosp, Aizuwakamatsu; Tohoku Univ, Sendai, Japan)
Radiology 178:433–439, 1991   1–4

Magnetic resonance imaging is useful in detecting cerebral infarction, but its utility in detecting an infarcted lesion within 24 hours of the ictus has not been established. A new MR sign of acute cerebral ischemia/infarction was identified.

Eight patients with acute cerebral ischemia/infarction were studied retrospectively (Fig 1–4). Each had undergone MRI within 26 hours of symptom onset and again 4–18 days after ictus. Abnormally contrast-enhanced curvilinear structures were demonstrated within 26 hours on contrast-enhanced, high-field-strength, T1-weighted, spin-echo images. The abnormal enhancement was thought to represent cortical arterial vessels of markedly slowed circulation in regions of underlying brain injury that would eventually progress to frank infarction. This was shown by CT and later MR evaluations. The degree of contrast enhancement of vessels generally appeared to be most intense in the proximal positions. The intensity of enhancement gradually declined in the more distal parts of those vessels as they pass over the convexities and finally disappeared.

Abnormally enhanced vessels observed in T1-weighted MR images represent an early sign of evolving cerebral ischemia/infarction. This sign appears to indicate marked slowing of the arterial circulation in the area of evolving ischemia/infarction. It may be seen immediately after a major

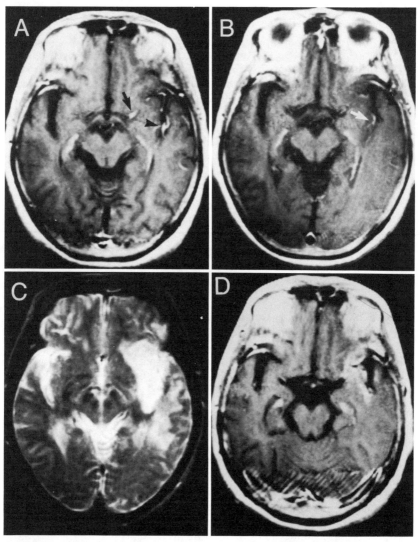

Fig 1–4.—Magnetic resonance images of cerebral ischemia/infarction in the frontotemporoparietal region and the basal ganglia. Contrast-enhance T1-weighted images obtained 2 hours after ictus. Abnormally enhanced curvilinear structures are seen along the surfaces of the insular-opercular region and temporoparieto-occipital region on the left *(arrowheads)*. The enhanced structures are considered to represent arterial vessels in those areas, and the degree of enhancement appears most intense in the proximal part along the insular-opercular region, gradually diminishing distally over higher parieto-temporo-occipital convexity. The proximal middle cerebral artery also appears enhanced *(arrow)*. (Courtesy of Sato A, Takahashi S, Soma Y, et al: *Radiology* 178:433–439, 1991.)

vessel is occluded. This sign should therefore be considered crucial for possible institution of thrombolytic treatment and/or surgical therapy for revascularization in patients in a hyperacute stage of cerebral ischemia/infarction.

▶ This looks like a neat trick. The small arterial vessels enhance in the region of infarction caused by slow flow. As MRI scans become more popular, this may be the preferred method of evaluating possible early infarction.— R.D. Currier, M.D.

Intracranial Aneurysms: Evaluation by MR Angiography

Ross JS, Masaryk TJ, Modic MT, Ruggieri PM, Haacke EM, Selman WR (Univ Hosps of Cleveland/Case Western Reserve Univ)
AJR 155:159–165, 1990   1–5

With 3-dimensional gradient echo sequence, MR angiography (MRA) provides an accurate anatomical depiction of intracranial vasculature and vascular pathology. The accuracy of volume gradient-echo MRA was compared with that of intra-arterial digital subtraction angiography (IA DSA). Of the 47 patients studied by MRA, 19 had saccular or giant intracranial aneurysms confirmed on IA DSA and 28 had no aneurysms and served as controls. Sensitivity and specificity were calculated for evaluation of the cine 3D reconstruction (cine MRA) only; cine MRA + inspection of the individual partitions; and cine MRA + individual partitions + spin-echo (SE) studies.

In the aneurysm group, MRA images were of diagnostic quality in 84% of the patients (Fig 1–5). For the 21 aneurysms, including 3 that were missed in 2 patients, the sensitivity varied from 67% for cine MRA only to 86% for the cine MRA + partitions + SE studies. For the 19 patients in whom it was assumed that the diagnosis of any 1 aneurysm would lead to angiography and detection of additional aneurysms, the

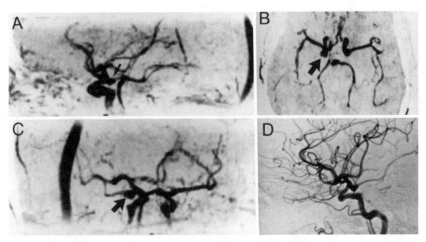

Fig 1–5.—Posterior communicating artery aneurysm. Lateral *(A)*, base *(B)*, and right anterior oblique *(C)* views of 3D MR angiogram show 6–mm right posterior communicating artery aneurysm *(arrows)* with good visualization of intracranial circulation. Lateral view *(D)* from intra-arterial digital subtraction angiogram also shows aneurysm, which measures 7 mm. (Courtesy of Ross JS, Masaryk TJ, Modic MT, et al: *AJR* 155:159–165, 1990.)

sensitivity varied from 73% for cine MRA only to 95% for the cine MRA + partitions + SE studies.

These findings suggest that MRA can define the circle of Willis sufficiently to allow detection of intracranial aneurysms as small as 3–4 mm. Magnetic resonance angiography is a promising noninvasive screening procedure for intracranial vasculature in patients at risk for aneurysm.

▶ Magnetic resonance angiography is almost equal to arteriography in showing aneurysms and perhaps some day will supplant the latter technique. When that day comes, I will be glad. I have always worried about the part played by the angiographic process and dye in the production of vasospasm. Will vasospasm decrease when MRA takes over?—R.D. Currier, M.D.

Contrast Enhancement of the Labyrinth on MR Scans in Patients With Sudden Hearing Loss and Vertigo: Evidence of Labyrinthine Disease
Seltzer S, Mark AS (George Washington Univ; Washington Hosp Ctr, Washington, DC)
AJNR 12:13–16, 1991   1–6

The sudden onset of hearing loss, with or without vertigo, is a diagnostic challenge. Labyrinthine enhancement was observed on gadopentetate dimeglumine-enhanced MRI in 5 patients with sudden hearing loss and/or vertigo. All 5 patients were studied with T2-weighted axial images through the whole brain, contrast-enhanced 3-mm axial T1-weighted images through the temporal bone, and enhanced T1-weighted sagittal images through the whole brain. Findings on MR were correlated with audiologic and electronystagmographic (ENG) studies. Three patients had recent or concurrent viral illness and 2 had leutic labyrinthitis.

Cochlear enhancement was present on the symptomatic side in 4 patients with unilateral hearing loss and in the profoundly deaf ear of 1 patient with bilateral but asymmetric hearing loss (Fig 1–6). Of 4 patients with vertigo, vestibular enhancement was present only in 3 with severe

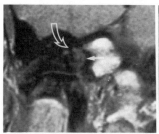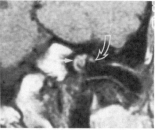

Fig 1–6.—T1-weighted enhanced images, 600/24/4, in patient with profound right-sided hearing loss, facial palsy on the right, moderate left-sided hearing loss, and positive CSF and blood serology for syphilis. Coronal image shows enhancement of right cochlea *(solid arrows)* and right facial nerve *(open arrows)*. Left cochlea and facial nerve are normal. (Courtesy of Seltzer S, Mark AS: *AJNR* 12:13–16, 1991.)

ENG abnormalities. In 2 patients, follow-up MR studies 4–6 months later showed resolution of the cochlear enhancement that correlated with resolution of symptoms. In contrast, labyrinthine enhancement was not seen in 30 controls or in 6 patients with acoustic neuromas studied with contrast-enhanced MR.

Enhancement of the labyrinth on contrast-enhanced MRI appears to be a highly specific sign of labyrinthine disease. Because abnormalities on ENG and audiograms are nonspecific and indicate only a sensorineural problem, contrast-enhanced MR scans may distinguish patients with retrocochlear lesions (e.g., acoustic neuromas) from those in whom the abnormal process is labyrinthine or intra-axial. It is important to carefully scrutinize the structures of the membranous labyrinth, in addition to the internal auditory canal, cerebellopontine angle, and the brain stem, when evaluating a patient with sudden hearing loss or vertigo.

▶ Sudden loss of hearing with vertigo is a diagnostic and therapeutic problem, and if the MRI scan with contrast enhancement shows the lesion of acute labyrinthitis, its use will become common. The authors don't state how soon the MRI changes appear, nor do they say that all patients with the syndrome have it, but one assumes that their series is consecutive. Now when we say to patients that they have "inner ear disease," we may be telling the truth.— R.D. Currier, M.D.

Contrast-Enhanced MR Imaging of the Facial Nerve in 11 Patients With Bell's Palsy

Tien R, Dillon WP, Jackler RK (Univ of California, San Francisco)
AJR 155:573–579, 1990   1–7

The clinical or radiographic diagnosis of idiopathic facial palsy (Bell's palsy) is usually by exclusion. Imaging is warranted when paralysis lasts longer than the 6–8 weeks typical of Bell's palsy or when symptoms are atypical. Recent reports have shown that the intratemporal part of the facial nerve is enhanced in MR images using gadopentetate dimeglumine (GPDG) in Bell's or postoperative facial palsy.

Five patients with acute Bell's palsy, 3 with chronic Bell's palsy, and 3 with facial palsies of other types were studied by pre- and postcontrast axial and coronal MRI of the temporal bone area. Contrast was achieved with GPDG, .1 mmol/kg, and T1-weighted images were obtained immediately. The intensity of the affected nerve was compared with that of the unaffected nerve in pre- and postcontrast images. In all of the Bell's palsy patients and 2 of the others, diffuse, uniform enhancement of the affected facial nerve was observed from the fallopian canal to the stylomastoid foramen, including the geniculate ganglion and upper and lower nerve segments (Fig 1–7).

The configuration of enhancement observed is compatible with the hy-

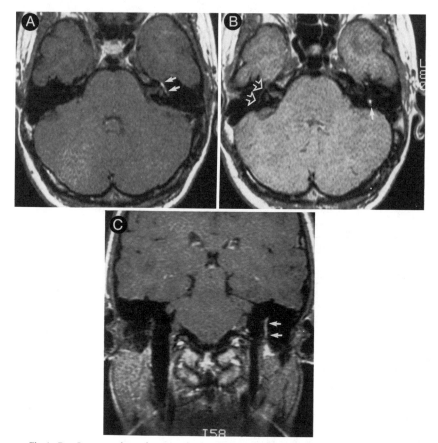

Fig 1–7.—Contrast-enhanced, 11-weighted MR images of 12-year-old boy with acute left Bell's palsy. **A,** axial image (600/20) shows intense enhancement of horizontal portion of facial nerve *(arrows)* and no enhancement of opposite, unaffected nerve. **B,** axial image 3 mm below previous image shows enhancement of affected descending portion of left facial nerve *(closed arrow).* Normal horizontal portion of right facial nerve does not enhance *(open arrows).* **C,** coronal image through temporal bone shows intense enhancement of descending portion of left facial nerve *(arrows).* (Courtesy of Tien R, Dillon WP, Jackler RK: *AJR* 155:573–579, 1990.)

pothesis that viral geniculate ganglionitis and nerve entrapment caused by subsequent swelling within the fallopian canal are responsible for Bell's palsy. With the positive diagnostic criteria described here for this relatively benign condition, patient fears of more sinister causes for their facial paralysis can promptly be set to rest, and therapy for viral neuritis can be started.

▶ I hope that these lesions of the affected facial nerves show up well in the Figure so you will be convinced that this is an excellent way to look at them. Enhanced MRI may permit a positive radiographic diagnosis of Bell's palsy. Another triumph for MR. Now the question is: Should we get an MR scan in every patient with Bell's palsy? I hope not.—R.D. Currier, M.D.

MR Imaging in Patients With Temporal Lobe Seizures: Correlation of Results With Pathologic Findings

Heinz ER, Crain BJ, Radtke RA, Burger PC, Friedman AH, Djang WT, Wilkinson WE (Duke Univ)
AJR 155:581–586, 1990   1–8

Drug therapy is often ineffective against seizures that arise from a focus in the mesial temporal lobe, whereas temporal lobectomy can result in a complete cure or significant improvement in seizure activity. In the past, EEG has provided the major data on the location of such seizures. A number of studies have shown MRI to be an excellent diagnostic method in temporal lobe epilepsy. Researchers report the use of MRI in 39 patients with complex partial seizures.

On the basis of pathologic findings after lobectomy, the patients were divided into 3 groups. Group 1 (13 patients) had neoplasms or other abnormal tissue; group 2 (13 patients) with classic mesial temporal sclerosis (MTS) had moderate to severe gliosis and neuronal loss; group 3 (14 patients) had incomplete pathologic data, although most probably had MTS.

In group 1, MRI revealed significant increases in signal intensity (3+) in 8 patients. In 4 of the remaining patients a moderate increase in signal intensity (2+) was observed, and in 1, a minimal increase (1+). Eight patients in group 2 had an abnormal MR signal in the temporal lobe; mass deformity or calcification was not established in any of these patients. In group 3, MR studies revealed a 1+ increase in signal in 5 patients; another had a 2+ signal. All of the 8 controls (scattered throughout the series) were normal.

The findings suggest that MRI can detect almost all tumors and a significant number of MTS lesions in patients with complex partial seizures. All of the patients in this series with very high signal intensity (3+) had neoplasms, and most with subtle but definite tissue signal abnormalities (1+) had either MTS or an incomplete pathologic examination.

▶ Magnetic resonance is a blessing when it comes to patients with temporal lobe seizures, and the yield from careful MR studies seems to be going up with further refinements.

The next article (Abstract 1–9) reinforces the thought, and Jackson et al. (1) in a study of 81 patients agree.— R.D. Currier, M.D.

Reference

1. Jackson GD, et al: *Neurology* 40:1869, 1990.

Temporal Lobe Seizures: Lateralization With MR Volume Measurements of the Hippocampal Formation

Jack CR Jr, Sharbrough FW, Twomey CK, Cascino GD, Hirschorn KA, Marsh WR, Zinsmeister AR, Scheithauer B (Mayo Clinic and Found, Rochester, Minn)
Radiology 175:423–429, 1990   1–9

At the study institution, patients who are surgical candidates for medically intractable temporal lobe epilepsy (TLE) undergo clinical and EEG evaluation to lateralize the seizure disorder. But the determination of which side to operate on is not always straightforward. The ability of each of 5 different MRI-based tests to lateralize the seizure disorder was assessed.

Forty-one right-handed patients with presumed mesial sclerosis underwent surgery for medically refractory TLE. All MR studies were performed at 1.5 T on a Signa unit (Fig 1–8). The 5 tests compared—in order of decreasing usefulness—were hippocampal formation (HF) volume measurements, visual grading of MR images for unilateral HF atrophy, anterior temporal lobe volume measurements, visual grading of MR images for unilateral anterior temporal lobe atrophy, and evidence of

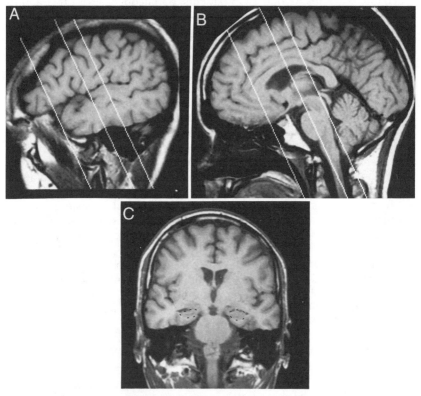

Fig 1–8.—Volume measurement in patient with right-side seizures. **A,** parasagittal image defines the orientation of the left temporal lobe. Cursors demarcate the orientation in which the oblique coronal images are acquired. **B,** midline sagittal image, with cursors demarcating the orientation of the oblique coronal images. From posterior to anterior, the 3 cursor lines depict the oblique coronal plane through the posterior commissure, which defines the posterior margin of both the HF and anterior temporal lobe (ATL), the most anterior section of the HF, and the most anterior section of the ATL. **C,** oblique coronal image in which the HFs are outlined *(dashes)* as they would be for volume measurements, on the normal *(left)* and atrophic *(right)* sides. (Courtesy of Jack CR Jr, Sharbrough FW, Twomey CK, et al: *Radiology* 175:423–429, 1990.)

unilateral medial temporal lobe signal intensity abnormalities on long repetition time MR images.

To quantify unilateral HF atrophy with a single number, a right-side minus left-side volume (DHF) was obtained. Whereas patients with right-sided seizures had a median DHF of $-.4$ cm^3, those with left-sided seizures had a median DHF of .8 cm^3. This finding was consistent with atrophy of the HF ipsilateral to the seizure disorder. Measurements of DHF had a sensitivity of 76% and a specificity of 100% when conservative volumetric threshold values ($-.2$ cm^3 and .6 cm^3) were used to separate individual DHF measurements into right-side abnormal, indeterminate, and left-side abnormal.

The "gold standard" in lateralization of the seizure disorder in these 41 patients was clinical and video-recorded EEG localizing criteria. Postoperative follow-up supported the accuracy of the clinical–EEG criteria for seizure lateralization. When quantitative MR evidence of HF atrophy does not correlate with this gold standard, chronic invasive electrophysiologic monitoring may be needed.

▶ These investigators very carefully measured the volume of the HF on MR slices and found that the method was 100% specific for correct lateralization of mesial temporal sclerosis. Quite impressive.— R.D. Currier, M.D.

Fourier Analysis of Cerebrospinal Fluid Flow Velocities: MR Imaging Study

Thomsen C, Ståhlberg F, Stubgaard M, Nordell B, and The Scandinavian Flow Group (Univ of Copenhagen; Univ of Lund; Univ of Stockholm)
Radiology 177:659–665, 1990   1–10

Magnetic resonance imaging phase methods have been used in measuring CSF flow. Because CSF is produced in the cerebral ventricles, there must be CSF outflow through the cerebral aqueduct. An MRI study was done to ascertain whether the phase method could measure flow in the cerebral aqueduct, find the peak velocity range, describe the frequency of flow by Fourier analysis, and estimate CSF production.

Volunteers for the study were 5 healthy adults, 24–45 years of age. The MRI technique was an interleaved pseudocinematographic fast low-angle shot sequence with additional pulsed gradients for flow encoding. Flow-encoded images were obtained by subtracting paired, differently encoded phase images (Fig 1–9). Using a calibration curve with the slope 26.5 radian $\cdot$ m^{-1} $\cdot$ sec, the resulting phase information was converted to flow velocity. Fourier analysis was done by transforming the velocity vs. time function and fitting a continuous curve to the data by means of the zeroth, first, second, and third harmonics.

Cerebral aqueduct outflow ranged from 6 to 51 mm/sec (mean, 23 mm/sec) and inflow ranged from -3 to -28 mm/sec (mean, -15 mm/sec). The average peak volume outflow was 155 µL/sec and the average peak volume inflow, -107 µL/sec. Production of CSF, calculated as the

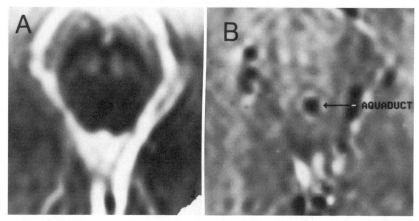

Fig 1–9.—**A**, modulus image, frame 2, 184 msec after R wave. Note the increased signal intensity in the cerebral aqueduct as a result of inflow enhancement. **B**, corresponding subtracted phase image. The phase in the aqueduct is positive, indicating a caudal flow (outflow). (Courtesy of Thomsen C., Ståhlberg F, Stubgaard M, et al: *Radiology* 177:659–665, 1990.)

difference between outflow and inflow, ranged from .6 to 1.2 L/day. The CSF pulse wave in the aqueduct was delayed about one fourth of the heart cycle.

In the cerebral aqueduct, CSF flow can be quickly and easily determined by MRI. This technique may prove useful in patients with abnormal CSF hydrodynamics or in patients receiving drugs that affect CSF flow or production.

▶ I hope this turns out to be useful in the long run, because it would solve the problem of detecting CSF flow in the brain and thus should make diagnosing occult hydrocephalus easier. When will we see a study of its usefulness in the clinical setting?—R.D. Currier, M.D.

Neurosarcoidosis: Gadolinium-Enhanced MR Imaging
Williams DW III, Elster AD, Kramer SI (Bowman Gray School of Medicine, Wake Forest Univ, Winston-Salem, NC)
J Comput Assist Tomogr 14:704–707, 1990   1–11

On noncontrast MRI the white matter lesions of neurosarcoidosis may be nonspecific or indistinguishable from those of multiple sclerosis. Two patients with neurosarcoidosis were studied by gadolinium-diethylenetri-amine pentaacetic acid (Gd-DTPA)-enhanced MRI.

In both patients, non–contrast MRI showed multiple periventricular and subcortical foci of increased signal on T2-weighted images. Administration of Gd-DTPA showed diffuse leptomeningeal enhancement immediately adjacent to the parenchymal abnormalities. Presumed perivascular spread of neurosarcoidosis along Virchow-Robin spaces was exquisitely demonstrated, as evidenced by contrast enhancement along the course of the vessels supplying some of the white matter abnormalities.

Gadolinium-DTPA-enhanced MRI provides a proper radiologic diagnosis of neurosarcoidosis, as well as demonstrating the full extent of intracranial abnormalities. Furthermore, Gd-DTPA-enhanced MRI may obviate the need for contrast-enhanced CT that other authors suggest as necessary and complementary to non–contrast MRI.

▶ The question of what sarcoid looks like on MRI scans is being answered. The changes along vessels seen with gadolinium enhancement are striking and should be of diagnostic help in this disorder.— R.D. Currier, M.D.

Noninvasive Detection of Occlusive Disease of the Carotid Siphon and Middle Cerebral Artery
Ley-Pozo J, Ringelstein EB (University Hosp, Aachen, Germany)
Ann Neurol 28:640–647, 1990   1–12

To determine how accurately transcranial Doppler (TCD) sonography detects stenosing or occluding lesions of cerebral arteries, a review was made of the findings in 133 consecutive patients who underwent both TCD sonography and selective cerebral arteriography after acute stroke or transient ischemia. Eighty-five patients had a completed stroke. Continuous-wave Doppler examination of the extracranial arteries was carried out along with TCD sonography and selective angiography of the common carotid artery.

In 133 of 139 arterial segments, TCD sonography and arteriography agreed. Sonography was a sensitive and specific means of detecting obstruction of the carotid siphon or the main stem of the middle cerebral artery. The diagnostic reliability of TCD sonography was affirmed by calculating a chance-corrected measure of agreement. One patient with middle cerebral arterial stenosis had a falsely negative angiogram. Transcranial Doppler sonography is a useful means of noninvasively detecting intracranial lesions of the carotid siphon and middle cerebral artery.

▶ Any information about intracranial arterial lesions that can be obtained noninvasively is worth having. Transcranial Doppler sonography is a new modality, the place of which is still being assessed. Here is one more report suggesting that it is both sensitive and specific in detecting stenosis or occlusion of the middle cerebral artery.— J.F. Toole, M.D.

A Comparison of Thermography and Electromyography in the Diagnosis of Cervical Radiculopathy
So YT, Olney RK, Aminoff MJ (Univ of California, San Francisco)
Muscle Nerve 13:1032–1036, 1990   1–13

The role of thermography in the clinical evaluation of patients with neuromuscular disorders is controversial. The diagnostic value of thermography was compared to that of electromyography in 14 patients with clinically unequivocal cervical radiculopathy and 20 asymptomatic controls. A quantitative analysis of thermograms was used. The average skin temperature was measured in designated regions over the neck, shoulder, and upper extremities. Also, skin temperature was measured between corresponding regions of the 2 limbs and between fingers innervated by different roots in the same hand. An abnormality was defined as an interside difference exceeding 3 SD from the normal mean.

Electromyography supported the clinical diagnosis of cervical radiculopathy in 10 of 14 patients (71%). Thermography was abnormal in 6 of 14 patients (43%). Thermographic abnormalities were seen only in the hands and fingers, and the pattern did not follow the dermatomal distribution of the clinically involved cervical root. Furthermore, when compared with electromyography, thermography provided no additional diagnostic information in patients with abnormal thermograms.

Thermography has limited localizing value in evaluation of patients with suspected cervical radiculopathy, even in those in whom the clinical diagnosis is not in doubt. Thermography does not have an established role in evaluation of patients with cervical radiculopathy.

▶ Here is another in the short but growing list of situations in which thermography does not seem to do as well as electromyography. Now let's hear from all you thermographers out there.—R.D. Currier, M.D.

Complications of Cerebral Angiography for Patients With Mild Carotid Territory Ischaemia Being Considered for Carotid Endarterectomy
Hankey GJ, Warlow CP, Molyneux AJ (Western Gen Hosp, Edinburgh; and Radcliffe Infirmary, Oxford, England)
J Neurol Neurosurg Psychiatry 53:542–548, 1990   1–14

It is necessary to image the carotid bifurcation in symptomatic patients with carotid ischemia who are under consideration for endarterectomy. Selective intra-arterial angiography is the best means of resolving disease, but this invasive procedure is associated with some risk, and this risk must be added to that of surgery in assessing overall efficacy.

A prospective study was made of 382 patients with mild symptoms of carotid ischemia who underwent cerebral angiography to image a potentially resectable bifurcation lesion. Thirteen patients had complications after 14 angiographic studies. Ten patients had neurologic complications (table). No particular risk factor pattern was evident in the 8 patients who sustained a stroke after angiography. The rate of stroke in 64 patients seen after the occurrence of a stroke was 6%.

Patients with symptomatic carotid ischemia have a 1% risk of permanent disability from stroke after cerebral angiography. This risk presum-

Postangiographic Stroke Rate for Symptomatic Carotid Ischemia
Post-angiogram stroke

Diagnosis	Patients	Reversible No	%	Permanent No	%	Total No	%	(95% CI)
TIA brain +/or eye	259	1		1		2	0·8	(0–1·8)
Retinal Infarct	59	0		2		2	3·4	(0–8·0)
Stroke	64	2		2		4	6·2	(0·3–12·1)
Total	382	3	0·8	5	1·3	8	2·1	(0·7–3·5)

(Courtesy of Hankey GJ, Warlow CP, Molyneux AJ: *J Neurol Neurosurg Psychiatry* 53:542–548, 1990.)

ably can be lowered by selecting physiologically younger patients without systemic illness who are neurologically stable and have definite symptoms of carotid ischemia, as well as a potentially operable lesion on duplex screening. The risk is further reduced if arch and/or selective cerebral angiography is done by an experienced radiologist using a transfemoral approach, small catheters, and minimal amounts of nonionic contrast medium.

▶ Complications of cerebral arteriography depend on the method used, the skill of the arteriographer, allergic reaction, and type of lesions being imaged. In this group of 382 patients with mild carotid ischemia, the rate of complications associated with arteriography was 3.4%; 10 complications (2.6%) were neurologic. This seems high to those of us on this side of the Atlantic, but no one can gainsay that arteriography is a safe procedure. All one can hope for is that the risk:benefit ratio will be strongly in the patient's favor.—J.F. Toole, M.D.

rCBF-SPECT in Brain Infarction: When Does It Predict Outcome?
Limburg M, van Royen EA, Hijdra A, Verbeeten B Jr (Academisch Medisch Centrum, Amsterdam)
J Nucl Med 32:382–387, 1991   1–15

Single-photon emission CT (SPECT) images of regional cerebral blood flow (rCBF) have not always consistently predicted the outcome after ischemic stroke, possibly because of the lack of a fixed interval between the onset of stroke and examination. Imaging with SPECT was carried out at fixed intervals after acute cerebral infarction in 26 consecutive patients with supratentorial cortical infarcts. The patients were older than 18 years of age and had stable or progressive signs of focal cerebral ischemia and hemiparesis.

Imaging was performed using [201]T-diethyldithiocarbamate within 24 hours of onset of stroke and was repeated after 2 weeks and 6 months. The flow deficit present at admission correlated with the outcome. The imaging findings at admission and at 6 months correlated with the clinical state, but the smaller flow deficits present at 2 weeks (Fig 1–10) did

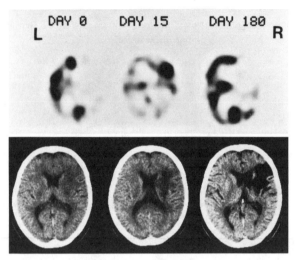

Fig 1–10.—Consecutive SPECT and CT scans from a 60-year-old woman with a severe left-sided hemiparesis. Initially, CT shows only slight hypodensity in the right frontoparietal region, but finally the full extent is evident. The initial flow deficit on SPECT after 2 weeks becomes "filled in" with mixed normal activity to hyperactivity. (Courtesy of Limburg M, van Royen EA, Verbeeten B Jr: *J Nucl Med* 32:382–387, 1991.)

not correlate with clinical parameters. The 9 patients who had smaller flow defects at 6 months had improved clinically more than 6 patients whose flow deficits had increased. More patients who improved had received the calcium-entry blocker flunarizine.

The results of SPECT studies of rCBF in acute ischemic stroke depend to an important degree on the interval between onset of stroke and time of examination. Images are not the sole product of regional cerebral perfusion, and the findings obtained 2 weeks after onset do not correlate closely with the patient's clinical condition.

▶ This study clarifies SPECT scanning of strokes. There is no flow immediately, but at 2 weeks there is hyperperfusion and later on the no-flow situation returns. The authors found the very early SPECT scan to be a good predictor of outcome. It may show the defect when the CT scan appears normal.

The MRC European Carotid Surgery Trial (1) has now reported the interim results of the largest randomized trial of any surgical procedure—2,518 patients randomized in the past 10 years (2). The results are clear for those with no to 29% carotid stenosis (leave it alone), and for those with 70% to 99% stenosis (do it in a good surgical center), but the results for the group with 30% to 69% stenosis are still uncertain and the trial continues. The editorialist comments that carotid endarterectomy will increase in the United Kingdom by threefold to fivefold and probably decrease in the United States.

A recent report by Meyer et al. from the Mayo Clinic (3) notes that it is safe even in the older population aged 70 to 90 years. Yes, in their hands and with patients selected by them (4).—R.D. Currier, M.D.

References

1. Warlow C: *Lancet* 337:1235, 1991.
2. Editorial, *Lancet* 337:1255, 1991.
3. Meyer FB, et al: *Mayo Clin Proc* 66:464, 1991.
4. Adams MP: *Mayo Clin Proc* 66:539, 1991.

SPECT in Patients With Epilepsia Partialis Continua

Katz A, Bose A, Lind SJ, Spencer SS (Yale Univ)
Neurology 40:1848–1850, 1990   1–16

Epilepsia partialis continua (EPC) may present a diagnostic problem when its clinical manifestations are subtle and EEG does not demonstrate an epileptic pattern. In such cases, single-photon emission CT (SPECT) may be useful. In 2 patients the diagnosis of EPC was facilitated by SPECT.

Man, 79, was hospitalized for worsening right facial weakness and difficulty in speaking. One month earlier he had sustained a left middle cerebral artery stroke with mild residual right facial weakness, right upper extremity apraxia, and expressive aphasia. He did not have a history of seizures. On his third day in the hospital, continuous activity of the right side of the face and arm began. An EEG obtained during seizure activity did not show any abnormality. A technetium hexamethylpropylene amine oxime (HMPAO) SPECT study showed a distinct area of hyperperfusion in the left prerolandic region (Fig 1–11). Hypoperfusion was seen in the rest of the left hemisphere. The patient responded well to intravenous lorazepam, with resolution of the partial motor seizures. On a repeat scan,

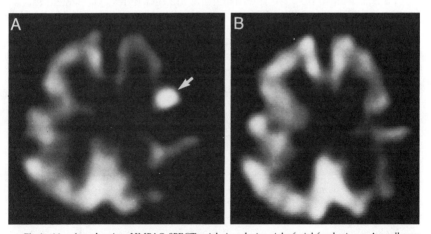

Fig 1–11.—A, technetium HMPAO SPECT axial view during right facial focal seizure. A small area of increased signal *(arrow)* can be seen at the left prerolandic cortex. A decreased signal is identified posteriorly as well as anteriorly. **B,** the same axial view following seizures. No area of increased signal can be seen. (Courtesy of Katz A, Bose A, Lind SJ, et al: *Neurology* 40:1848–1850, 1990.)

the left hemisphere hypoperfusion defect persisted, but the area of increased signal intensity was gone.

The 2 patients described had a discrete area of hyperperfusion on HMPAO SPECT that resolved when the clinical seizure activity subsided. This technique is a valuable in the assessment of patients with EPC.

▶ The finding of increased uptake at the point of increased cerebral activity during EPC may be helpful clinically in those peculiar cases that don't have an EEG abnormality. Single-photon emission CT of the brain is now available at most places in the United States and is becoming useful.—R.D. Currier, M.D.

A Study of Immunoglobulin G in the Cerebrospinal Fluid of 1007 Patients With Suspected Neurological Disease Using Isoelectric Focusing and the Log IgG-Index: A Comparison and Diagnostic Applications

McLean BN, Luxton RW, Thompton EJ (Inst of Neurology, Queen Square, London)

Brain 113:1269–1289, 1990   1–17

An overview of the neurologic abnormalities associated with altered CSF immunoglobulins was undertaken in 1,007 patients hospitalized in a 30-month period. Isoelectric focusing (IEF) was carried out, and the immunoglobulin G content estimated in the serum and CSF using a "monorocket" technique.

Isoelectric focusing to detect oligoclonal banding had a much higher yield than measuring IgG and albumin to estimate a log IgG index (table). Not only did more patients exhibit local synthesis by isoelectric focusing, but the test was more specific—no false positive results compared with a 3.5% false positive rate using the log IgG index. Isoelectric focusing was positive in 95% of patients with clinically definite multiple sclerosis, whereas the log IgG index was positive in only 67% of this group.

Isoelectric focusing compares favorably with MRI in detecting abnormality in multiple sclerosis, and performs better than evoked potential recording. Isoelectric focusing is the best approach to detecting IgG abnormalities in the CSF. The quantitative approach is much less useful, especially for screening purposes.

▶ This careful study shows that isoelectric focusing of CSF oligoclonal banding is more sensitive than the IgG index in detecting multiple sclerosis. The au-

Summary of Results of IgG Analysis for 1,007 Patients

	IEF	Log-Index	Both
Local synthesis	282	225	163
No local synthesis	725	782	663
Total	1007	1007	826

(Courtesy of McLean BN, Luxton RW, Thompson EJ: *Brain* 113:1269–1289, 1990.)

thors found a 90% detection rate overall, with a 95% positive rate for what they called definite cases. What is a "definite" case of multiple sclerosis? In this series the definition did not include a positive MRI scan. One wonders whether this technique in definite cases, as defined by both clinical and MRI criteria, would not be even higher than 95%—perhaps close to 100%.—R.D. Currier, M.D.

2 Localization Aphasia and Behavior

Left Handedness and Immune Disorders
McKeever WF, Rich DA (Northern Arizona Univ, Flagstaff; Bowling Green State Univ, Ohio)
Cortex 26:33–40, 1990   2–1

The incidence of immune system disorders in left- and right-handed persons has been under direct investigation for nearly 10 years, but the findings of such research have been inconsistent. The hypothesis that immune disorder is more common in left-handed than in right-handed persons was investigated.

A sample of 3,080 college students from 2 universities was tested on a self-report instrument. For each of a list of immune disorders, the subjects indicated whether they had no reason to believe they had the disorder, thought they might have the disorder, had the disorder diagnosed by a physician, or had the disorder diagnosed and treated by a physician.

Women reported significantly more immune disorders than men did. The distribution of responses across the 4 response categories was not different for left-handed and right-handed women. However, immune disorders were reported in significantly higher frequency by left-handed women when only the extreme response categories were considered. Handedness had no effect across the 4 categories among men, even when only the extreme categories were considered. Laterality quotients and immune disorders were not related in either sex.

These findings provide no support whatever for an association of immune system disorders and left-handedness in men. Although there is a modicum of support for the hypothesis among women, it is weak and somewhat equivocal.

► In studies on the association between handedness and any other trait, it is important to think of the full spectrum of handedness from −100 through +100. Many interesting associations exist for the middle group lying between 0 and +60. If these are clumped with the right-handed group, it tends to abolish interesting findings. Furthermore, the distribution of handedness in the population is not normal but rather J-shaped, so the word "mean" loses its meaning and more appropriate statistics need be done. Unfortunately, most studies on this topic do not pay sufficient attention to these caveats, so it is still unknown whether associations are or are not present.—A.M. Galaburda, M.D.

MRI Evaluation of the Size and Symmetry of the Planum Temporale in Adolescents With Developmental Dyslexia

Larsen JP, Høien T, Lundberg I, Ødegaard H (Central Hosp of Rogalnad, Stavanger, Teacher College; Univ of Umeå, Sweden)
Brain Lang 39:289–301, 1990   2–2

The planum temporale is an anatomical structure in the sylvian fissure located posterior to the transverse auditory gyrus of Heschl on the superior surface of the temporal lobe. Pathologic studies indicate asymmetry in the anatomical size of the planum temporale in normal subjects, but autopsy studies in persons with developmental dyslexia show an unexpected symmetry of this structure. Magnetic resonance imaging was used to examine the size and symmetry of the plana temporales in 19 dyslexic students in grade 8 and in 17 closely matched controls.

Of the 19 dyslexic patients, the plana temporales were of equal size in 13 (Fig 2–1) and larger on the left in 6. In contrast, 12 of 17 control subjects had asymmetry on the left. The association between plana symmetry and dyslexia was significant, with symmetry of the plana being the dominant pattern in the dyslexic group. Calculation of the mean length of the right and left plana temporales showed that a larger right planum temporale was the cause of symmetry of the plana in dyslexics.

There was no clear association between symmetry/asymmetry of planum temporale and handedness. Word-reading strategies among the dyslexics and controls were investigated with computerized tasks in which accuracy and naming latency were recorded. All dyslexic subjects with pure phonological deficits in reading had symmetric plana temporales. In addition, 2 of 3 controls with pure phonological deficiency had symmetric plana temporales.

Symmetry of the plana is significantly more likely to occur in dyslexic adolescents. The close relationship between symmetry and specific deficiency in the phonological route of word decoding suggests a possible neuroanatomical basis for a characteristic symptom of linguistic processing deficiency in developmental dyslexia.

▶ Morphometric studies of the brain for relating brain structure and behavior are more possible than ever before because of the advent of MRI. The planum temporale, which has been associated with language and language disorders in the past, can now be assessed in living subjects by this technique. The process of reconstruction of the planum takes some experience and has been done relatively well in the present study. The reader is also referred to the work of Steinmetz and colleagues in Düsseldorf who have achieved a great degree of precision in reconstructing the planum temporale (1).—A.M. Galaburda, M.D.

Reference

1. Steinmetz J, et al: *Ann Neurol* 29:315, 1991.

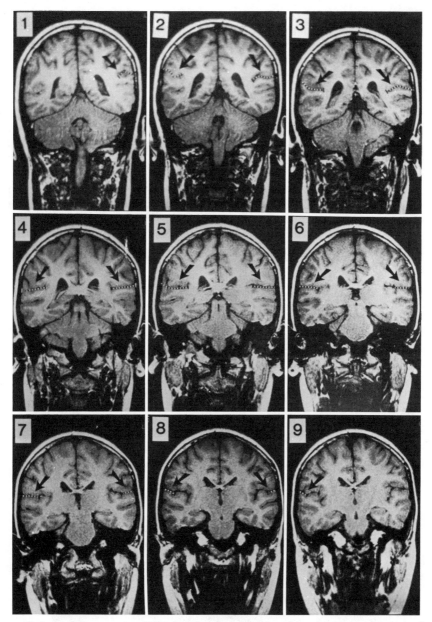

Fig 2–1.—Subsequent coronal MRI slices through posterior part of the sylvian fissure of the brain of a 15-year-old girl with developmental dyslexia. Slice 1 is the most posterior section and slice 9 is the most anterior section of the brain. The slice numbers are indicated in the upper left corner of each slice image. The extent of the right and left planum temporale in each slice is marked with a dotted line. The MRI images are T1-weighted and with a slice thickness of 3 mm. (Courtesy of Larsen JP, Høien T, Lundberg I, et al: *Brain Lang* 39:289–301, 1990.)

Auditory Hallucinations and Smaller Superior Temporal Gyral Volume in Schizophrenia

Barta PE, Pearlson GD, Powers RE, Richards SS, Tune LE (Johns Hopkins Univ; Univ of Alabama, Birmingham)

Am J Psychiatry 147:1457–1462, 1990   2–3

The cause of auditory hallucinations in schizophrenia is unknown. Recent studies, however, suggest that abnormalities in the temporal lobe may be associated with auditory hallucinations in schizophrenic patients. Temporal lobe structures were examined by MRI to examine the hypothesis that the volumes of these structures would be smaller in schizophrenic patients than in controls.

The patient group included 15 men (mean age, 30.6 years). Fifteen controls matched individually to the patients as to age, sex, race, years of education, and parental socioeconomic status. A neuropathologist familiar with temporal lobe anatomy and blind to the diagnoses assessed the MRI scans for target regions (superior temporal gyrus, amygdala volume, and third ventricle volume) and control regions (midbrain area, pons area, midsagittal area, whole temporal lobe, and overall brain volume).

When compared with controls, the schizophrenic patients had smaller superior temporal gyri bilaterally, smaller left amygdalas, and larger third ventricles on MRI (Fig 2–2). In nontarget regions, only the right temporal lobe was significantly different, and this difference ceased to exist after the Bonferroni correction. The whole brain was 2% smaller in patients than in controls, the left temporal lobe was 7.7% smaller, and the right temporal lobe was 10% smaller.

The smaller size of the overall brain or temporal lobe in patients did

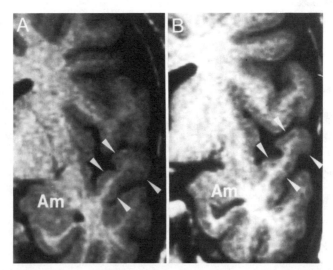

Fig 2–2.—Portions of T1-weighted coronal MRIs of brains of a control (**A**) and a schizophrenic patient (**B**). The superior temporal gyrus *(arrowheads)* is measured at the level of the amygdala *(AM)*. (Courtesy of Barta PE, Pearlson GD, Powers RE, et al: *Am J Psychiatry* 147:1457–1462, 1990.)

not account for the smaller size of the left superior temporal gyrus and left amygdala. Studies have found an association between the superior temporal gyrus and auditory response, and shrinkage of the left superior temporal gyrus in schizophrenia is strongly and selectively correlated with the severity of auditory hallucinations.

▶ This interesting study confirms and expands on previous findings by the authors and others. There are still some unresolved questions. First, it is well known that patients who lose hearing may experience auditory hallucinations, which raises questions about hearing in schizophrenics, particularly in view of the changes in the superior temporal gyrus. Second, the lesion that produces Wernicke's aphasia injuries mainly the left superior temporal gyrus, which sheds new light on the schizophrenic jargon that these patients often produce, which is often difficult to distinguish from the aphasic jargon of patients with Wernicke's disease. Third, bilateral superior temporal gyrus lesions might be associated with the syndrome of pure word deafness, whereby written comprehension is preserved relative to oral comprehension. To my knowledge, this has not been checked in schizophrenics.—A.M. Galaburda, M.D.

The Lateralization of Language Comprehension Using Event-Related Potentials

Nelson CA, Collins PF, Torres F (Univ of Minnesota)
Brain Cognition 14:92–112, 1990   2–4

There may be left hemisphere vs. right hemisphere differences in processing of language stimuli. Long-latency event-related potentials (ERPs) can sometimes demonstrate laterality differences in the processing of linguistic and other cognitive events. A study was done to ascertain whether left- and right-handed subjects differed in ERP responses to language and non–language visual stimuli presented to the left and right hemispheres, respectively.

Ten adults—5 left-handed and 5 right-handed—were studied. Event-related potentials were recorded over the occipital and parietal scalp areas. The subjects were presented with a language stimulus (the word "bat") and a non–language stimulus (a set of Chinese characters). A divided field, "oddball" paradigm was used. Stimuli were presented separately to the left and right hemispheres as ERPs were recorded.

The P300 component of the ERP was larger over the left than the right hemisphere of right-handed subjects when the language stimulus was presented to the left hemisphere. In left-handed subjects no hemispheric differences were observed regardless of the field of presentation. Right-handers tended to have longer P3 latencies than left-handers. With both stimuli, left-handers had greater correlations between N200 latencies and reaction times, but right-handers and the greatest overall correlations for P300 latencies to the linguistic stimulus.

Right-handers' P300 responses to language stimuli differ both from their ERPs to non–language stimuli and from left-handers' ERPs to either stimulus. Lateralized ERP correlates of hemispheric dominance for language processing can be recorded, although more direct study would be useful. Left-handers may have greater homogeneity as to hemispheric dominance.

▶ Event-related potentials are a tremendous tool for analyzing brain function. No longer constrained to simple reaction time measurements, psychophysiologists are teasing apart the intricacies of cognition with markers of neuronal population activity. Studies such as this support our current theories of cortical localization. If we can ever solve the "inverse problem" (what structures inside the cranium contribute to a scalp field potential), we'll be well on our way to understanding how the brain thinks.—Eric Undesser, M.D., Assistant Professor of Neurology, University of Mississippi

---

Memory for the Temporal Order of Events in Patients With Frontal Lobe Lesions and Amnesic Patients
Shimamura AP, Janowsky JS, Squire LR (VA Med Ctr, San Diego; Univ of California, San Diego)
Neuropsychologia 28:803–813, 1990   2–5

Research on patients with memory disorders has provided useful data on the organization and structure of normal memory functions. The temporal order memory deficit documented in patients with Korsakoff's syndrome is out of proportion with their deficits in other memory aspects. This impairment may be the result of frontal lobe damage. Performance on tests of item memory was compared with performance on tests of temporal order memory in patients with frontal lobe lesions.

Patients with frontal lobe lesions, amnesic patients with Korsakoff's syndrome, non–Korsakoff amnesic patients, and controls were tested. In the first experiment, subjects were given a list of 15 words and asked to reproduce the list order from a random array of words. They were then asked to arrange in chronological order a random display of 15 factual events occurring between 1941 and 1985. In both experiments, patients with frontal lobe lesions were impaired in their placement of items in the correct temporal order, even though item memory was normal. The 2 groups of amnesic patients demonstrated impaired memory for temporal order and impaired item memory. Patients with Korsakoff's syndrome had poorer temporal order memory than other amnesic patients, even though they had similar levels of item memory.

These results indicate that patients with frontal lobe lesions have difficulty in organizing information temporally. Korsakoff patients with both diencephalic and frontal damage have memory impairment, together with a disproportionate deficit in memory for temporal order.

▶ In this paper, patients with frontal lobe lesions had abnormal temporal order of memory items. Compared with the paper on frontal lobe and memory in which recognition was impaired (Abstract 2–6), these patients had preserved recognition. However, we are not given the exact location of their frontal lobe lesions. I would estimate that recognition might be impaired with dorsal lesions, whereas temporal order problems might arise from inferior prefrontal involvements.—A.M. Galaburda, M.D.

Preserved Recall Versus Impaired Recognition: A Case Study
Delbecq-Derouesné J, Beauvois MF, Shallice T (Hôp de la Salpêtrière, Paris; MRC Applied Psychology Unit, Cambridge, England)
Brain 113:1045–1074, 1990   2–6

The principle of modularity postulates the functional independence of modules, namely, hypothetical subsystems engaged in certain types of tasks. According to this principle, a cerebral lesion could destroy or disorganize an isolated cognitive subsystem without necessarily disturbing the functioning of other subsystems involved in the same task. A dissociation not reported previously was seen.

Man, 46, underwent surgery for an aneurysm of the anterior communicating artery. About 8 years after the operation, he was reexamined. Neuropsychological assessment revealed a dissociation between very poor performance on recognition tests, on which the patient's performance was as poor as that of classic amnesic patients, and normal performance in recall, estimated by the number of correct responses. The patient was able to achieve a number of difficult learning tasks, at times normally. The relearning of one of these tasks after 1 hour was perfectly normal (Fig 2–3).

The pattern of dissociation seen in this case is the reverse of that observed in normal subjects and amnesic patients. This patient's recognition

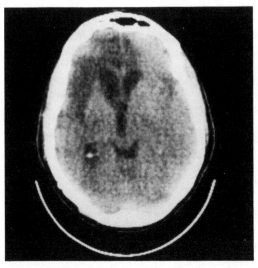

Fig 2–3.—Computed tomographic scan. (Courtesy of Delbecq-Derouesné J, Beauvois MF, Shallice T: *Brain* 113:1045–1074, 1990.)

failure suggests that memory performance results from an interaction between knowledge and the subjective experience of remembering.

▶ This complex paper reports a finding that is not wholly intuitive. It is difficult to visualize a patient who could recall a fact but not recognize it. But the reader is reminded that dorsomedial frontal lesions are known to produce that type of dissociation. Take, for instance, the echolalia that can occur with such lesions: A patient is often seen to repeat long sentences without having any understanding of them. Think of it as the hyperreflexia of some hemiplegias; the limb moves on being struck, but volitional movement is impossible. Modularity has been recognized in neuropsychologic processes for a long time.—A.M. Galaburda, M.D.

Stereo Perception in Callosal Agenesis and Partial Callosotomy
Jeeves MA (Univ of St Andrews, St Andrews, Scotland)
Neuropsychologia 29:19–34, 1991   2–7

The perception of stereopsis requires a comparison of the images of each eye. Most binocular interactions occur intrahemispherically, but those close to the vertical meridian of the field may involve interhemispheric connections. Midline stereopsis was investigated in 2 acallosal patients and 2 patients who had partial callosotomy. In addition, 3 normal persons were tested. Apart from comparing midline stereopsis with peripheral presentations, 4 disparities were used to test fine and coarse stereopsis.

All 3 patients lacking a splenium had midline deficits, making few uncrossed midline responses (Fig 2–4). A patient who underwent partial callosal section whose splenium was mostly spared performed better at the midline than in the periphery. All degrees of disconnection, however, led to some overall loss of performance.

The specific problems experienced by acallosal patients in handling uncrossed disparities may reflect a marked reduction or absence of *far* neurons in the acallosal brain. An important role for the anterior commis-

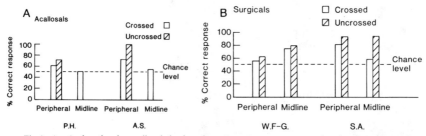

Fig 2–4.—**A,** data for the acallosals broken down into responses to crossed and uncrossed stimulus presentations at the midline and in the periphery using Richard's methods of calculation. **B,** data for the surgical patients broken down into responses to crossed and uncrossed stimulus presentations at the midline and in the periphery using Richard's method of calculation. (Courtesy of Jeeves MA: *Neuropsychologia* 29:19–34, 1991.)

sure in efficiently integrating cross disparity may explain the relative success achieved by acallosal patients in making crossed disparity judgments. Normal persons exhibit some variation in performance and, not surprisingly, greater variation is evident in acallosal patients.

▶ Partial or total section of the corpus callosum is an accepted form of therapy for some forms of intractable epilepsy. It is important, therefore, to be familiar with the perceptual and cognitive deficits associated with these forms of surgery. Here is one: perception of depth. For this function there is a complementarity between functions of the corpus callosum and those of the anterior commissure, with significant functional preservation remaining when the latter is spared, as it is in most acallosal and surgical cases.—A.M. Galaburda, M.D.

Frontal Systems Impairment Following Multiple Lacunar Infarcts
Wolfe N, Linn R, Babikian VK, Knoefel JE, Albert ML (Boston Univ; Boston VA Med Ctr)
Arch Neurol 47:129–132, 1990   2–8

The cognitive impairment associated with multiple subcortical lacunar infarcts (lacunes) has not been fully described. In a prospective study, the neuropsychological performance of 11 subjects with multiple lacunes (mean, 3.1) on CT was compared with that of 11 medical controls matched for age and education and with no clinical or CT evidence of infarction. Subjects were tested at least 1 month after the most recent lacunar infarction.

Patients with multiple lacunes scored significantly lower than did controls on overall cognitive performance, although only 27% met the criteria for a clinical diagnosis of dementia. Patients with multiple lacunes scored significantly lower on specific tests sensitive to frontal lobe dysfunction, such as deficits in shifting mental set, response inhibition, and executive function. In addition, these patients often displayed apathetic behavior. Patients with multiple lacunes were not more impaired on all tasks but, rather, exhibited a pattern of dysfunction consistent with subcortical pathologic findings. The number of lacunes did not correlate with the degree of impairment on frontal lobe tests.

These data suggest a continuum of cognitive impairment in lacunar states, ranging from frontal systems impairment to dementia.

▶ This study shows that multiple lacunes are associated with (often subclinical) abnormalities in frontal function. However, it is not possible to tell from the article whether the lacunes predominantly affect the frontal lobes and their connections. My guess is that they do not, but that they are less well tolerated when they affect frontal networks than posterior ones, particularly early on in the lacunar disorder. This hypothesis could be checked directly in future studies.—A.M. Galaburda, M.D.

Mood Disorders in Long-Term Survivors of Stroke: Associations With Brain Lesion Location and Volume

Sharpe M, Hawton K, House A, Molyneux A, Sandercock P, Bamford J, Warlow C (Univ of Oxford, England)
Psychol Med 20:815–828, 1990   2–9

Several reports suggest a high rate of depression following stroke, but these studies have many shortcomings. The relationship between stroke and mood disorders was examined in 60 surviving patients who were interviewed a mean of 45 months after the stroke. The patients had widely varying degrees of disability; more than 50% were fully independent, whereas 25% were severely disabled.

Seventeen of the 60 patients (28%) met *DSM-III-R* criteria for major depression at some time since the stroke; none had experienced major depression just before the event. Depression was most prevalent in the first 6 months. Five patients had received antidepressants, but none was referred to the psychiatric service. Although symptom scores correlated with lesion volume, the presence of depression was unrelated to the type of pathology or to the occurrence of a left hemispheric or left anterior lesion.

Major depression probably is less frequent in long-term stroke survivors than previous studies suggest. The site of the lesion is probably not an important factor in depression. Future studies of mood disorder after stroke will have to include large community-based samples of patients or focus on high-risk groups. In contrast to depression, anxiety disorders are relatively frequent after stroke.

▶ The answer to the question of whether depression follows stroke in general and certain types of strokes in particular remains elusive. Some patients after stroke may become depressed, others may become unconcerned, and still others (those with lesions in Wernicke's area) may become euphoric. It has been argued that only the latter 2 reactions are abnormal, because a disability causing stroke *should* appropriately cause depressive symptoms. More recently, it has been reported that left anterior lesions produce depression comparatively out of proportion to disability. The present study's findings may differ because of the long interim period between stroke and evaluation for presence or absence of depression.—A.M. Galaburda, M.D.

Progressive Aphasia Without Generalized Dementia

Northern B, Hopcutt B, Griffiths H (Manchester Royal Infirmary, England)
Aphasiology 4:55–65, 1990   2–10

Aphasia in primary degenerative dementia of the Alzheimer type is common, as are aphasic syndromes in patients with focal dominant hemisphere lesions. Language disturbance arising from subcortical lesions has also been well described. However, slowly progressive aphasia in the absence of other cognitive deficits is rare. Progressive aphasia in the absence of generalized dementia was observed.

Man, 64, right-handed, was first seen with an 18-month history of progressive deterioration in his linguistic ability and tremor of his right hand. Except for the tremor, no other neurologic signs were found on initial examination. There was no evidence of vascular disease. Computed tomography showed involutionary changes in the left hemisphere with prominence of the left lateral ventricle and sylvian fissure. No definitive diagnosis could be made. The patient was referred for speech therapy. Further assessment performed 6 months later showed a normal EEG and normal findings on carotid angiography. Neuropsychological assessment confirmed that the patient had a selective language disorder. In contrast to the progressive deterioration in the patient's linguistic skills, his praxis, perception, spatial and navigational abilities, and memory were largely preserved. Single-photon emission tomography performed 2 years after presentation demonstrated a striking reduction of uptake in the left frontal, temporal, and parietal regions and in the left subcortex, whereas the right hemisphere uptake was still normal. Repeat CT performed 1 year later demonstrated increasing atrophy and ventricular dilatation of the left side and the appearance of mild right-sided involutional changes (Fig 2–5). His speech was by then limited to arbitrary production of "yes" and "no." During a 5-year follow-up period, the patient gradually lost the ability to communicate. His continued physical decline necessitated transfer to a nursing home, where he has been unable to communicate with the staff.

The language disorder in this patient could not be classified under any of the major syndromes contained in the Boston classification of aphasia. Although the patient's language impairment initially was consistent with a cortical aphasic syndrome arising from a dominant hemisphere lesion,

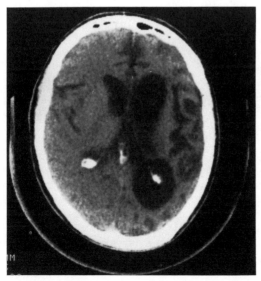

Fig 2–5.—Computed tomographic scan shows marked dilatation of the left lateral ventricle and enlargement of the left sylvian fissure. (Courtesy of Northern B, Hopcutt B, Griffiths H: *Aphasiology* 4:55–65, 1990.)

vascular disease was excluded by neurologic investigation. This patient, therefore, was assigned the diagnosis of progressive aphasia without impairment of cognitive abilities, with the most likely etiology being localized cerebral atrophy affecting the dominant hemisphere.

▶ In 1982 Mesulam reported 6 patients similar to the present one. In 1 of Mesulam's patients the deficits were first noted at the age of 17 years! In view of the young age at onset in some of these patients, one has to wonder whether the syndrome represents truly a "developmental" disorder. Thus it would be important to know whether these patients exhibited language impairment/delay as children.—A.M. Galaburda, M.D.

Reversed Lateralization of Cognitive Functions in Right Handers: Exceptions to Classical Aphasiology
Fischer RS, Alexander MP, Gabriel C, Gould E, Milione J (Boston Univ)
Brain 114:245–261, 1991   2–11

Anomalous cases must be explained when attempting to formulate comprehensive theories about the cerebral organization of language or cognitive functions. Four right-handed patients with left hemispheric lesions exhibited dissociations between neuropsychological functions usually considered to be lateralized to the left hemisphere. They also had totally reversed lateralization of functions ostensibly associated with the right hemisphere.

Woman, 62, who abruptly experienced right-sided weakness was found to have paroxysmal atrial fibrillation. She considered herself to be primarily right-handed, although some unimanual tasks were done with the left hand, reportedly because the patient had been taught them by a left-handed person. Severe spastic right hemiparesis was present with marked right-sided sensory loss and right-sided inattention. Affect prosody was severely reduced. Computed tomography revealed a large left hemispheric infarct (Fig 2–6). No language abnormality was apparent when the Western Aphasia Battery was given 2 weeks after the onset. Testing at 6 weeks showed deficits in attention, spatial function, insight, and higher-level functioning. The verbal and performance IQ values were 109 and 87, respectively. Visuoperceptual function was mildly impaired. The patient did poorly on tests of attention and her affect was extremely flat.

Other similar patients in this study had minimal aphasia. Two patients had severe buccofacial and limb apraxia, expected in right-handed persons who have left hemispheric lesions. These patients and 1 other had severe visuospatial deficits and exhibited right-sided neglect. Attention was impaired in all cases. All 4 patients had poor affective prosody and reduced overall emotional expression. All denied or minimized the extent of their deficits. "Exceptions" such as these may be explained in part by viewing language operations as among the most flexibly organized cognitive operations.

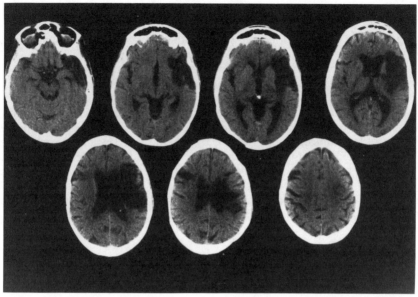

Fig 2–6.—Computed tomography was performed 5 weeks post onset. There is a large infarct involving much of the territory of the left middle cerebral artery, extensively damaging the frontal operculum, lower motor cortex, posterior middle frontal gyrus, inferior parietal lobe, anterior temporal lobe, insula, lateral putamen, and entire periventricular white matter. (Courtesy of Fischer RS, Alexander MP, Gabriel C, et al: *Brain* 114:245–261, 1991.)

▶ Despite the exceptions presented in this paper, we should be guided by 2 rules of thumb: (1) If aphasia does not occur in righthanders from the appropriate left hemisphere lesions, we should consider that the patient has mixed dominance, or that there is a family history of non–right-handedness; and (2) if a patient has a "right hemisphere" syndrome attributable to a left hemisphere lesion, we should look carefully for a toxic or metabolic cause of a confusional state, which can and often does mask as a right hemisphere syndrome.—A.M. Galaburda, M.D.

Development of Language in Six Hemispherectomized Patients
Vargha-Khadem F, Isaacs EB, Papaleloudi H, Polkey CE, Wilson J (Inst of Child Health; Hosp for Sick Children; Maudsley Hosp, London)
Brain 114:473–495, 1991   2–12

The ability of the right hemisphere for language is best assessed when right-sided processing is independent of left-sided input. Previous studies of hemidecorticated patients suggest that, despite an early cerebral insult leading to right hemispheric mediation of speech and language functions, residual deficits in syntactic comprehension predominate. Left hemidecorticated patients reportedly have difficulty comprehending passive negative constructions.

Three patients underwent left, and 3 right, hemispherectomy because of intractable epilepsy. Two patients each were injured in early, middle, and late childhood. Control groups included normal children, children having left temporal lobectomy, and others who incurred a unilateral, nonprogressive cerebral insult congenitally or perinatally.

Language processing was severely impaired at all stages of development in patients having left hemispherectomy. Right hemispherectomy had more limited effects, which were most apparent when a lesion was acquired in early childhood. Gross language functions can be adequately subserved by the isolated right hemisphere, but this site does not provide efficient lexical access. The isolated right hemisphere is deficient when using degraded semantic or syntactic cues to produce correct inflections. Language functions are largely intact if right hemispherectomy is done at ages 5–6 years or afterward. Development of language function in childhood may depend on the combined effects of age at the time of injury, the side of hemispheric insult, and the presence or absence of diffuse seizures.

▶ The perceived folklore is that the right hemisphere is perfectly capable of taking over language function when the left one is damaged early in life. However, a variety of considerations based on findings from developmental neurobiology would suggest otherwise, and the present paper supports this suggestion. Brain asymmetries are present at least from the middle of gestation, and perfect equipotentiality would seem unlikely. In fairness to previous reports, however, we should consider the possibility that recovery of language from the right hemisphere after early left hemisphere injury may be dampened if the underlying diagnosis is epilepsy, which as we know can cryptically involve both hemispheres.—A.M. Galaburda, M.D.

Crossed Aphasia in Chinese: A Clinical Survey
Yu-huan H, Ying-guan Q, Gui-qing Z (Shihezi Med College, Xinjiang, People's Republic of China)
Brain Lang 39:347–356, 1990   2–13

Theories of cerebral laterality of language function still prevail in Western countries. Most believe that dextrals have language function localized to the left side of the brain, and that aphasia is more frequent in dextrals with lesions on the left side of the brain. Aphasia in left hemiplegic dextrals (crossed aphasia after damage to the right side of the brain) is considered to be rare.

In China, crossed aphasia is seen much more often among stroke victims who are members of the Han, the largest ethnic group in the country, than in members of the Uighur-Kazaks. Motor aphasia is most frequent in Han patients, and pure sensory or posterior aphasia is rare. Among 367 pure Han dextrals were 57 cases of crossed aphasia (15.5%). Forty-nine of the 57 patients (86%) had motor aphasia.

There is no definite Wernicke's area on the left side of the brain of the Chinese. It seems likely that in the Han, language function is localized to the right side of the brain or to both hemispheres, and that theories of cerebral laterality of language function are not universally applicable.

▶ This is an interesting double dissociation, but not a surprising one given the clinical evidence. Language comprehension and production, usually affected by left but not right hemisphere lesions, depend on rapid temporal transitions of sound, wherein most of the information is stored. For instance, the difference between "ball" and "pall" is all in the first few milliseconds of sound, where most of the meaning of the syllable is stored. On the other hand, pitch differences attribute to the words prosody and music, best implemented in the "all" part of the syllable. The latter also conveys a certain kind of nonlinguistic meaning, which is disrupted usually by right hemisphere lesions. It is clear that both hemispheres participate in language, although in different ways.—A.M. Galaburda, M.D.

Auditory Perception of Temporal and Spectral Events in Patients With Focal Left and Right Cerebral Lesions
Robin DA, Tranel D, Damasio H (Univ of Iowa)
Brain Lang 39:539–555, 1990   2–14

Most studies agree that aphasic patients have impaired auditory temporal perception, but it is not clear whether this defect is causal. The perception of temporal and spectral auditory events was examined in 10 right-handed subjects with focal left and right cerebral hemispheric lesions. All of the patients had temporoparietal lesions.

Temporal tasks included a gap detection test in which subjects had to detect a silent interval between 2 tones, and 2 complex pattern perception tasks in which they had to identify placement of the 2 closest tones within a sequence of 6 tones. The spectral tasks involved pitch matching and frequency discrimination.

Patients with left-sided lesions were impaired in their ability to perceive temporal information, but they perceived spectral information normally. In contrast, those with right-sided lesions were impaired in their ability to perceive spectral information, but they perceived temporal information normally.

It appears that left temporoparietal lesions disrupt the perception of temporal elements in auditory signals, whereas right hemispheric lesions impair the perception of spectral information. Temporal changes are used to process speech and prosodic information. Patients with left hemispheric lesions and language or prosodic impairment, or both, may be unable to execute or decode speech and language information rapidly enough to process it meaningfully.

▶ This is a remarkable study that needs to be replicated before we restructure our understanding of language organization in the brain. One possibility for these findings is that the gross definition of dextral and sinistral is insufficient for identifying individuals with mixed handedness (a laterality score would be more useful). In that case, crossed aphasia may be more common simply because of a greater prevalence of mixed handedness in the population, which itself would be interesting. Another interpretation could have to do with the structure of the written language, which may bias the brain toward greater right hemisphere participation, even in oral language. There is precedent for this in illiterates, who show more anomia from right hemisphere lesions than do literates. Such an interpretation would be boosted if the crossed aphasics were all literate, but we are not told. Still, much needs to be learned about genetic and environmental influences on brain organization and lateralization for language, which is clearly less rigid than previously suspected.—A.M. Galaburda, M.D.

3 Alzheimer's Disease

Genetic Linkage Studies Suggest That Alzheimer's Disease Is Not a Single Homogeneous Disorder
St George-Hyslop PH, Haines JL, Farrer LA, Polinsky R, Van Broeckhoven C, Goate A, Crapper McLachlan DR, Orr H, Bruni AC, Sorbi S, Rainero I, Foncin J-F, Pollen D, Cantu J-M, Tupler R, Voskresenskaya N, Mayeux R, Growdon J, Fried VA, Myers RH, Nee L, Backhovens H, Martin J-J, Rossor M, Owen MJ, Mullan M, Percy ME, Karlinsky H, Rich S, Heston L, Montesi M, Mortilla M, Nacmias N, Gusella JF, Hardy JA, and other members of the FAD Collaborative Study Group (Massachusetts Gen Hosp, Boston; Boston Univ; Natl Inst of Neurological Disorders and Stroke, Bethesda, Md; Born Bunge Found, Antwerp; St Mary's Hosp Med School, London; et al)
Nature 347:194–197, 1990   3–1

Alzheimer's disease is usually considered a single disorder, but recent studies have suggested genetic heterogeneity. The inheritance of 5 polymorphic DNA markers from the proximal long arm of chromosome 21 was investigated in 48 pedigrees with familial Alzheimer's disease. The data were analyzed using both the maximum likelihood and affected pedigree member methods.

There was evidence that Alzheimer's disease results from genetic defects in chromosome 21 and also from other genetic or nongenetic factors. There was significant overall evidence of linkage, but not all of the pedigrees contributed positively to this finding. Linkage was evident for presenile-onset pedigrees, but neither the maximum likelihood nor the affected pedigree member method demonstrated positive evidence for linkage in senile-onset kindreds.

There appears to be more than one cause of Alzheimer's disease. Apart from a defect in chromosome 21, the disease may result from other monogenic or polygenic genetic defects, nongenetic agents, or a combination of genetic and environmental factors.

▶ Much discussion has centered around the question of whether a majority of Alzheimer's disease cases are inherited, or whether a significant number may be attributable to nongenetic causes. With respect to the inherited disorders, early genetic studies suggested that Alzheimer's disease may be caused by a gene localized to the proximal long arm of chromosome 21. Recent studies such as the one described in the present paper suggest that the assignment to chromosome 21 is more likely in presenile-onset pedigrees, whereas there is little evidence for linkage in senile-onset pedigrees. What is now becoming more clear is the presence of genetic heterogeneity and the fact that many different single gene defects, or even multiple gene defects, may be responsible for Alzheimer's disease. Even within early-onset Alzheimer's disease there may be nonallelic heterogeneity.—S.H. Appel, M.D.

Neurotrophic and Neurotoxic Effects of Amyloid β Protein: Reversal by Tachykinin Neuropeptides
Yankner BA, Duffy LK, Kirschner DA (Harvard Med School; Children's Hosp, Boston; Univ of Alaska, Fairbanks)
Science 250:279–282, 1990   3–2

Amyloid β protein is found in the brains of patients with Alzheimer's disease, but its pathogenic role, if any, is uncertain. The effects of amyloid β protein on neuronal viability in cultures of hippocampal cells from embryonic rates were examined.

Amyloid β protein proved to be neurotrophic for undifferentiated hippocampal neurons in low concentrations but was neurotoxic for mature neurons at higher concentrations. In differentiated neurons, exposure to the protein led to dendritic and axonal retraction and neuronal death. A segment of the protein from amino acids 25–35 mediated both the trophic and toxic effects. This segment exhibited homology with tachykinin neuropeptides such as eledoisin. Specific tachykinin neuropeptides selectively reversed the early neurotrophic and late neurotoxic effects of amyloid β protein.

It is possible that amyloid β protein normally acts at low concentrations as a neurotrophic factor for immature differentiating neurons in the CNS. Accumulation of high concentrations of the protein in the differentiated CNS, as in Alzheimer's disease, could lead to neuronal degeneration. If this is so, tachykinins might prove useful in reversing neurotoxicity.

▶ One of the important questions with respect to the pathogenesis of Alzheimer's disease is whether β amyloid proteins are a primary or secondary factor in neuronal destruction. If they are secondary, then neuronal destruction may have already occurred and the β amyloid deposition may be a consequence of this neuronal death. Alternatively, deposition of β amyloid could be an early event in the pathogenesis of Alzheimer's disease. As a result, understanding exactly how the β amyloid protein may cause neuronal death could lead to effective therapies in the future. Yankner et al. noted that an amino acid sequence contained within the 43 amino acids of the β amyloid protein exhibits homology with tachykinin neuropeptides. They documented that tachykinin antagonists could mimic the toxic effects of β peptide. If these results can be reproduced in other laboratories, the toxic effects of β amyloid might be offset by various tachykinin analogues. Such an approach, if validated, could pave the way for a new era in therapy of Alzheimer's disease.—S.H. Appel, M.D.

Segregation of a Missense Mutation in the Amyloid Precursor Protein Gene With Familial Alzheimer's Disease
Goate A, Chartier-Harlin M-C, Mullan M, Brown J, Crawford F, Fidani L, Giuffra

L, Haynes A, Irving N, James L, Mant R, Newton P, Rooke K, Roques P, Talbot C, Pericak-Vance M, Roses A, Williamson R, Rossor M, Owen M, Hardy J (St Mary's Hosp, London; Yale Univ; Duke Univ; Univ of Wales, Cardiff)
Nature 349:704–706, 1991 3–3

A recent genetic analysis of a large number of families with Alzheimer's disease suggests that the disease is heterogeneous. In families with late-onset Alzheimer's disease, linkage to chromosome 21 markers is not observed; such markers were shown previously to segregate with familial Alzheimer's disease close to the amyloid precursor protein (APP) gene. Similarly, in some families with early-onset Alzheimer's there is no linkage with chromosome markers, although this is observed in other families. These findings suggest that there is a nonallelic heterogeneity even within early-onset familial Alzheimer's disease.

In a single family with early-onset Alzheimer's disease confirmed at autopsy, segregation of polymorphic DNA markers along the long arm of chromosome 21 was investigated. These markers covered the genetic distance in which the Alzheimer's disease locus has been mapped. The APP gene in an affected individual was analyzed by polymerase chain reaction (PCR) direct sequencing using intronic primers. An autoradiograph of a sequencing gel from part of exon 17 of the APP gene showed a C to T transition causing an amino acid substitution of a valine by an isoleucine at codon 717. The substitution created a *Bcl*/I restriction site that allowed detection of the corresponding polymorphism within the PCR product. Linkage analysis showed that the polymorphism cosegregated with Alzheimer's disease.

The *Bcl*/I restriction site was also detected in 2 affected individuals from a second unrelated family in which this variant occurred. This substitution was not detected during screening by PCR of 100 unrelated normal population controls and 14 affected individuals from 9 families with familial late-onset disease. These findings suggest that some cases of Alzheimer's disease could be caused by mutations in the APP gene.

▶ Given the increasing evidence for genetic heterogeneity in Alzheimer's disease, it becomes extremely important to attempt to define the genetic defects and to understand how they may cause the characteristic neurodegeneration. Deposition of β amyloid is increasingly recognized as an early event in the pathogenesis of Alzheimer's disease, and abnormal processing of the amyloid precursor protein that gives rise to β amyloid is a likely explanation. In a kindred showing linkage to chromosome 21 markers, a point mutation was found in the APP gene that substituted valine for isoleucine 2 amino acids beyond the carboxylterminus of the β amyloid within the membrane domain. Genetic data documented that the disease locus was linked to this missense mutation but did not prove causation. Nevertheless, this polymorphism was not noted in 200 normal chromosomes, suggesting that it may well be pathogenic. Such data provide important documentation that β amyloid peptide deposition may be the central event in the pathogenesis of Alzheimer's disease.— S.H. Appel, M.D.

Cortical Senile Plaques in Coronary Artery Disease, Aging and Alzheimer's Disease

Sparks DL, Hunsaker JC III, Scheff SW, Kryscio RJ, Henson JL, Markesbery WR (Univ of Kentucky; Kentucky Justice Cabinet, Lexington)
Neurobiol Aging 11:601–607, 1990   3–4

The most consistent neuropathologic feature of Alzheimer's disease is the presence of senile plaques (SPs). Numerous forms of SPs have been reported at autopsy in Alzheimer's patients, and the cognitive changes in this disease have been correlated to the characteristic pathologic lesions in the brain. A number of studies, however, have reported age-related increases in the number of SPs in the brains of cognitively normal individuals. An attempt was made to clarify the relationship between critical coronary artery disease (cCAD) and the presence of SPs.

Included in the study were 20 nondemented individuals who died of cCAD or in whom cCAD was an incidental finding at autopsy, 16 nondemented individuals who died of causes other than heart disease, and 17

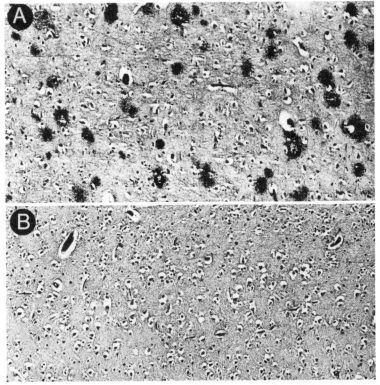

Fig 3–1.—Sections of PHG from nondemented patients. **A,** 71-year-old patient with cCAD, multiple SPs observed; **B,** 74-year-old patient without AD; SPs not found in this typical field. Bielschowsky method; calibration bar = 100 μm. (Courtesy of Sparks DL, Hunsaker JC III, Scheff SW, et al: *Neurobiol Aging* 11:601–607, 1990.)

individuals with clinical evidence and pathological confirmation of Alzheimer's disease. The cause of death was known in only 4 of 17 persons with Alzheimer's disease; 2 had died of cCAD. Seven of the 20 cCAD patients died of non–heart-disease trauma.

Brain weight differed significantly between groups, those of the patients with Alzheimer's being significantly lower than those of both non–heart-disease and cCAD groups. The presence or absence of SPs did not affect brain weight. Whereas SPs were observed in either the frontal pole (FP) or parahippocampal gyrus (PHG) in 15 of 20 cCAD subjects, only 2 of 16 non–heart-disease subjects had similar findings (Fig 3–1). The Alzheimer's disease group had a greater prevalence of SP than did the cCAD group. Neurofibrillary tangles, characteristic of Alzheimer's disease, were rarely found in either cCAD subjects or non–heart-disease controls.

The finding that many nondemented individuals dying with or as a result of cCAD have abundant SP formation in the cerebral cortex suggests a possible pathogenic relationship between cCAD and SPs. Chronic disease alone does not appear to be a factor in SP formation, as a number of the non–heart-disease subjects without SP died after a prolonged illness. The SPs in Alzheimer's brain may be an accompaniment of, but not causally related to, dementia. Alternatively, there may be a relationship between the presence of SPs and cognitive alterations in both cCAD and Alzheimer's disease.

▶ Here's a surprise. These SPs seem to accompany coronary artery disease death in nondemented patients. Would dementia have followed if the patients had lived? A suggestion for future study: Is there a connection between blood flow and Alzheimer's disease? I recall a paper years ago by a well-known cerebrovascular expert on a single Alzheimer's patient with bilateral carotid artery occlusion. That was heresy at the time but should the possibility again be considered?—R.D. Currier, M.D.

Myoclonus, Seizures, and Paratonia in Alzheimer Disease
Risse SC, Lampe TH, Bird TD, Nochlin D, Sumi SM, Keenan T, Cubberley L, Peskind E, Raskind MA (American Lake VA Med Ctr, Tacoma, Wash; VA Med Ctr, Seattle; Univ of Washington)
Alzheimer Dis Assoc Disord 4:217–225, 1990   3–5

The incidence of myclonus, seizures, and paratonia in Alzheimer's disease was studied in 28 patients with the clinical diagnosis of Alzheimer's disease who were followed longitudinally until death. Only 22 of the 28 patients fulfilled the pathologic criteria for Alzheimer's disease when autopsied; the remaining 6 had other degenerative neurologic diseases. Myoclonus was present in 12 patients with Alzheimer's disease, 7 of whom manifested symptoms within a year of death. Myoclonus was not found in the patients who did not have Alzheimer's. Similarly, seizures were more frequent in patients with Alzheimer's disease (64%) than in the others (17%). Paratonia was common in both groups of patients (about 83% to 86%). Myoclonus, seizures, and paratonia usually developed late in the course of the illness, with the mean onset of symptoms occurring 2, 3, and 3 years, respectively, before death.

The incidence of myoclonus, seizures, and paratonia in this series is higher than reported in most previous studies. The findings suggest that the diagnosis of Alzheimer's disease is most likely when myoclonus and seizures are evident late in the course of a dementing illness.

▶ So, seizures particularly late in the course are typical in those with Alzheimer's disease but not in the other quarter or so of the group who turned out in the long run not to have the disease. In addition, the authors found that paratonia (which you and I call gegenhalten) is typical in Alzheimer's disease.—R.D. Currier, M.D.

4 Stroke

Slowdown in the Decline of Stroke Mortality in the United States, 1978–1986
Cooper R, Sempos C, Hsieh S-C, Kovar MG (Loyola Univ Stritch School of Medicine, Maywood, Ill; Natl Ctr for Health Statistics, Hyattsville, Md)
Stroke 21:1274–1279, 1990   4–1

There has been a gradual decline in the stroke mortality rate in the United States since the 1970s. Mortality data for the years 1968 to 1986, as reported by the National Center for Health Statistics, were studied to assess the trends in stroke mortality rates and examine the causes of these changing trends.

Three distinct periods were identified (Fig 4–1). Period I, 1960–1972 for whites and 1960–1967 for blacks, was a period of slow decline in the stroke mortality rate. Period II, 1973–1978 for whites and 1968–1978 for blacks, was a period of rapid decline. During this period, the rate of decline in the stroke mortality rate accelerated markedly by almost 50%, so that the United States then had one of the lowest stroke mortality rates in the world. Period III, 1979–1986 for both races, was a period of gradual decline. Compared with the previous decade, period III was characterized by a 57% slowing of the absolute rate of decline for white men, 58% for white women, 44% for black men, and 62% for black women. If the decline in the 1980s had continued at the rate observed in period II, there would have been 131,000 fewer stroke deaths during period III. This deceleration in the rate of decline occurred while

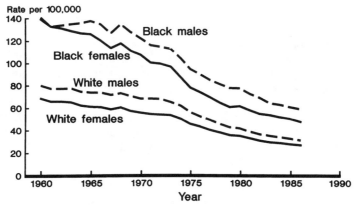

Fig 4–1.—Graph of trends in age-adjusted stroke mortality rates in the United States by sex-race group, 1960–1986. Rates for blacks are not available for 1962 and 1963. Data derived by linear interpolation. National Center for Health Statistics, National Vital Statistics System, 1960–1986. (Courtesy of Cooper R, Sempos C, Hsieh S-C, et al: *Stroke* 21:1274–1279, 1990.)

mortality rates associated with coronary heart disease and all causes were leveling off.

During the past decade, the rate of decline in stroke mortality in the United States slowed by more than 50% in all major sex–race groups, except in the case of black men. The reasons for this slowdown are unknown. The corresponding trends in the treatment and control of hypertension do not provide a satisfactory explanation for the decline.

▶ This is the other side of the argument about the imperfect relationship of the control of hypertension and decline of stroke mortality. Several years ago, the question was raised as to why the decline in stroke mortality seemed to be greater and occurred sooner than the control of hypertension nationwide. Now hypertension is better controlled and stroke mortality is leveling off. An assumption made in some papers is that hypertension is the only pertinent risk factor. Although it is the greatest, other risk factors are also changing with time, including control of diabetes, decreased smoking and alcohol consumption, monitoring of the cholesterol intake, use of birth control pills, and better heart disease treatment, but there must be a bottom to the effects of all.

An article by Kittner et al. (1) on black–white differences in stroke incidence points out that, even considering all of the above risk factors, there is a greater stroke prevalence in blacks than would be expected. The question arises as to whether there is an unknown factor in blacks that may lead to greater tendency for strokes and heart disease.

What else is new in stroke? Sohn et al. (2) point out that in the lacunar syndromes, not only the location but also the size of infarcts is an important factor in the clinical picture. Sensorimotor syndromes had the largest infarcts and dysarthria–clumsy hand syndrome the smallest. This is something I suppose we all knew subliminally, but it's nice to have it pointed out.

Drake et al. (3) treated 2 men in whom a manic state developed after the occurrence of relatively small ventral unilateral pontine infarctions, as shown by MRI scan. Both patients responded to lithium and were well within 18 months. It's a shame that pictures of the lesions were not included in the article. The authors can't explain it. Food for thought.

Along the same line, House et al. of Great Britain (4), in an analysis of mood disorders after stroke, lay low the previous studies showing that left-sided lesions do this, right-sided lesions do that, and frontal lesions do something else. The authors identified 73 consecutive stroke patients and studied them with psychological, psychiatric, and CT evaluations. They explain the failure to confirm that left-sided lesions were associated with more consistent depressive symptoms, and that right-sided lesions were associated with hypomania, on the basis that other reported populations were selected and they used different conventions for the definition and measurement of psychiatric disorders.— R.D. Currier, M.D.

References

1. Kittner SJ, et al: *JAMA* 264:1267, 1990.
2. Sohn YH, et al: *Stroke* 21:1258, 1990.

3. Drake ME Jr, et al: *Clin Neurosci* 2:322, 1990.
4. House A, et al: *Brain* 113:1113, 1990.

International Trends in Stroke Mortality: 1970–1985
Bonita R, Stewart A, Beaglehole R (Univ of Auckland, New Zealand)
Stroke 21:989–992, 1990   4–2

Mortality from coronary heart disease (CHD) in many industrialized countries has declined in recent decades. However, there has been an even more dramatic decline in mortality from stroke, which in many countries antedated the decline in CHD. The rates of decline of stroke mortality and CHD mortality during a 15-year period were compared for 27 countries.

Age-standardized mortality rates for the period 1970–1985 for men and women aged 40–69 years were obtained from the World Health Organization databank for stroke and CHD. A regression model was used to calculate the annual percentage of decline in stroke mortality and CHD mortality by sex for each country.

Stroke mortality rates declined in 21 countries for men and in 25 countries for women. The highest stroke mortality rates occurred in Bulgaria and the lowest in Switzerland. In 23 countries the decline in stroke mortality in women was greater than that in men. Rates for men were 23% to 115% higher than those for women in all countries. The greatest disparities between men and women were found in countries with low stroke mortality rates, namely, France, Austria, and Switzerland. Eastern European countries had the highest stroke mortality rates, experiencing either an increase or virtually no change during the years examined.

Except for Japan, the rank order of countries remained about the same throughout the 15-year study period. Japan had the highest stroke mortality for both sexes in 1970 but ranked only eleventh highest in 1985. The 7% annual decline in stroke mortality in Japan was the highest. For both sexes, countries with the highest stroke mortality rates were also those with the least favorable secular trend. The rate of stroke mortality decline was greater than that of CHD mortality in those countries that experienced a decline in both stroke and CHD.

Similar patterns were noted for CHD mortality rates. However, in contrast to stroke mortality rates, there was a tenfold difference in CHD mortality rates between the highest- and lowest-ranked countries, and the rates in men were 3–4 times those in women. Singapore was the only country to experience a decline in stroke mortality but an increase in CHD mortality.

Whereas the changes in stroke mortality from 1970 to 1985 varied widely among the 27 countries studied, the patterns within countries, between the sexes, and between stroke and CHD remained remarkably consistent. Overall, the decline in stroke mortality was greater than that in CHD. The Eastern European countries experienced increases in both stroke mortality and CHD mortality. International comparisons of risk factor levels over time are required to explain these striking differences among countries.

▶ Here are some fascinating data comparing mortality from CHD and stroke in 27 different countries. What is most remarkable is the continuing decline in death rates associated with stroke during this epoch. This is the case for men in 21 countries and for women in 25 countries, but there is a great disparity between this trend in the Western and Eastern European blocks. In the latter, there was actually some increase in stroke mortality rates. Whether this is a consequence of differences in national health care delivery systems, different risk factors, or risk factor management is not known, but it is food for future population-based epidemiologic investigations.

Recently, I returned from an extensive trip through the Soviet Union and, without a doubt, their health care delivery system is primitive and their risk factor reduction measures minimal. Cigarette smoking is rampant, and the diet is high in fat. I saw no evidence of programs for the evaluation of asymptomatic hypertension. Therefore, one might guess that the continued excess mortality in Eastern Europe reflects a lack of attention to risk factors rather than a difference among the populations.

An important question that is not addressed in the report by Bonita and colleagues is whether the decline in mortality has been accompanied by a similar decline in morbidity, or whether we are being left with an increasing pool of individuals disabled by stroke.—J.F. Toole, M.D.

Silent Cerebrovascular Disease in the Elderly: Correlation With Ambulatory Pressure
Shimada K, Kawamoto A, Matsubayashi K, Ozawa T (Kochi Med School, Japan)
Hypertension 16:692–699, 1990   4–3

Previous studies indicate that ambulatory blood pressure measurements, rather than readings obtained in the clinic, correlate with left ventricular hypertrophy and hypertensive retinopathy. Whether average daily blood pressure correlates with hypertensive cerebrovascular disease has not been clearly studied.

Two abnormal findings on MRI of the brain are suggestive of hypertensive cerebrovascular disease, namely, low intense foci (lacunae) and periventricular hyperintense lesions on T1- and T2-weighted images. The presence of these abnormalities was correlated with office and average daily blood pressure recordings in 73 healthy normotensive and hypertensive elderly subjects. The mean age was 70 years. Ambulatory blood pressure was monitored noninvasively for 24 hours and during awake and asleep periods.

Thirty-four patients (47%) had at least 1 lacuna (maximum number, 19) located in the basal ganglia (54%), deep white matter (34%), or brain stem (12%). The number of lacunae correlated significantly with advancing age and the average ambulatory blood pressures, but not with casual office blood pressures. Similarly, the grade of periventricular hyperintensities correlated significantly with advancing age and average ambulatory systolic blood pressures, particularly during sleep, but not with office pressures. Among the normotensive, "office hypertensive," and hypertensive subgroups, MRI abnormalities were more appropriate to the level of the 24-hour blood pressure than the office blood pressure. In hypertensive patients, MRI abnormalities were also associated with ECG evidence of left ventricular hypertrophy.

Lesions suggestive of hypertensive cerebrovascular disease seen on MRI are unexpectedly common in healthy elderly individuals, including those with mild to moderate essential hypertension. Ambulatory blood pressure monitoring is superior to casual office blood pressure measurements in predicting latent cerebrovascular disease.

▶ A close relative who has had many deep basal ganglia internal capsule lacunar strokes in the past several years objects to that diagnosis because he has not been found consistently to be hypertensive. This study shows that one can be hypertensive when monitored but not by the casual office measurement. I suppose the practical thing to take home from this is that if the blood pressure is found to be elevated on 1 test but not on the next 3 or 4, the patient still should be considered to have hypertension. And may have strokes. And Binswanger's disease.—R.D. Currier, M.D.

Transient Ischaemic Attacks in Young Patients: A Thromboembolic or Migrainous Manifestation? A 10-Year Follow-Up Study of 46 Patients
Larsen BH, Sørensen PS, Marquardsen J (Rigshospitalet, Copenhagen; Bispebjerg Hosp, Copenhagen; Ålborg Hosp, Ålborg, Denmark)
J Neurol Neurosurg Psychiatry 53:1029–1033, 1990   4–4

Some transient ischemic attacks (TIAs) occur in younger patients without heart disease or hypertension and may represent a relatively benign vascular disorder, probably a type of vasomotor disturbance. Data were reviewed on 46 patients aged 18–39 years seen during a 10-year period with TIAs. Two thirds were women, and the mean age was 29 years.

Twenty-five patients had headache as part of their attacks and 7 had a history of common migraine. Only 4 of 27 angiograms were abnormal; no patient had an operable carotid artery lesion. All 4 patients with major cerebrovascular risk factors, but only 2 of the other 42 patients, had a stroke or myocardial infarction during a mean follow-up of 10 years. Migraine developed in 8 patients during follow-up. No major vascular events occurred in the 15 patients with migraine.

Most TIAs in young persons, especially women, are not caused by thromboembolism but by flow disorders related to the underlying migraine. Angiograms are nearly always normal in these patients. The long-term outlook is excellent except in the small number of patients in whom TIAs are caused by thromboembolism. Angiography is most appropriate for these patients, chiefly males, who have cardiovascular risk factors.

▶ This authoritative report is a very important one regarding transitory episodes of neurologic deficit in young persons. This is the most vexing group of all. If the noninvasive studies are normal, should one obtain an angiogram? No one knows for sure, but the authors have given us some guidelines for consideration. One element not considered in detail by them is the possibility of paradoxical embolism resulting from a patent foramen ovale, but this is not a major oversight. Those who take care of young patients with transitory neurologic deficits are well advised to read the full-length article.—J.F. Toole, M.D.

Circadian Variation in Onset of Acute Ischemic Stroke
Marsh EE III, Biller J, Adams HP Jr, Marler JR, Hulbert JR, Love BB, Gordon DL (Univ of Iowa; Natl Inst of Neurological Disorders and Stroke, Bethesda, Md)
Arch Neurol 47:1178–1180, 1990   4–5

Little is known about the events leading to ischemic stroke in patients with previously asymptomatic disease, but some clinical observations suggest that a circadian component may be relevant. Prospective data from 151 patients having acute ischemic stroke were analyzed. All of the patients were seen within 24 hours of onset of stroke. The median age was 63 years.

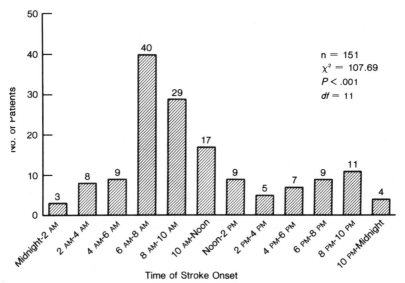

Fig 4–2.—Time of stroke onset for all patients with ischemic stroke. $P < .001$; n = 151; χ^2 = 107.69; df = 11. (Courtesy of Marsh EE III, Biller J, Adams HP Jr, et al: *Arch Neurol* 47:1178–1180, 1990.)

Most strokes occurred between 6 AM and noon (Fig 4–2). There was little chance that this pattern could result from random distribution. The pattern persisted after redistributing the patients who had stroke on awakening. Use of aspirin did not appear to influence the temporal pattern of stroke occurrence.

All subtypes of stroke have a tendency to occur more often in the early morning than at other times of day. The first hour after awakening may be the most critical period. It is not likely that a single factor explains the morning peak of stroke onset. Possible factors include circadian variation in thrombotic/antithrombotic balance and variation in the susceptibility of the brain to ischemia.

▶ Just as with myocardial infarction, stroke has a circadian distribution, occurring more often in the early morning than at other times of the day. The authors note that the first hour after awakening may be the most critical period, and it is a question as to whether these are strokes that are present at the time of awakening or occur after one is up on one's feet. The distinction is very important. In the former case, a stroke could have occurred at any time during the night and could be related to a variety of factors, even up to and including malposition of the head on the neck, which might kink arteries. If a stroke occurs after the patient arises, it could be caused by changes in circulation dynamics. Which is the culprit? We await further news.—J.F. Toole, M.D.

Racial Differences in the Anterior Circulation in Cerebrovascular Disease: How Much Can Be Explained by Risk Factors?
Inzitari D, Hachinski VC, Taylor DW, Barnett HJM (Univ of Florence, Italy; Univ of Western Ontario, London; McMaster Univ, Hamilton, Ont)
Arch Neurol 47:1080–1084, 1990   4–6

Studies have suggested that intracranial segments in white persons are involved less often by cerebrovascular disease than they are in Orientals or blacks, for reasons that are not clear. An attempt was made, by analyzing data on 1,367 patients enrolled in the Extracranial/Intracranial Bypass Study, to learn whether risk factors and race independently affect the site of cerebrovascular lesions in various ethnic groups.

Blacks in this population were more likely to be hypertensive and diabetic and to smoke cigarettes, whereas whites had higher systolic pressures and hemoglobin values. Vascular risk factors were least prevalent in Orientals. Nevertheless, race was a strong independent predictor of the location of cerebrovascular lesions. Both intermittent claudication and ischemic heart disease, like internal carotid artery lesions, were least frequent in Orientals and most prevalent in whites.

These findings affirm a role for race in determining the site of cerebrovascular lesions. Pathologic studies indicate that the intracranial and extracranial vessels are anatomically distinct, and that atherosclerosis may differ in these types of vessels. Furthermore, the chemical constitution of cerebral vessel walls may differ with race.

▶ In analyzing a cohort of 1,367 individuals in the Extracranial/Intracranial Bypass Study, 586 were Caucasians from North America, 472 Caucasians from Europe, 86 blacks from North America, and 220 Orientals. The authors conclude that there is a different racial propensity to and distribution of cerebral circulatory abnormalities, but their data do not permit them to reach any conclusions as to why.

Some suspect diet, as, for example, in Orientals in whom there is very little atherosclerosis and an excess of the complications of sustained hypertension, both probably related to life-long nutritional habits.—J.F. Toole, M.D.

Deteriorating Ischemic Stroke: Risk Factors and Prognosis
Dávalos A, Cendra E, Teruel J, Martinez M, Genis D (Hosp of Girona, Spain)
Neurology 40:1865–1869, 1990   4–7

Forming unified criteria to define progressive stroke has been difficult. The definition of deteriorating stroke covers patients in whom the neurologic dysfunction increases gradually over several hours. To determine the frequency of neurologic deterioration in cerebral infarction and to define a deterioration risk profile in patients examined within the first 8 hours of cerebral ischemia, clinical and radiologic data were reviewed concerning 98 patients. The Canadian Neurological Scale Score and Barthel index were recorded during a 3-month follow-up.

Overall, 41% of the patients deteriorated neurologically in the first 48 hours. According to logistic regression analysis, high systolic blood pressure, an increased blood sugar concentration at admission, and carotid territory involvement were independently related to deterioration. Strokes were fatal in 35% of those with deteriorating infarcts and in 8.6% of those with stable infarcts. At the end of the study, functional capacity was lower in patients with deteriorating infarcts. However, the 2 groups showed parallel improvement from the fourth day onward.

There appears to be a group of variables having independent predictive power in deteriorating ischemic stroke. However, an early risk profile of deterioration could not be established, as these variables allowed correct classification in only 67% of the patients. The discouraging prognosis for deteriorating cerebral infarct indicates that the search must continue for new drugs that can stop or prevent progression in the first hours of cerebral ischemia.

▶ How to predict the course when the stroke patient first appears? After a number of years you get a feel for these things and are able to make some sort of a prediction, but this study is helpful. High blood pressure, high blood sugar, and carotid territory involvement make it more likely that the patient will deteriorate in the first 48 hours. The next question is, how are we supposed to treat him?

During the recent annual stroke meeting of the American Heart Association in San Francisco, 2 interesting findings were reported. One is that patients with markedly stenotic carotids do better with operation, and the other is that smoking is a high-grade risk factor for ruptured berry aneurysms. The first is no surprise despite the clouds of confusion caused by those who have been operating for all degrees of narrowing. The second finding was not as obvious: An 11 times greater risk in smokers of ruptured aneurysms is something to keep in mind when exhorting those who still smoke.—R.D. Currier, M.D.

Stroke Recurrence Within 2 Years After Ischemic Infarction
Hier DB, Foulkes MA, Swiontoniowski M, Sacco RL, Gorelick PB, Mohr JP, Price TR, Wolf PA (Univ of Illinois, Chicago; Michael Reese Hosp and Med Ctr, Chicago; Natl Inst of Neurological Disorders and Stroke, Bethesda, Md; Columbia-Presbyterian Med Ctr, New York; Univ of Maryland; et al)
Stroke 22:155–161, 1991   4–8

The risk factors for recurrence of stroke are not firmly established. A large number of patients were followed prospectively in an attempt to identify prognostic indicators of stroke recurrence. The study sample comprised 1,273 patients who had an initial stroke diagnosed as cerebral infarction. Follow-up information was gathered by direct contact, telephone, or mail at 3, 6, 12, and 24 months after the stroke. Recurrent stroke was defined as an event producing a different neurologic deficit, occurring in a different anatomical site or vascular territory, or fitting into a different stroke subtype than the initial stroke. The median follow-up time was 13 months.

A recurrent stroke developed in 129 patients, a rate of 10.1% (Fig 4–3). For all patients the estimated 2-year cumulative recurrence rate was 14.1%. Age, race, and sex were not associated with stroke recurrence. A history of diabetes and stroke was associated with recurrence, whereas a history of atrial fibrillation, myocardial infarction, congestive heart failure, angina, and transient ischemic attack were not. Hypertension at the initial examination was predictive of recurrence, but discharge with aspirin or anticoagulant therapy was not.

When the subtype of the recurrent stroke was known, most proved to be the same as the initial stroke. Univariate analysis showed that a history of stroke, stroke subtype, history of diabetes, initial blood pressure, abnormal initial CT scan, history of hypertension, and initial blood glucose level were significant predictors of stroke recurrence. A patient with diabetes, hypertension, previous stroke, and any infarct of known cause was estimated to have a risk of recurrent stroke 2.9 times higher than that in a nondiabetic, normotensive patient with no previous stroke but

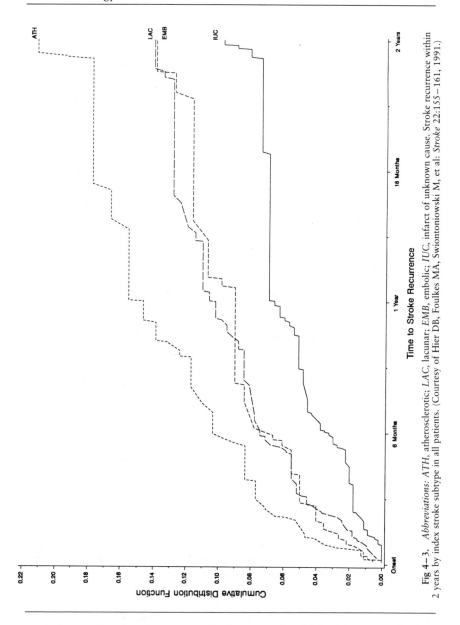

Fig 4–3. *Abbreviations: ATH,* atherosclerotic; *LAC,* lacunar; *EMB,* embolic; *IUC,* infarct of unknown cause. Stroke recurrence within 2 years by index stroke subtype in all patients. (Courtesy of Hier DB, Foulkes MA, Swiontoniowski M, et al: *Stroke* 22:155–161, 1991.)

an infarct of unknown cause. Patients in the high-risk group had a 24.5% incidence of recurrent stroke, compared to 9.5% for patients in the low-risk group.

The relative risk ratios for predictors of stroke recurrence at 2 years are modest but significant. It may be difficult to identify patient subgroups at high risk.

► Large numbers of patients followed prospectively can yield interesting information regarding where to put one's time and energy. The fact that the recurrence rate of stroke is about 10% suggests that secondary preventive measures with interventions to reduce modifiable risk factors might be useful. It is not surprising that the authors found elevated blood pressure and a history of diabetes to be associated with an increased risk of stroke recurrence but, unexpectedly, atrial fibrillation and transient ischemic attacks (TIAs) were not associated with increased risk. These 2 factors have been the subject of intense investigation by many researchers who have found that patients with atrial fibrillation and the risk of cardioembolic embolism to the brain respond dramatically to the use of aspirin and long-term anticoagulants, and that TIAs and stroke can be prevented by endarterectomy in appropriate patients. That neither is associated with an increased risk of stroke is such a surprise that I have reservations about these data.—J.F. Toole, M.D.

Transient Ischemic Attacks and Small-Vessel Disease
Kappelle LJ, van Latum JC, Koudstaal PJ, van Gijn J, for the Dutch TIA Study Group (Univ Dept of Neurology, Utrecht; Univ Hosp Dijkzigt, Rotterdam)
Lancet 337:339–341, 1991   4–9

Small-vessel disease may account for 20% to 25% of all ischemic strokes, but its role in transient ischemic attacks (TIAs) is less certain. Data were reviewed on 606 patients in whom transient cerebral ischemia developed with symptoms lasting for less than 24 hours. None had episodes suggestive of posterior fossa ischemia. The median age was 65 years.

A relevant supratentorial infarct was demonstrated on CT in 79 patients (13%). Forty-six patients had a lacunar infarct and 33 had cortical lesions—25 in the end zone and 8 in the boundary zone. Forty-six other patients had evidence of an old infarct that in 33 of them was of the lacunar type. Thirty-two of the 46 patients with a recent lacunar infarct and 11 of the 33 with a relevant recent cortical infarct had a unilateral neurologic deficit without cortical symptoms. A history of no previous cortical symptoms was obtained from 54% of all patients with a recent infarct and from 64% of those without CT evidence of a relevant infarct.

Lacunar TIAs may have a better prognosis than cortical TIAs, or they may often precede cortical attacks. Alternatively, many cortical infarcts may occur without warning. Small-vessel disease probably is the most common cause of TIAs.

► The Dutch TIA Study Group has come up with another interesting and very important finding—small vessel intracranial arterial disease can result in TIAs. The authors aver that these small infarcts have a better prognosis than those emanating from larger arteries. Of course, the management options are different as well and include administration of platelet antiaggregants, anticoagulants, and hemorheologic agents.—J.F. Toole, M.D.

Clinical–Computed Tomographic Correlations of Lacunar Infarction in the Stroke Data Bank
Chamorro A, Sacco RL, Mohr JP, Foulkes MA, Kase CS, Tatemichi TK, Wolf PA, Price TR, Hier DB (Neurological Inst of New York; Natl Inst of Neurological Disorders and Stroke, Bethesda, Md; Boston Univ; Univ of Maryland; Michael Reese Hosp and Med Ctr, Chicago)
Stroke 22:175–181, 1991   4–10

Data were reviewed concerning 1,273 cerebral infarctions registered in the Stroke Data Bank. Lacunar stroke accounted for 337 cases, or 26% of the total. The median age of patients with lacunar infarction was 66 years. Most (316 patients) had classic lacunar syndromes. Hypertension and diabetes were more frequent in patients with lacunar infarction than in those with cardioembolic infarction. Stroke risk factors are given for recognized lacunar syndromes in the table.

Computed tomography demonstrated a lesion in 35% of patients with lacunar stroke, most often in the internal capsule and corona radiata. The mean infarct volume was greatest in patients with pure hemiparesis or a sensorimotor syndrome. Among patients with pure hemiparesis and an infarct in the posterior limb of the internal capsule, lesion volume correlated with the severity of hemiparesis. Infarcts involving the lowest part of the internal capsule were an exception, producing a severe deficit regardless of their volume. Lesions in the corona radiata produced a variety of hemiparesis syndromes. Lesions underlying sensorimotor syndrome were mainly in the posterior limb of the internal capsule and corona radiata. The site and volume of a lacunar infarct are not reliable predictors of the form of clinical deficit.

Stroke Risk Factors by Lacunar Syndrome Subgroup

Risk factor	Lacunar syndrome				
	PMH ($n=181$)	SMS ($n=63$)	AH ($n=33$)	PSS ($n=21$)	DCH ($n=18$)
Hypertension (1)	76	71	67	80	78
Diabetes	30	14	30	24	17
Claudication (2)	27	33	18	19	28
Previous TIA (12)	12	9	6	33	24
Previous stroke (5)	17	20	21	19	22

Abbreviations: PMH, pure motor hemiparesis; *SMS,* sensorimotor syndrome; *AH,* ataxic hemiparesis; *PSS,* pure sensory syndrome; *DCH,* Dysarthria-clumsy hand syndrome; *TIA* transient ischemic attacks; ( ), missing data among all 5 subgroups. Data are percent.
(Courtesy of Chamorro A, Sacco RL, Mohr JP, et al: *Stroke* 22:175–181, 1991.)

Lacunar Transient Ischemic Attacks: A Clinically Useful Concept?
Hankey GJ, Warlow CP (Western Gen Hosp, Edinburgh)
Lancet 337:335–338, 1991   4–11

Because lacunar ischemic stroke syndromes are distinct from cortical ischemic stroke, the question arose of whether cerebrovascular transient ischemic attacks (TIAs) are similarly heterogeneous. Prospective studies were made in 130 patients with TIAs, including 71 who underwent carotid angiography.

Twenty-five patients (19%) had a lacunar TIA and 81% had cortical TIAs. Lacunar attacks were purely motor in most instances. A lacunar TIA was present in 24% of the 71 patients having cerebral angiography; 76% had a cortical TIA. The extracranial carotid was significantly more stenosed in patients with cortical attacks (Fig 4–4). Twenty patients with cortical TIAs and 3 with lacunar TIAs had ischemic stroke during follow-up. Two of the 3 latter patients had a lacunar stroke.

These findings support an association between cortical TIAs and ipsilateral extracranial internal carotid disease. Patients with lacunar TIAs, in contrast, are more likely to have disease of small intracranial vessels. Patients with cortical TIAs may benefit from angiography and endarterectomy. Further study may show whether small-vessel occlusion or hemorrhagic stroke develops in those with lacunar TIAs.

Cerebrovascular Accidents Related to Chiropractic Care: Further Considerations
Lädermann J-P (Geneva, Switzerland)
Eur J Chiropractic 38:63–68, 1990   4–12

So-called iatrogenic brain stem syndromes occurring after chiropractic treatment have received more publicity than their true frequency war-

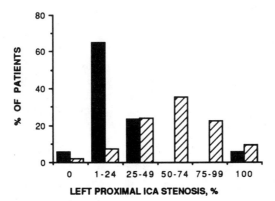

Fig 4–4.—Angiographic findings in left internal carotid artery *(ICA)*. *Filled columns* indicate lacunar TIAs (n = 17), and *hatched columns* indicate cortical TIAs (n = 54). (Courtesy of Hankey GJ, Warlow CP: *Lancet* 337:335–338, 1991.)

rants. About 100 such cases have been recorded in the past 50 years, half of them fatal; 12 cases involved chiropractors, and these probably are recorded more systematically than others.

Conditions that have followed manipulative treatment include the Wallenberg syndrome (Horner syndrome, vocal cord paralysis, trigeminal deficits), the "locked-in" syndrome, internuclear ophthalmoplegia, sensorineural hearing loss, and a global brain stem and cerebellar syndrome rapidly producing fatal coma. A vascular insult is responsible for these disorders.

Warning symptoms may include tinnitus, nausea and vomiting, lightheadedness, vertigo, incoordination, difficulty in walking, slurred speech, numbness, and loss of consciousness. A disorder may develop immediately after spinal manipulation or after a period of days.

Screening measures might protect against malpractice but cannot be relied on to avoid these complications. Spinal manipulation can provoke some brain stem lesions. It is not really an iatrogenic situation if this implies that adverse effects would not have occurred had sound therapeutic procedures been followed. Occasionally, a brain stem syndrome is induced by rational, widely accepted, properly administered chiropractic treatment.

▶ It's difficult to understand what is meant by "rational" chiropractic treatment. That aside, it is no surprise that any form of therapy, no matter how well intentioned, should occasionally result in complications. What is interesting is that this problem is mentioned in the chiropractic literature. The author alleges no clear cause and effect relationship, apparently giving no weight to traumatic vertebral artery dissection. Carotid and vertebral dissections occurring with head turns are hardly news, and the forced, rapid head turns associated with chiropractic manipulation occasionally injure these vessels.—J.J. Corbett, M.D.

A Prognostic System for Transient Ischemia or Minor Stroke
Kernan WN, Horwitz RI, Brass LM, Viscoli CM, Taylor KJW (Yale Univ)
Ann Intern Med 114:552–557, 1991   4–13

An attempt was made to develop a better way of assigning risk to patients with carotid transient ischemia or minor stroke. In all, 142 patients hospitalized between 1984 and 1987 within 1 month of a first episode were included in the trial and followed for at least 2 years.

Within 2 years of the initial episode, 38 patients died or had a stroke. Thirteen patients died without having had a stroke, and 4 died after having a stroke. Application of a proportional hazards model identified age over 65, diabetes, and severe hypertension as significant risk factors for stroke or death. Three risk groups were well differentiated when coronary heart disease and a distinction between transient ischemia and stroke were incorporated into the prognostic system (Fig 4–5). Older age and diabetes were slightly more heavily weighted than hypertension. The predictive system performed well when tested in a cohort of patients en-

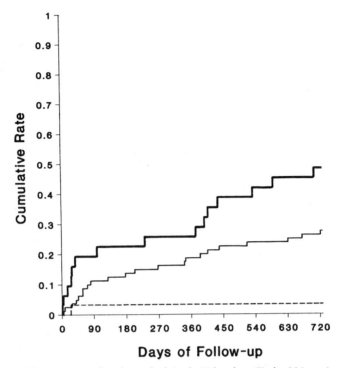

Days of Follow-up

Fig 4–5.—The occurrence of stroke or death in the Yale cohort (Kaplan-Meier estimates). The length of follow-up was measured from study entry. Risk group 1 is indicated by a *dashed line*, risk group 2, a *normal-type line*, and risk group 3, a *boldface line*. Each patient's risk group status was determined by his or her total point score for 5 factors: age of more than 65 years (3 points), diabetes (3 points), hypertension (2 points), the distinction between stroke and transient ischemia (2 points for stroke), and coronary heart disease (1 point). (*P* < .001 by the log-rank test.) (Courtesy of Kernan WN, Horwitz RI, Brass LM, et al: *Ann Intern Med* 114:552–557, 1991.)

rolled in a trial of aspirin and sulfinpyrazone for threatened stroke. Nevertheless, there is much room for refining this system.

▶ This study delineates the predictors for stroke in a population of patients with transient ischemic attacks or minor stroke. One must be wary of the results, however, because the numbers are so few. Based on this study of 142 patients hospitalized within a month of the first episode, the authors developed a proportional hazards model that was used to determine significant risk factors. Aside from the fact that this was a select population of hospitalized patients, the numbers are too few to allow firm conclusions. As with the report by Hier et al. (Abstract 4–8) of modifiable risk factors, only diabetes mellitus and severe hypertension reached statistical significance.

What is surprising to me is that the use of aspirin and the presence of internal carotid artery plaque (not described by degree of severity and/or stenosis) were not of significance. The fact that one of the criteria for inclusion in this study was the presence of bilateral internal carotid artery plaque is a puzzle, because one is interested in the presence of severe stenosis, not the presence or absence of bilaterality. In this particular study, bilateral plaque had a relative risk of 1.5, whereas carotid obstruction demarcated by lumen reduction exceeding 75% had a relative risk of only .9. Like the Hier et al.'s study, this one also flies in the face both of logic and the data coming a variety of sources detailing how increasing stenosis vastly increases the risk of stroke distal to the obstruction. I suspect that we may be dealing with a statistical artifact rather than data about which we can generalize.—J.F. Toole, M.D.

Mechanism of Stroke in Patients Taking Aspirin
Chimowitz MI, Furlan AJ, Nayak S, Sila CA (Cleveland Clin Found)
Neurology 40:1682–1685, 1990   4–14

Aspirin appears to reduce, but not eliminate, the risk of stroke in patients with transient ischemic attacks (TIAs) or minor stroke. The criteria for the use of aspirin based on the causal mechanisms of TIA or stroke, however, have not been closely studied, making it difficult to determine which patients are most likely to benefit from aspirin treatment. To determine the mechanisms of ischemic stroke in patients taking aspirin, 47 patients sustaining a cerebral infarction while taking aspirin were studied prospectively over 1 year.

The mechanism of stroke was undetermined in 26% of the patients. In the remaining 35 patients, 39 potential mechanisms were identified, including large-artery atherosclerosis in 40%, cardioembolism in 32%, and small-vessel occlusive disease in 11%. Of 11 patients who sustained carotid atherosclerosis and stroke, 82% had more than 90% carotid stenosis or occlusion. Of 12 patients with strokes of undetermined mechanism, 83% had a previous stroke, with 8 being of undetermined mechanisms. In 57% of the patients, disability after stroke was moderate or severe.

These findings suggest that stroke in patients taking aspirin has a variety of etiologies. Such strokes frequently cause moderate or severe disability. Patients with carotid disease in whom aspirin therapy fails often have high-grade carotid stenosis or occlusion. Stroke of undetermined mechanism may recur more often than other stroke subtypes in patients taking aspirin.

▶ Here is a disconcerting article describing the mechanism and severity of breakthrough stroke in patients taking aspirin to reduce the risk of cerebral infarction. The authors categorized patients by various mechanisms of stroke, including cardioembolism, small-vessel disease, large artery plaque with distal embolism, carotid stenosis or occlusion, and so on. In all, aspirin had been prescribed for primary or secondary prevention.

Not only did breakthrough strokes occur, the resultant disability was, in some cases, severe. Of particular importance is that patients with high-grade carotid stenosis are still at excess risk despite the use of aspirin.—J.F. Toole, M.D.

The Syndrome of Bilateral Hemispheric Border Zone Ischemia

Sloan MA, Haley EC Jr (Univ of Virginia, Charlottesville)
Stroke 21:1668–1673, 1990   4–15

Patients with unilateral or bilateral carotid occlusive disease have also been known to have symptoms compatible with vertebrobasilar ischemia. Intracranial steal phenomena may explain these symptoms. The spectrum of symptoms compatible with published criteria for vertebrobasilar transient ischemic attacks (TIAs) was examined in 54 patients with severe bilateral carotid occlusive disease; the symptoms were correlated with angiographic lesions, patterns of collateral flow, and CT data.

Eight patients had symptoms suggesting vertebrobasilar insufficiency; 5 were identified retrospectively and 3, prospectively. Various combinations of hemodynamically mediated, transient bilateral motor, sensory, or visual impairment were seen. Generally, there was no dysarthria, dysphagia, or diplopia. Each patient also had additional symptoms compatible with transient hemispheric or retinal ischemia. The anatomical areas subserving the bilateral vertebrobasilar-like symptoms were correlated with angiographically estimated arterial border zones in both hemispheres.

Subtle changes in perfusion pressure in patients with severe hemodynamic lesions of both internal carotid arteries may provoke simultaneous bilateral border zone ischemia, a syndrome of bilateral motor and/or sensory symptoms with facial sparing, gait disturbances, or bilateral visual phenomena but no intrinsic brain stem symptoms. The correlation of symptoms and their mechanisms with the angiographic vascular anatomy suggests the possible hemispheric origin of such vertebrobasilar-like symptoms.

▶ For those of us who have been rather rigid in our criteria for the diagnosis of carotid and vertebrobasilar artery TIAs, this is a very disturbing report and amplifies those of others, particularly Bogousslavsky and Regli (1), who report that symptoms heretofore accepted as characteristic of vertebrobasilar artery TIAs can in reality represent bilateral carotid artery syndrome. This will make we who have considered the vertebrobasilar artery syndrome to be a well-defined entity for which surgical intervention is not mandated rethink our position. For example, many patients who are thought to have vertebrobasilar TIAs are not subjected to noninvasive imaging, much less arteriography. Now we discover that some patients who apparently have a vertebrobasilar TIA have bilateral carotid artery disease. Explanations for this occurrence have, in the past, been attributed to a "steal" from the vertebrobasilar to the carotid systems. Sloan and Haley now suggest that these are bilateral carotid TIAs that simulate vertebral-basilar phenomena because of ischemia in the border zone between the carotid and vertebrobasilar systems. This is one more nail in the coffin of the rigidly defined TIA concept.—J.F. Toole, M.D.

Reference

1. Bogousslavsky J, Regli F: *Arch Neurol* 42:64, 1985.

Cerebral Blood Flow and Oxygen Metabolism in Patients With Vascular Dementia of the Binswanger Type

Yao H, Sadoshima S, Kuwabara Y, Ichiya Y, Fujishima M (Kyushu Univ, Fukuoka, Japan)
Stroke 21:1694–1699, 1990
4–16

Binswanger's disease, recently described as a type of vascular dementia, is characterized by slowly progressive dementia and periventricular white matter lesions. Patients with vascular dementia often experience intellectual decline in association with ischemic brain damage in the form of white matter lesions with multiple lacunes. It is therefore important to measure the cerebral blood flow (CBF) and brain metabolism in patients with Binswanger-type dementia.

Clinical and neuroradiologic studies, including positron emission tomography, were done in 5 patients with Binswanger-type vascular dementia. These patients had slowly progressive dementia, vascular risk factors (e.g., hypertension), often a history of minor stroke, and characteristic white matter lesions observed on brain CT or MRI. No occlusive lesions in any patient were found on digital subtraction angiography of the cervical and intracranial arteries. Both CBF and the cerebral metabolic rate for oxygen were greatly decreased in the white matter, as well as in the parietal, frontal, and temporal cortices, where no abnormalities were detected by brain CT or MRI. Vascular dementia of the Binswanger type may be caused by disconnection between the cerebral cortex and subcortical structures because of ischemic damage in the white matter.

▶ This is further confirmation that Binswanger's disease is associated with vascular disease. The flow is markedly reduced. Whether flow reduction is secondary to the disease or is the cause is not yet clear. As for the cause of the radiopathologic changes, Leys et al. (1) believe that wallerian degeneration in the white matter may be partially responsible because it also occurs in those diseases with primary neuronal loss, e.g., Alzheimer's.—R.D. Currier, M.D.

Reference

1. Leys D, et al: *J Neurol Neurosurg Psychiatry* 54:46, 1991.

Relation of Leukoaraiosis to Lesion Type in Stroke Patients

Hijdra A, Verbeeten B Jr, Verhulst JAPM (Academisch Medisch Centrum, Amsterdam)
Stroke 21:890–894, 1990
4–17

Leukoaraiosis is characterized by periventricular white matter lucencies observed on CT scans in the absence of hydrocephalus or well-defined white matter diseases. It may be more common in patients with the types of lesions associated mainly with small-vessel disease than in those with cortical infarcts or hemorrhages from arteriovenous malformations

(AVMs). To test this hypothesis, 367 patients with ischemic or hemorrhagic stroke underwent CT.

Leukoaraiosis was found in 141, or 38%. Patients with leukoaraiosis were significantly older than patients without it. They were also significantly more likely to have hypertension, diabetes mellitus, general vascular disease, and lacunar infarcts observed on CT, but less likely to have cortical infarcts than were those without leukoaraiosis. Logistic regression analysis found increasing age, lacunar infarcts, and hemorrhages to be significant determinants of leukoaraiosis. Cortical infarcts had a significant negative correlation with the disease. Patients with hemorrhages had leukoaraiosis significantly more often when aneurysms or AVMs were not present.

These observations suggest that leukoaraiosis is associated with small-vessel disease in patients with cerebrovascular disorders. The prognosis for stroke outcome in such patients may be worse than in those without leukoaraiosis.

▶ It is hard to keep up with the evolving concepts and the burgeoning literature related to leukoaraiosis. It seems that it is an asymptomatic MRI entity in most individuals. Whether it is accompanied by pathology that can be identified post mortem is problematic. Some believe that it is caused by focal edema, but it is not accompanied by changes in the permeability of the blood-brain barrier.

Leukoaraiosis correlates with hypertension and with the vascular consequences of hypertension, e.g., lacunar infarction, microvascular disease, and cerebral hemorrhage. Some believe that these vascular disorders per se cause leukoaraiosis; others think that it is a combination of arteriolar disease plus hypoperfusion of the white matter.

As of now, leukoaraiosis is an entity visible on MRI, but whether it is a disease and what causes it remain to be determined.—J.F. Toole, M.D.

Randomised, Double-Blind, Placebo-Controlled Trial of Nimodipine in Acute Stroke

Trust Study Group (Univ Hosp, Nottingham, England)
Lancet 336:1205–1209, 1990   4–18

Nimodipine, a dihydropyridine calcium channel blocker, is a cerebral vasodilator that increases blood flow within the infarcted area in acute stroke. Nimodipine also exerts a cytoprotective effect by limiting intracellular calcium flux. Its role in the treatment of acute stroke was studied in a randomized, double-blind, placebo-controlled multicenter trial of 1,215 patients older than 40 years. The patients had become hemiparetic in the previous 48 hours, were conscious and able to swallow, and were living independently before the stroke. Nimodipine, 120 mg/day, was given orally to 607 patients for 21 days, 608 patients were given placebo. The primary end point was functional independence after 6 months, which was defined as a score of 60 or higher on the activities of daily living scale, the Berthel index.

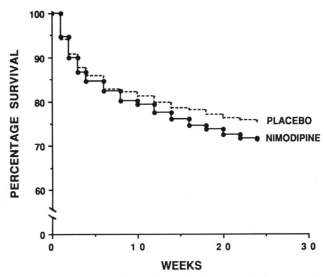

Fig 4–6.—Survival curves for nimodipine and placebo. Generalized Breslow comparison, $P = .17$. (Courtesy of Trust Study Group: *Lancet* 336:1205–1209, 1990.)

At 6 months, 55% of the group given nimodipine and 58% of those given placebo functioned independently. The odds ratio for patients given nimodipine was .88, and for death during nimodipine therapy, 1.22. The difference in mortality began to appear between weeks 3 and 24, when the death rate increased from 12% at week 3 to 25% at week 24 in the placebo-treated group and from 13% to 29%, respectively, in the nimodipine-treated group (Fig 4–6). The mortality rate was not affected even when nimodipine was given within 24 or 48 hours of entry into the study. There was a trend toward delayed recovery in the nimodipine-treated patients at week 3. Contrary to earlier reports, this study shows that nimodipine, 120 mg/day, administered orally within 48 hours of the stroke does not improve functional recovery in patients with acute stroke in a general hospital setting.

▶ The onomatopoeic words *randomized, double-blind, placebo-controlled trial* with appropriately placed commas and hyphens suggest powerful results. When first I read this now recurring title in journals, I believed the bottom line from each trial, but now that I am seeing them sometimes come up with conflicting results (e.g., the Physicians Health Study in the United States vs. the outcome of the United Kingdom Physicians Trial concerning the use of aspirin for prevention of myocardial infarction and stroke) I am approaching these well-sounding phrases with a more sophisticated, and perhaps jaundiced eye. This publication is one more example of a study fatally marred by methodological defects that only the careful reader would note. For example, this study is a clinical one purporting to show that nimodipine is not effective in patients with hemiparetic stroke. A CT was done, when possible, between days 7 and 14. However, of the 1,215 patients, only 24% underwent CT. Therefore, we are dealing with a mixed bag of clinical patients who may have had a variety of etiologies for stroke.

Furthermore, the entry window was 48 hours, and it is well known that in order to reverse or halt the evolution of a cerebral event, one must intervene within no more than several hours and, preferably, within 60 minutes. Lastly, nimodipine was given orally at an arbitrary dosage without determination of blood levels or an attempt to assess absorption and efficacy. Patients who are ill have a variety of absorptive problems in the gastrointestinal tract that could have an effect on outcomes.

It is the hope of statisticians and clinicians that the aggregation of large numbers will overcome methodological defects, and sometimes they may be right. However, they may also be wrong, so that I conclude that this particular study is a draw. There is no need to discuss type I and type II errors and other nuances. One hopes that in the future, when researchers go by such sophisticated names as Trust Study Group and when the trial is billed as randomized, double-blind, and placebo-controlled, journals will be more critical of the methodology before they publish inconclusive trials such as this.—J.F. Toole, M.D.

Predicting the Appropriate Use of Carotid Endarterectomy, Upper Gastrointestinal Endoscopy, and Coronary Angiography
Brook RH, Park RE, Chassin MR, Solomon DH, Keesey J, Kosecoff J (Rand Corp, Santa Monica, Calif; Value Health Sciences, Santa Monica, Calif; Univ of California, Los Angeles)
N Engl J Med 323:1173–1177, 1990   4–19

In a previous study of Medicare patients aged 65 years or older living in 1 of 5 states, about 25% of coronary angiographies and upper gastrointestinal endoscopies and 67% of carotid endarterectomies were performed for reasons that were less than medically appropriate. Whether the appropriateness of each procedure can be predicted from easily obtainable data on the characteristics of patients, physicians, or hospitals was investigated. Measurements of appropriateness included the patient's age, sex, and race; the physician's age, board-certification status, and experience with the procedure; and the hospital's teaching status, profit-making status, and size.

In general, less than 4% of the variance in medical appropriateness could be attributed to easily observable characteristics of patients, physicians, or hospitals. However, for all 3 procedures, appropriateness increased in a teaching hospital, particularly in the case of carotid endarterectomy. Older or more affluent patients were more likely to undergo angiographies for appropriate reasons. The likelihood of undergoing an appropriate carotic endarterectomy decreased by almost one third, from 40% to 28%, among patients treated by a surgeon who performed a high, rather than a low, volume of procedures. This was because surgeons performing many endarterectomies operated on patients with less severe stenosis and with no previous carotid symptoms.

The medical appropriateness of a procedure cannot clearly be predicted from the easily obtainable data on characteristics of patients, physicians, or hospitals. These findings suggest that, if the level of appropriateness is to improve, it must be assessed directly at the level of each patient, hospital, and physician.

▶ The surgeon who does the most and is therefore presumably the best at an operation has a lower likelihood of appropriateness of procedure. Teaching hospitals were more likely to perform endarterectomy appropriately than nonteaching hospitals. So I suppose you need to find a surgeon in a teaching hospital who doesn't do too many endarterectomies or whatever, but those he does perform are done very well. There are such. Good luck!

The question of whether carotid endarterectomy in symptomatic patients is worthwhile was answered in part by the North American Symptomatic Carotid Endarterectomy Trial group at the recent stroke conference (February 1991) in San Francisco. The procedure is beneficial in centers with "documented surgical and neurological expertise" for patients with 70% to 90% carotid stenosis. At "18 months 12% of medical patients but only 5% of surgical patients had experienced major or fatal stroke in any territory or death from any cause." The greater the stenosis, the greater the operative benefit—so the plan is next to study 30% to 69% stenosis (1).—R.D. Currier, M.D.

Reference

1. *NINDS Clinical Alert* Feb 1991.

Prospective Study of the Effectiveness and Durability of Carotid Endarterectomy
Sundt TM Jr, Whisnant JP, Houser OW, Fode NC (Mayo Clinic and Found, Rochester, Minn)
Mayo Clin Proc 65:625–635, 1990   4–20

Recently, the medical community has expressed justifiable concern that treatment with carotid endarterectomy may be worse than the disease. When digital subtraction angiography (DSA) became available, a prospective study was initiated to correlate postoperative DSA and follow-up DSA findings with clinical results in a group of 252 patients who had undergone 282 carotid endarterectomies. The patients were followed for 2–6 years. Digital subtraction angiography was done after surgery in 95% of the patients, and follow-up DSA was done in 66%.

The overall rate of operative minor morbidity was 1%; there was no major morbidity, and the mortality rate was .7%. Complications were well correlated with the patient's preoperative risk category. During follow-up, 10 minor strokes occurred, only 1 of which was attributable to the reconstructed artery. Ten transient ischemic attacks also occurred, 3 of which were thought to be related to recurrent stenosis. Asymptomatic mild to moderate restenosis of the internal carotid or common carotid artery was detected in 10% of the follow-up DSAs, severe stenosis or occlusion was identified in 3%.

In 48 cases (26%) stenosis in the opposite common carotid or internal carotid artery progressed. Ten of these became symptomatic. According to actuarial analysis of patients who had endarterectomy, the cumulative probability of ipsilateral stroke was 1.5% at 1 month and 2% at 5 years. The cumulative probability of transient ischemic attack, ipsilateral stroke, or reversible ischemic neurologic deficit was 4% at 1 month and 8% at 5 years.

Digital subtraction angiography is an excellent method for visualizing the carotid bifurcation postoperatively and assessing the adequacy of endarterectomy. The results of endarterectomy in this series compared favorably with the 6% annual risk of stroke after a transient ischemic attack for patients treated with anticoagulant and aspirin therapy.

▶ This must be one of the cleanest studies of the effect of carotid endarterectomy. I always get that feeling when I look at things the Mayo Clinic does. Their cumulative probability of stroke, transient ischemic attack, or reversible ischemic neurologic deficit of 8% at 5 years is difficult to fault. Yet, in a discussion of the same issue, Matchar is not as carried away with the results and points out many possible sources of bias and error.

Along the same line, Rautenberg et al. (1) followed patients with asymptomatic internal carotid artery occlusion for 44 months. The stroke and TIA rate was 28%. I had always glibly swallowed the notion that, once the carotid was totally occluded, that side of the brain was safe, but it doesn't look so. The authors conclude: "This may favor carotid endarterectomy for selected patients in the preocclusive state because medical treatment has not been shown to prevent progression to occlusion."—R.D. Currier, M.D.

Reference

1. Rautenberg W, et al: *J Neurol Sci* 98:213, 1990.

^{99}Tc^m-HM-PAO Brain SPECT in Subarachnoid Haemorrhage

Maini CL, Castellano G, Benech F, Podio V, Cornaglia G, Fontanella M (Univ of Ancona; Univ of Torino, Italy)
Nucl Med Commun 11:491–502, 1990   4–21

Xenon-133 has been used in many studies of cerebral blood flow (CBF) in subarachnoid hemorrhage. Single-photon emission CT (SPECT) using HM-PAO is much easier to perform, but true quantitative data are not available, and different diagnostic criteria must be used. To clarify the role of HM-PAO SPECT in subarachnoid hemorrhage, 26 HM-PAO SPECT studies in 24 patients were analyzed. Fifteen patients were in Hunter and Hess clinical grades I and II. The remaining 9 were in grades III, IV, and V.

Sixteen patients had derangements of brain perfusion on HM-PAO

SPECT. Focal hypoperfusion was noted in 15 cases and focal hyperperfusion in 1. One patient, who was studied twice, had a diffuse hypoperfusion in the first study and focal hypoperfusion in the second study. In identifying complications in the first week and in the first 2 weeks after hemorrhage, HM-PAO SPECT was more sensitive than transmission CT. Also, HM-PAO SPECT demonstrated changed tissue perfusion in 4 patients in whom CT, angiography, and transcranial Doppler flowmetry results were normal.

Derangements of CBF appear to occur in a high percentage of patients with subarachnoid hemorrhage. This percentage is higher among those with more severe disease, with focal hypoperfusion being the most common finding. In assessing ischemic complications, HM-PAO SPECT is more sensitive than CT. It can show ischemia even if no complicating factor, as assessed by the usual neuroradiologic techniques, is present; also, HM-PAO results are associated with prognosis.

▶ The authors report that SPECT is of value both for the diagnosis and prognosis of patients with subarachnoid hemorrhage. They believe that this modality will delineate vasospasm earlier than other methods, but, in my opinion, it remains to be seen whether transcranial Doppler or SPECT will be the better test.

The important message in this study is that SPECT, and in the not-too-distant future, positron emission tomography (PET), will begin to take increasingly important places in the management of patients with cerebrovascular disorders. Until now, they have been rather exotic and academic modalities, but I predict that they will become standard components of the diagnostic evaluation of patients with serious intracranial disorders.—J.F. Toole, M.D.

The Natural History of Symptomatic Arteriovenous Malformations of the Brain: A 24-Year Follow-Up Assessment

Ondra SL, Troupp H, George ED, Schwab K (Walter Reed Army Med Ctr, Washington, DC; Helsinki Univ, Finland)
J Neurosurg 73:387–391, 1990   4–22

The indications for therapeutic intervention in cerebral arteriovenous malformations (AVMs) remain controversial because of the lack of understanding of their natural history. In a prospective series, 166 of 262 patients with symptomatic AVMs had had no therapeutic intervention, and 160 (96%) were followed for a mean of 23.7 years (range, 12–45 years). Of these, 71% had hemorrhage, 24% had seizures, and 5% had headaches, asymptomatic bruits, or vague neurologic complaints when first seen.

The rate of major rebleeding was 4% per year, and this rate remained constant during the follow-up period. The mean interval between hemorrhagic events was 7.7 years (range, 6 weeks to 22 years). The combined incidence of morbidity and mortality was 2.7% per year, and 85% of those who had hemorrhage initially sustained major morbidity or died.

The mortality rate was 1% per year, regardless of the manner of presentation. Death was caused by an AVM hemorrhage in 23%, and the number of deaths attributable to AVM hemorrhage remained constant during the study period. The mean age at death in the group dying of AVM hemorrhage was significantly lower (44.4 years) than that in the group dying of other causes (59.4 years) and was much lower than that of the general Finnish population (73 years).

This population provides a unique opportunity to better define the natural history of cerebral AVM. It appears that the clinical course of all symptomatic patients with cerebral AVMs is the same regardless of the manner of presentation.

▶ Although in this large and long-studied series there was some preselection by the surgeons, this seems to be a superb analysis of the long-term outlook for AVMs of the brain. It may be as close to the truth in this matter as we will get. The lesions are not benign. A 4% repeat bleeding rate per year is considerable.

Several groups now embolize and then resect these AVMs, and a recent report by Fox et al. (1) of 38 treated patients described 25 with no deficit, or no change in deficit, after treatment; 11 patients had worsening of the neurologic syndrome, and there were 2 deaths. No doubt, as we learn more about the proper way of handling these patients, treatment will become even more efficient.

Magnetic resonance angiography is coming on fast, and several reports, including that by Marchal et al. (2), can be found in the current literature. Such reports illustrate both benefits and a few problems with the technique. The fast flow in AVMs sometimes leads to incomplete demonstration of the vessels.— R.D. Currier, M.D.

References

1. Fox AJ, et al: *Radiology* 177:51, 1990.
2. Marchal G, et al: *Radiology* 175:443, 1990.

Reduced Stroke Incidence With Structured Hypertension Care: The Skaraborg Hypertension Project
Lindblad U, Råastam L, Rydén L, Ranstam J, Berglund G, Isacsson S-O (Lund Univ, Malmö; Karolinska Institute, Stockholm)
J Hypertension 8:1147–1153, 1990   4–23

Structured care increases the efficacy of blood pressure treatment. Whether this also reduces the incidence of hypertensive complications (e.g., stroke) was investigated in a geographically defined population.

The Skaraborg Hypertension Project, conducted from 1977 to 1981, was implemented in half of the county of Skaraborg, Sweden. The other half served as a control. In the study area, all treated hypertensive patients had improved blood pressure control. Blood pressure reduction av-

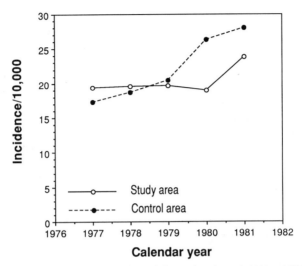

Fig 4–7.—Annual stroke incidence per 10,000 inhabitants born between 1908 and 1941 in the study *(open circle)* and control *(closed circle)* areas. (Courtesy of Lindblad U, Råastam L, Rydén L, et al: *J Hypertension* 8:1147–1153, 1990.)

eraged 2–5 mm Hg. Patients sustaining fatal and nonfatal strokes were identified from local and national mortality and morbidity registers. Diagnoses were validated using medical records.

Of 1,169 cases reported, 1,097 were true stroke victims after validation. There was a statistically significant difference in stroke incidence trends, both fatal and nonfatal, between the study and control populations (Fig 4–7). Improved hypertension control in the study area is the most likely explanation for the relative decrease in stroke incidence there.

▶ I am happy that the Swedes were able to carry this out. They set up hypertension control clinics in half of the county of Skaraborg and not in the other half. This was an open trial, and one wonders whether permission would have been granted by institutional review boards in the United States. The only disease targeted was hypertension, which was treated to a moderate degree, so it took 3 years for the change to show up in the treated population.—R.D. Currier, M.D.

Natural History of Progressive Ischemic Stroke in a Population Treated With Heparin
Slivka A, Levy D (New York Hosp-Cornell Med Ctr, New York)
Stroke 21:1657–1662, 1990   4–24

To define the acute course of patients treated with heparin for progressive stroke, the charts of 69 patients identified through the Cornell Neurology Database from 1979 to 1985 were reviewed. The charts were analyzed to determine whether further clinical deterioration or hemorrhagic complications were associated with readily identifiable clinical or laboratory variables. Overall, 36% of the patients continued to deteriorate while taking heparin, 3% worsened because of intracerebral hemorrhage, and 14% had bleeding complications. Patients who were likely to benefit from heparin therapy had no distinguishing clinical features or heparin dosing regimens. Neither clinical progression nor hemorrhage correlated with the level of anticoagulation as measured by the average heparin dose per day or the mean partial thromboplastin time.

Without unequivocal evidence showing that heparin is ineffective in patients with progressive stroke, many clinicians will continue to use it in such cases. This decision should not be governed by clinical features (e.g., patient age or sex), or by the vascular distribution of the stroke. Because the partial thromboplastin time does not correlate with outcome, its frequent measurement and overzealous efforts to adjust it may be unnecessary.

▶ This report thumps the drum once more for anticoagulants, but it is a single beat and not a very loud one at that. The authors report: "Without unequivocal evidence demonstrating heparin's ineffectiveness for progressive stroke, many clinicians managing such patients will continue to use heparin." Therefore, those of us with a gut feeling that anticoagulants are useful for halting the progress of ischemic infarction have a modicum of support for our position. In this day and age, however, gut feelings are as useless as card-sorting machines and until a prospective randomized trial of patients classified accurately by appropriate visualization is done, we are flying blind without instruments. Pending this, those of us who prefer to give anticoagulants to our patients with evolving infarction may continue to do so without feeling guilty.—J.F. Toole, M.D.

The Effect of Low-Dose Warfarin on the Risk of Stroke in Patients With Nonrheumatic Atrial Fibrillation

The Boston Area Anticoagulation Trial for Atrial Fibrillation Investigators (Kistler JP, Massachusetts Gen Hosp, Boston)
N Engl J Med 323:1505–1511, 1990   4–25

The Framingham study indicated a fivefold increase of stroke in patients with nonrheumatic atrial fibrillation (Fig 4–8). The efficacy and risk of long-term anticoagulant therapy has not been determined. Therefore, to assess the efficacy of low-dose warfarin in preventing strokes associated with nonrheumatic atrial fibrillation, 420 patients were enrolled in a randomized controlled trial and followed for 2.2 years. Of these patients, 212 were assigned to receive warfarin and 208 served as controls. The control group could choose to take aspirin.

In the warfarin-treated group the mean weekly dose was 29.7 mg. Prothrombin-time ratios were within target range during 83% of the trial. There were 2 strokes in the group given warfarin, compared with 13 in the control group. The warfarin group had an 86% reduction in risk of

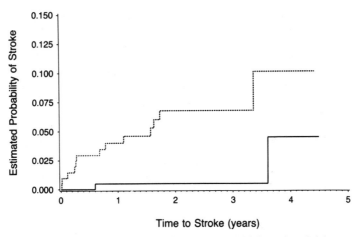

Fig 4–8.—Cumulative probability of stroke during the course of the trial. Probabilities were estimated by the Kaplan-Meier method. The *dotted line* represents the control group and the *solid line* represents the warfarin group. The large steps in probability as a result of late strokes are imprecisely estimated because of the small numbers of patients who were followed for such long periods. (Courtesy of The Boston Area Anticoagulation Trial for Atrial Fibrillation Investigators: *N Engl J Med* 323:1505–1511, 1990.)

stroke. Of the 37 patients who died, 11 were in the warfarin-treated group and 26 in the control group. Nineteen deaths were of cardiac origin and 18 deaths were noncardiac; fatal hemorrhage occurred in 2 patients and a fatal stroke in another. One fatal hemorrhage occurred in each group; the frequency of other bleeding events was essentially the same in both groups. The rate of minor hemorrhage was higher in the warfarin-treated group.

There was an 86% reduction in the rate of stroke, and the death rate was markedly lower in the warfarin-treated group. With careful monitoring, low-dose warfarin therapy was safe and highly effective in preventing stroke in patients with nonrheumatic atrial fibrillation.

▶ It looks as though low-dose warfarin is the right thing to give patients with nonrheumatic atrial fibrillation. Only half of the control group chose to take aspirin. Warfarin was remarkably safe in this series because of low dosage and careful handling. So one presumes we will enter a new era of anticoagulation for this particular type of stroke.

An accompanying editorial in the same issue of the *New England Journal of Medicine* (1) discusses the paper in relation to previous similar studies and is good reading for those about to initiate its use in a patient.—R.D. Currier, M.D.

Reference

1. Chesebro JH, et al: *N Engl J Med* 323:1557, 1990.

5 Pediatric Neurology

Delayed Central Nervous System Myelination in the Sudden Infant Death Syndrome
Kinney HC, Brody BA, Finkelstein DM, Vawter GF, Mandell F, Gilles FH (Children's Hosp, Boston; Harvard Med School; Harvard School of Public Health)
J Neuropathol Exp Neurol 50:29–48, 1991   5–1

Sudden infant death syndrome (SIDS) is the leading cause of death in young infants, but its etiology remains unknown. Most instances of SIDS occur at ages 1–6 months, peaking at 2–4 months. Evidence of subtle prenatal and postnatal growth retardation in SIDS victims suggests something that makes these infants vulnerable to dying suddenly in the first months of life. Myelination, a good marker of CNS development, was evaluated in 61 cases of SIDS and 89 autopsy controls. Myelination was graded in myelin-stained histologic sections at 62 sites. The control group included several infants who died of congenital heart disease.

In nearly half of the sites evaluated, the SIDS victims had significantly delayed myelination. Hypomyelination was a feature of systems developing both before and after birth. The pyramidal, cerebellar, and prefrontal-temporal-limbic systems all were affected. Hypomyelination, however, did not correlate with individual clinicopathologic variables in SIDS cases. Body growth and brain weight were greater in the SIDS group than in controls. Hypomyelination did not relate to a history of apnea or to a family history of SIDS.

This study presents anatomical evidence that myelination is delayed in SIDS. The current search for abnormalities in areas related to arousal and cardiorespiratory function should extent to somatomotor and visceromotor regions in the cerebellum and the prefrontal-temporal-limbic system.

▶ Sudden infant death syndrome is a very perplexing phenomenon. An apparently healthy infant is found dead without explanation for the family or physician. The syndrome occurs in approximately 2 of every 1,000 live births. Siblings of SIDS cases have 5 times the usual risk. However, monozygotic twins are at no greater risk than dizygotic twins. Epidemiologic studies suggest that pre- and postnatal environmental factors are involved. This lessens the likelihood of an inborn error of metabolism related to myelination as a cause for SIDS. Given the lack of evidence of other causes of delayed myelination, SIDS remains an enigma. This study should be confirmed by other investigations to focus research accurately on this leading cause of infant mortality.—O.B. Evans, M.D.

The UCLA-University of Utah Epidemiologic Survey of Autism: The Etiologic Role of Rare Diseases

Ritvo ER, Mason-Brothers A, Freeman BJ, Pingree C, Jenson WR, McMahon WM, Petersen PB, Jorde LB, Mo A, Ritvo A (Univ of California, Los Angeles; Univ of Utah)
Am J Psychiatry 147:1614–1621, 1990   5–2

Autism is a behaviorally defined syndrome that has occasionally been associated with a number of uncommon disorders (table). Clinical surveys and case reports do not indicate whether these diseases cause autism or are merely randomly associated with it. An epidemiologic survey of the entire state of Utah yielded 233 autistic probands, 26 of whom (11%) had 12 different rare diseases known to cause CNS pathology.

Six patients had suspected or documented congenital viral infection and 2 had *Hemophilus influenzae* meningitis. Two male patients had fragile X syndrome and 5 others had trisomy 21. Four male and 3 female patients had metabolic disorders including mucopolysaccharidosis III and congenital hypothyroidism. Four female patients had symptoms of Rett's syndrome.

The developmental delay and symptoms used to diagnose autism may be a direct result of various diseases that affect the CNS by different means. If, in fact, certain rare diseases produce CNS pathology and, in turn, autism, the symptoms of autism would represent a final common pathway of various causative agents.

▶ Autism is a severe disorder of children. The proper description is that of a pervasive developmental disorder that affects primarily those parts of the brain associated with social interactions. Communication and interpersonal relationships are perhaps the most obvious impairments in these children. It is not surprising that a survey such as the one reported here reveals a significant number with diagnosed underlying medical disorders, e.g., congenital infections, chromosomopathies, and the relatively recent disorder of Rett's syndrome. Human behavior is the product of neurobiology. Injuries to the developing nervous system can produce motor deficits, as seen in cerebral palsy, mental retardation, epilepsy, and other signs that may be associated with specific neuropathology. Autism is obviously another example of such a relationship. The table of known diseases reported to occur with autism is very useful. The clinician should find this helpful in evaluating such patients.—O.B. Evans, M.D.

Brain Morphology in Developmental Dyslexia and Attention Deficit Disorder/Hyperactivity

Hynd GW, Semrud-Clikeman M, Lorys AR, Novey ES, Eliopulos D (Univ of Georgia, Athens; Athens Magnetic Imaging, Athens, Ga)
Arch Neurol 47:919–926, 1990   5–3

Some 3% to 6% of all school-aged children are thought to have developmental dyslexia, defined as a rare form of reading retardation associ-

Diseases Reported to Occur With Autism

Viral, Bacterial, and Parasitic Infections
Rubella
Cytomegalovirus
Herpes
Varicella
Rubeola
Toxoplasmosis
Syphilis (lues)
Mumps
Hemophilus influenza

Chromosome and Genetic Abnormalities
Fragile-X
Down's syndrome (trisomy 21)
Sex chromosome aneuploidy (XXX, XXY XYY, XXYY)
Autosomal abnormalities of chromosomes 1, 2, 3,
    5, 6, 9, 13, 16, 17, 22
Oculocutaneous albinism
Tuberous sclerosis (chromosome 9)
Neurofibromatosis (chromosome 17)
Retinoblastoma (chromosome 13)

Metabolic Diseases
Phenylketonuria
Hyperlactatemia
Histidinemia
Lipidosis
Addison's diseases
Hyperuricosuria
Hurler's syndrome
Hyper- and hypothyroidism
Celiac disease
Adrenoleukodystrophy
Purine metabolism

Congenital Diseases
Microcephaly
Hydrocephalus
Moebius syndrome
Dandy-Walker syndrome
Cornelia de Lange syndrome

Related Diseases
Rett's syndrome
Tourette's syndrome

Other Diseases
Lead ingestion
Infantile spasms
Vascular occlusion

(Courtesy of Ritvo ER, Mason-Brothers A, Freeman BJ, et al: *Am J Psychiatry* 147:1614–1621, 1990.)

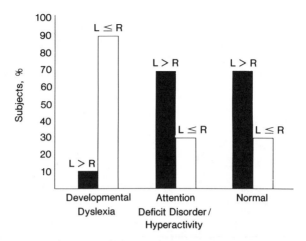

Patterns of Plana Morphology

Fig 5–1.—Percent of subjects by group with left-right asymmetry or symmetry of plana length. L > R indicates left greater than right; L ≤ R, left less than or equal to right. (Courtesy of Hynd GW, Semrud-Clikeman M, Lorys AR, et al: *Arch Neurol* 47:919–926, 1990.)

ated with CNS dysfunction. Although it is rare, it is also definable and diagnosable. To determine whether deviations in patterns of normal brain asymmetry characterize the brains of dyslexics, studies were made in 10 dyslexic children, 10 with attention deficit disorder/hyperactivity (ADD/H), and 10 normal age- and sex-matched controls. Patterns of normal brain asymmetry on MRI were analyzed.

Region of interest measurements for left and right anterior and posterior width and area, length of the bilateral insular region, and length of the bilateral planum temporale had excellent reliability values. The dyslexic and ADD/H children had significantly smaller right anterior-width measurements compared with normal children. Dyslexic children also had a bilaterally smaller insular area and significantly smaller left planum temporale than did normal children. Seventy percent of the normal and ADD/H children had the expected left greater than right pattern of plana asymmetry, compared with only 10% of the dyslexics. Although significantly more dyslexic children were left-handed compared with the other 2 groups, there were no significant relationships between left-handedness, incidence of allergies or familial autoimmune disease, and variability in indexes of brain morphological findings (Fig 5–1).

The significant increase in the incidence of plana symmetry or reversed asymmetry appears to be unique to dyslexia. It may be related to deviations in normal patterns of corticogenesis. In 70% of the normal and ADD/H children, the finding of left greater than right patterns of asymmetry in the region of the plana is consistent with similar findings reported by other researchers who used CT and MRI.

► This fascinating study has promise for establishing a possible organic basis for one of the developmental learning disabilities. Most pediatric neurologists, unless they have a specific interest in behavioral neurology, avoid developmental learning disabilities. They are difficult to diagnose without the aid of psychologists, and they are impossible to treat without special educators. The neurologist is thus relegated to screening for the rare child who has a seizure disorder, metabolic or degenerative disease, or acquired encephalopathy that might be characterized by learning impairments. Yet, neurologist should know more about the brain and its workings than any profession.

This study demonstrates anatomical differences in the brains of children with developmental dyslexia compared to controls. If verified by more extensive studies, such measurements may give the neurologist a diagnostic tool for evaluation of children with learning disabilities. More importantly, such studies stimulate research into the etiology and treatment of developmental learning disabilities.—O.B. Evans, M.D.

Prenatal Prediction of Risk of the Fetal Hydantoin Syndrome
Buehler BA, Delimont D, van Waes M, Finnell RH (Univ of Nebraska, Omaha; Washington State Univ, Pullman)
N Engl J Med 322:1567–1572, 1990   5–4

It has long been suspected that the teratogenicity of phenytoin and other anticonvulsant drugs is the result of an elevated level of toxic intermediary oxidative metabolites that are normally eliminated by the enzyme epoxide hydrolase. An attempt was made to determine whether the prenatal measurement of epoxide hydrolase activity can identify infants at risk for congenital malformations induced by anticonvulsant drugs.

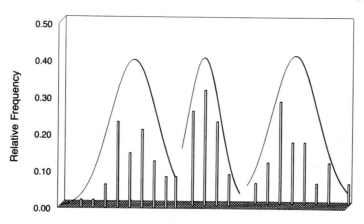

Epoxide Hydrolase Activity (% of standard)

Fig 5–2.—Distribution of epoxide hydrolase activity in the normal population. The relative frequency of low, moderate, and high epoxide hydrolase activity in the randomly selected control population is indicated by the *bars*. The normalized curves are indicated by the *continuous lines*. The normal population was arbitrarily divided into three subgroups. Bars are higher than in Figure 1 because denominators were subgroups instead of the total group; slight differences between the figures in relative bar heights reflect differences in numerical rounding of midrange values. (Courtesy of Buehler BA, Delimont D, van Waes M, et al: *N Engl J Med* 322:1567–1572, May 1990.)

In the first part of the study, thin-layer chromatography was used to measure epoxide hydrolase activity in a sample of amniocytes obtained from 100 randomly selected normal pregnant women. The assay indicated that enzyme activity values were not distributed normally; rather, they had a trimodal distribution (Fig 5–2). Further analysis of the 3 subgroups revealed that fetuses with low microsomal epoxide enzyme activity would be at increased risk for fetal hydantoin syndrome if exposed to anticonvulsant drugs.

In the second part of the study, epoxide hydrolase activity was measured in amniocytes obtained from 19 pregnant women with epilepsy who were being treated with phenytoin monotherapy and were prospectively monitored by amniocentesis. The assay identified 4 fetuses with low epoxide hydrolase activity. All 4 infants had clinical findings compatible with the fetal hydantoin syndrome after birth. The other 15 fetuses who had normal epoxide hydrolase activity were considered clinically normal at birth. Epoxide hydrolase activity appears to be a useful enzymatic biomarker for identifying fetuses at increased risk for congenital malformations induced by maternal anticonvulsant drug use.

▶ This fascinating study shows that enzymatic biomarkers may be used to identify infants who are at increased risk for congenital malformations induced by anticonvulsant drugs. I wonder if this might be extended to other complications of phenytoin therapy, e.g., the gingival and other somatic effects. At least identifying mothers at risk would simplify anticonvulsant therapy during pregnancy.— O.B. Evans, M.D.

Cerebrospinal Fluid Values in the Very Low Birth Weight Infant
Rodriguez AF, Kaplan SL, Mason EO Jr (Baylor College of Medicine, Houston; Texas Children's Hosp, Houston)
J Pediatr 116:971–974, 1990   5–5

Very-low-birth-weight (VLBW) infants are at risk for contracting serious systemic infections. An essential part of evaluating suspected infection is analysis of the CSF. Therefore, it is necessary to know the normal chemical values and changes of the leukocyte count in such infants. The CSF values were determined in 43 infants weighing 1,500 g or less.

All of the infants had birth weights appropriate for their gestational age. Their CSF cultures were negative for bacteria, and, according to head ultrasound examination, there was no evidence of intracranial bleeding in any. The infants had a mean birth weight of 1,002 g (range, 550–1,500 g). Their mean gestational age was 27 weeks (range, 24–33 weeks). Their CSF leukocyte counts ranged from 0 to 44 cells per mm^3 (mean, 5 cells per mm^3). The leukocyte differential was 7% polymorphonuclear leukocytes and 85% mononuclear leukocytes, with ranges of up to 66% and 13% to 100%, respectively. The mean protein concentration was 142 mg/dL (range, 45–370 mg/dL), and the mean glucose level was 60 mg/dL (range, 29–217 mg/dL) (table).

Cerebrospinal Fluid Values in VLBW Infants on Basis of Birth Weight

	Group 1 (≤1000 gm) (n = 38*)		Group 2 (1001-1500 gm) (n = 33*)		
	Mean ± SD	Range	Mean	Range	p
Birth weight (gm)	763 ± 115	550-980	1278 ± 152	1020-1500	
Gestational age (wk)	26 ± 1.3	24-28	29 ± 1.4	27-33	
Leukocytes/mm³	4 ± 3	0-14	6 ± 9	0-44	NS
Erythrocytes/mm³	1027 ± 3270	0-19,050	786 ± 1879	0-9750	
PMN leukocytes (%)	6 ± 15	0-66	9 ± 17	0-60	NS
MN leukocytes (%)	86 ± 30	34-100	85 ± 28	13-100	
Glucose (mg/dl)	61 ± 34	29-217	59 ± 21	31-109	NS
Protein (mg/dl)	150 ± 56	95-370	132 ± 43	45-227	NS

NS = not significant ($P > .05$); MN = mononuclear.
*Number of CSF specimens.
(Courtesy of Rodriguez AF, Kaplan SL, Mason EO Jr: *J Pediatr* 116:971–974, 1990.)

These measurements should help clinicians to better interpret the CSF values of VLBW infants undergoing examination for a CNS disorder. These findings are consistent with the theory of changed permeability in the blood-brain barrier for macromolecules in VLBW premature infants.

▶ Interpretation of CSF values in infants can be difficult because of their higher protein concentrations and often xanthochromic appearance at birth. The values usually fall toward the normal range within several months. This study extends our knowledge to the VLBW infant. The range of white blood cells is similar to that in term infants, but the protein values are somewhat higher. Unfortunately, using the limits of normal in this study, an infant with CSF values of 44 white blood cells with 66% neutrophils, a protein content of 370 mg/dL, and a glucose level of 29 mg/dL may or may not have bacterial meningitis. Clinical suspicion of sepsis and meningitis is perhaps still our most sensitive indicator.—O.B. Evans, M.D.

Measurement of Progressive Cerebral Ventriculomegaly in Infants After Grades III and IV Intraventricular Hemorrhages

Brann BS IV, Qualls C, Papile L, Wells L, Werner S (Univ of New Mexico, Albuquerque)
J Pediatr 117:615–621, 1990   5–6

The clinical management of posthemorrhagic ventricular dilation after intraventricular hemorrhage (IVH) in preterm infants is problematic. Physicians must ascertain whether the ventricle size is static or increasing and requires intervention. Guidelines to help predict which infants with severe IVH will require intervention were developed.

Serial cranial sonograms were obtained to measure the rate of growth of cerebral ventricular volumes in 48 preterm infants with and without IVH. The infants were divided into 3 groups: 22 with no IVH, 13 with IVH and acute ventricular dilation, and 13 with IVH with progressive

Clinical Characteristics and Rate of Growth of Lateral
Cerebral Ventricles and TVV, by Group, in All Infants

	Group		
	I **(n = 13)**	**NI** **(n = 13)**	**C** **(n = 22)**
Gestational age (wk)	28 ± 3	28 ± 2	30 ± 3
Birth weight (gm)	1177 ± 361	1170 ± 351	1385 ± 559
No. of infants with IVH			
Grade III	3	13	0
Grade IV	10	0	0
Total lateral ventricular volume growth (ml/day)	4.2 ± 3.3*,†	0.0 ± 0.2	0.0 ± 0.1
Total lateral ventricular volume (ml)	56.5 ± 19.9*,†	10.1 ± 7.5*	2.2 ± 1.0

Note: Values (except number of infants with grade III or IV IVH) are expressed as mean ± SD.

Abbreviations: I, intervention group; NI, no-intervention group; C, control group (no IVH).

*Significance: $P < .001$ vs. control group.

†Significance: $P < .001$ vs. no-intervention group.

(Courtesy of Brann BS IV, Qualls C, Papile L, et al: *J Pediatr* 117:615–621, 1990.)

ventricular dilation requiring intervention (table). Clinical criteria and the subjective assessment of increasing ventricular size on weekly cranial sonograms were the basis of the decision to intervene. The rate of cerebral ventricular volume growth in infants with IVH who required intervention was greater than that in infants without IVH and in those with IVH and acute ventricular dilation. Guidelines were generated and confirmed in 10 infants.

The simplest guideline for predicting the need for intervention is the single volume measure. At some point, the ventricular volume will be so large that there is little doubt about whether hydrocephalus will develop. If the total lateral cerebral ventricular volume (TVV) reaches 30 mL by age 21 days, there is almost a 90% certainty that the infant will require intervention. If the volume is 30 mL within 28 days, there is a greater than 90% chance. Using the fronto-occipital circumference (FOC) as an indirect measure of intracranial volume and dividing the TVV by the FOC improves predictive power. A TVV/FOC ratio of .9 mL/cm by age 17 days suggests with 90% certainty that an infant will require intervention. A stricter guideline with better predictive capability involves determining the rate at which the lateral cerebral ventricles are enlarging.

▶ The treatment of posthemorrhagic hydrocephalus in premature infants with IVH has always been problematic. A variety of medical therapies, including administration of diuretics and acetazolamide, serial lumbar punctures, and expectant observation, have all had their advocates. None is without risk to the infant. Regardless of therapy, approximately 50% of these infants will require a ventricular peritoneal shunt. Often, medical therapy is used to defer the need of a shunt in very small infants. Newer neurosurgical techniques have allowed the surgeons to place the shunts at earlier ages.

The design of this study has some flaws. The daily ventricular volume growth in the control group was zero, plus or minus .1 mL/day; that in infants with acute ventricular dilatation was zero, plus or minus .2 mL/day. One would assume that the ventricular ultrasound essentially showed no changes from week to week. On the other hand, those requiring intervention had a daily increase of 4.2 mL/day. This would be clearly evident from the ultrasound images. In other words, infants who required intervention had steadily enlarging ventricular sizes; those who did not require intervention did not have enlargement. It is unclear whether digitalizing these data and calculating volumes would add much to the clinical impression of increasing ventricular size on serial ultrasound images.—O.B. Evans, M.D.

Stroke in Pediatric Acquired Immunodeficiency Syndrome

Park YD, Belman AL, Kim T-S, Kure K, Llena JF, Lantos G, Bernstein L, Dickson DW (Albert Einstein College of Medicine, Bronx; State Univ of New York, Stony Brook)
Ann Neurol 28:303–311, 1990   5–7

Human immunodeficiency virus infection is often complicated by neurologic dysfunction. Although stroke is not uncommon in adults with AIDS, it has not often been reported in children with AIDS. The occurrence of stroke in pediatric AIDS was investigated in 68 children in a longitudinal study of neurologic complications of HIV infection. Four children had clinical and/or neurologic evidence of stroke. The clinical incidence of stroke in this population was 1.3% per year. During the 4½-year study, 32 children died. Permission for autopsy was granted in 18 cases, including 3 of the 4 with stroke.

The prevalence of cerebrovascular pathologic findings was higher in the autopsy series than the clinical incidence. Cerebrovascular disease was documented in 6 of 25 children (24%) with HIV infection. All 3 children who had clinical evidence of stroke had documented cerebrovascular disease. Four children had intracerebral hemorrhages; 6, nonhemorrhagic infarcts; and 3, both intracerebral hemorrhages and nonhemorrhagic infarcts. Hemorrhage was catastrophic in 1 child and clinically silent in 3; all had immune thrombocytopenia. In 1 child, arteriopathy affected the meningocerebral arteries. In another case, the arteries of the circle of Willis were dilated aneurysmally. Two children had cardiomyopathy as well as subacute necrotizing encephalomyelopathy with vascular proliferation (Fig 5–3).

Stroke must be considered when children with AIDS have focal neurologic signs. Hemorrhagic strokes usually occur in the presence of immune

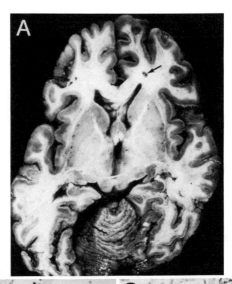

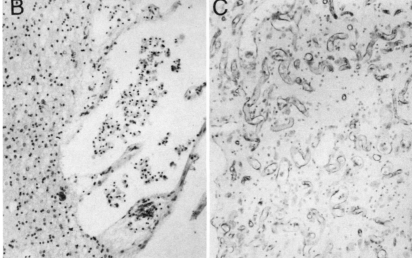

Fig 5–3.—A, the brain of a child with cardiomyopathy and subacute necrotizing encephalopathy shows focal periventricular white matter cystic lesions *(arrow).* **B,** the microscopic sections from these lesions show cystic encephalomalacia with gliovascular strands and surrounding gliosis. Hematoxylin-eosin; original magnification, ×80. **C,** *Ulex europaeus* type I (UEA-I) lectin histochemistry demonstrates proliferation and dilatation of the brain microvasculature analogous to that seen in Leigh's disease (UEA-I peroxidase stain with hematoxylin in counterstain; original magnification, ×1,000. (Courtesy of Park YD, Belman AL, Kim T-S, et al: *Ann Neurol* 28:303–311, 1990.)

thrombocytopenia. Cerebral arteriopathy or subacute necrotizing encephalopathy may be associated with nonhemorrhagic stroke.

▶ None of the patients in this series had a cerebrovascular event as the initial presenting sign of AIDS. All were known to have AIDS, and most had preexisting neurologic complications. However, should one test for HIV in the child or young adult with ischemic cerebrovascular disease without other evidence of AIDS? I probably will. Similarly, the children with lesions of subacute necrotizing encephalomyelitis (SNE) are of interest. The 2 children with SNE at autopsy did not appear to have the typical clinical features of SNE, although the clinical descriptions were abbreviated. These lesions are usually associated with thiamine deficiency, Leigh's disease, and mitochondrial cytopathies. Are there children with AIDS who will present initially only with signs and symptoms of Leigh's syndrome? Perhaps.—O.B. Evans, M.D.

High Risk of Recurrent Stroke After Discontinuance of Five to Twelve Years of Transfusion Therapy in Patients With Sickle Cell Disease
Wang WC, Kovnar EH, Tonkin IL, Mulhern RK, Langston JW, Day SW, Schell MJ, Wilimas JA (St Jude Children's Research Hosp, Memphis; Univ of Tennessee, Memphis)
J Pediatr 118:377–382, 1991   5–8

From 5% to 17% of patients with sickle cell disease have cerebrovascular complications, usually cerebral infarction. Infarction is most prevalent in children younger than 15 years of age and often produces death or serious neurologic sequelae. Long-term transfusion treatment may limit the occurrence of neurologic sequelae, but itself carries significant risks.

Transfusions were withdrawn prospectively from 10 patients having sickle cell disease. They had received transfusion therapy for a median time of 9½ years after a stroke, and all had received transfusions for at least 5 years. All of the patients had hemoglobin SS. Initial stroke occurred at a median age of 7 years. A pretransfusion hemoglobin S level below 30% was maintained by transfusions at 4-week intervals.

Five of the 10 patients experienced an ischemic event within a year of cessation of transfusion therapy. Two patients had massive intracranial bleeding, and another died suddenly of unknown causes. Three patients without sequelae chose not to resume transfusions and were relatively well after at least 18 months.

It is not safe to stop transfusion therapy abruptly in children with sickle cell disease who have had stroke. It may be safe, however, to transfuse patients less intensely, allowing a hemoglobin S level as high as 50%. Antisickling agents may prove helpful when transfusions are lessened or withdrawn. Raising the hemoglobin S level with hydroxyurea might be an acceptable alternative to long-term transfusion therapy.

▶ Children with sickle cell disease (SSD) who sustain a cerebral vascular accident (CVA) are at greater risk of a subsequent CVA than those SSD patients without such a history. Arteriographic and pathologic studies show a vasculopathy in many patients. The pathophysiology of the vasculopathy is unclear, but it does resolve in many patients with transfusion therapy. This study shows that there is a high risk of recurrent stroke after abrupt discontinuance of long-term transfusion therapy. Most physicians who treat children with SSD have observed this phenomenon. I have encountered several patients who sustained cerebrovascular accidents within weeks after a missed transfusion. I suspect that susceptible patients have a confounding predisposition to vascular disease that is expressed by SSD.

Despite the proven efficacy of transfusion therapy, it is surprising how little is known about how to administer it. The duration of therapy, safe concentrations of hemoglobin S, and use of iron chelation to prevent iron overload are treatment questions that should be resolved.—O.B. Evans, M.D.

New Ultrasound Evidence Appears to Link Prenatal Brain Damage, Cerebral Palsy
Skolnick A (Chicago)
JAMA 265:948–949, 1991   5–9

Cerebral palsy has been generally thought to result from brain asphyxia caused by intrapartum events. However, despite improvements in obstetric and neonatal care and a reduced incidence of perinatal asphyxia, there has been no consistent decrease in the frequency of cerebral palsy in the past 2 decades.

There is increasing evidence that cerebral palsy results from brain damage that occurs, at least 2 weeks before birth, rather than from mismanaged delivery or other birth trauma. Recently, Belfar and colleagues reported on their study of 512 premature infants who had intracranial ultrasound within a week of birth. Eleven infants had periventricular leukomalacia and 3 had porencephalic cysts, indicating that these infants had intraparenchymal destructions prenatally (Fig 5–4). Furthermore, these lesions were associated with the development of cerebral palsy. These findings confirm the theory first expressed by Bejar and colleagues in 1988 that destructive processes in the brain may predate delivery by several weeks and produce cystic brain structures that can be observed on the first day of life.

It appears that less is known about the etiology of cerebral palsy than previously thought. These recent findings provide new evidence linking prenatal brain damage with cerebral palsy.

▶ This is helpful in the continuing attempt to delineate the causes of cerebral palsy and presents a nice look at the future. As this report points out, it will probably help to calm the medical-legal waters.—R.D. Currier, M.D.

The Sequelae of *Haemophilus influenzae* Meningitis in School-Age Children
Taylor HG, Mills EL, Ciampi A, du Berger R, Watters GV, Gold R, MacDonald N, Michaels RH (Case Western Reverse Univ; McGill Univ; Children's Hosp of

Eastern Ontario, Ottawa; Hosp for Sick Children, Toronto; Children's Hosp of Pittsburgh)
N Engl J Med 323:1657–1663, 1990   5–10

Previous reports on the developmental sequelae of *Hemophilus influenzae* type b meningitis are inconsistent. Using a protocol for the comprehensive assessment of neuropsychological function, studies were made in 97 school-aged children recruited from a sample of 519 children treated for *H. influenzae* type b meningitis between 1972 and 1984. The mean age of the patients was 17 months at the time of illness and 9.3 years at the time of testing. Cognitive, academic, and behavioral measures were compared between index children and their siblings nearest in age. Forty-

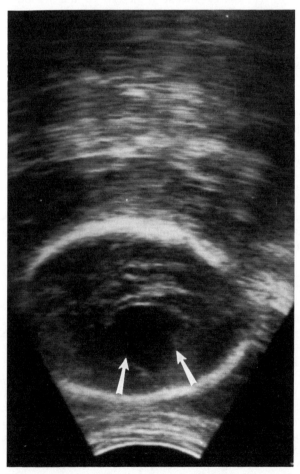

Fig 5–4.—Ultrasound image of a fetal brain shows destruction of white matter in the form of a porencephalic cyst *(white arrows)*. Cerebral palsy developed in this infant during his first year. Photo courtesy of H. Belfar, Magee-Women's Hosp, Pittsburgh. (Courtesy of Skolnick A: *JAMA* 265:948–949, 1991.)

one children had acute neurologic complications at the time of illness.

Only 14 children (14%) had persistent neurologic sequelae, including sensorineural hearing loss in 11, seizures in 2, and hemiplegia and mental retardation in 1. All of these children had complications during the acute phase. As a whole, index children scored lower on reading ability and were more likely to be receiving special educational assistance than were their siblings. However, the differences were small, and the differences on all measures were uniformly nonsignificant when the 58% of children without acute-phase complications were compared with their siblings. Behavioral problems were more common in index boys than index girls and in those who were older at the time of testing, but neither sex nor age was related to cognitive or academic sequelae. Lower socioeconomic status and a lower ratio of glucose in the CSF to that in blood at the time of illness were also associated with sequelae. In contrast to previous reports, the present data suggest a favorable prognosis for most children treated for *H. influenzae* type b meningitis.

▶ The prognosis for meningitis appears to be improving or is perhaps not as bad as previously thought. Earlier recognition and prompt therapy no doubt have improved statistics. This study showed only 14% of the patients to have persistent neurologic defects. This is about half of what was quoted previously. The most important finding was that all of the children with persistent problems had neurologic complications during the acute illness. Children appearing normal at discharge are unlikely to have later significant neurologic problems.— O.B. Evans, M.D.

Cerebrospinal Fluid Prostaglandins, Interleukin 1β, and Tumor Necrosis Factor in Bacterial Meningitis: Clinical and Laboratory Correlations in Placebo-Treated and Dexamethasone-Treated Patients
Mustafa MM, Ramilo O, Sáez-Llorens X, Olsen KD, Magness RR, McCracken GH Jr (Univ of Texas, Dallas)
Am J Dis Child 144:883–887, 1990   5–11

Meningeal inflammatory reactions are mediated by prostaglandins (PGs), interleukin 1β (IL-1β), and tumor necrosis factor α (TNFα). Levels of PGE_2, PGI_2, IL-1β, and TNF were determined in paired CSF samples from infants and children with bacterial meningitis.

Samples of CSF were obtained from 80 infants and children on admission and within 18–30 hours later. Forty children were given dexamethasone sodium, .6 mg/kg/day in 4 intravenous doses, and 40 were given an intravenous saline placebo. In the first CSF sample, PGE_2, PGT_2, IL-1β, and TNF were found in 90%, 56%, 98%, and 71% of specimens, respectively. The mean concentrations were 462, 377, 1,266, and 799 pg/mL, respectively. Concentrations of PGE_2 were significantly correlated with PGI_2, IL-1β, TNF, and lactate and inversely correlated with glucose levels in the first CSF specimen.

In CSF specimens from placebo-treated children, PGE_2, PGI_2, IL-1β, and TNF were still present in 40%, 18%, 97%, and 60%, respectively. Compared with children with detectable PGI$_2$ or TNFα concentrations in the second CSF sample, placebo-treated children with no detectable PGI$_2$ or TNFα activity in the second specimen had a lower incidence of neurologic sequelae. Children treated with dexamethasone had significantly lower PGE$_2$, IL-1β, and lactate concentrations and higher glucose levels in the CSF 18–30 hours later, a shorter duration of fever and a lower incidence of neurologic sequelae than did children given placebo.

These findings suggest a possible molecular basis for the CSF inflammatory response in patients with bacterial meningitis. There appears to be a correlation between dexamethasone administration and lower CSF concentrations of inflammatory mediators. It is not known yet whether the beneficial effects of this drug are principally a result of the reduction in inflammation and in the concentrations of mediators in CSF.

▶ Despite the ever-increasing numbers of new antibiotics for the treatment of meningitis, this infection continues to be the most serious one in childhood. Mortality is approximately 5%, and neurologic morbidity is as high as 20% in survivors. Recently, the use of steroids has shown a reduction of deafness in children with meningitis. This study supports the use of the drug in lowering mediators that stimulate the inflammatory response. Extension of this work may alter our therapy of meningitis in the future not only to eliminate the infectious agent, but also to lessen the harmful effects of inflammation that may mediate the actual injury to the brain. Scientific studies and carefully planned clinical trials support the experience of pediatricians and neurologists a generation ago when steroids were commonly used as adjunctive therapy.—O.B. Evans, M.D.

Seizures and Other Neurologic Sequelae of Bacterial Meningitis in Children
Pomeroy SL, Holmes SJ, Dodge PR, Feigin RD (Washington Univ; Baylor College of Medicine, Houston)
N Engl J Med 323:1651–1657, 1990   5–12

To determine late seizures and other neurologic sequelae of bacterial meningitis in children, 185 infants and children were prospectively followed during and after acute bacterial meningitis (mean follow-up, 8.9 years). In the first 6 years, standard neurologic assessments were performed; telephone interviews were conducted thereafter.

Neurologic sequelae occurred in 69 (37%) children 1 month after meningitis. Many of these effects resolved within 1 year, leaving only 26 (14%) children with persistent deficits; 18 (10%) had sensorineural hearing loss only and 8 (4%) had multiple neurologic deficits. One or more late seizures unassociated with fever occurred in 13 children (7%). Most late seizures occurred within 2 years, although 1 patient did not have seizures until 8 years later (Fig 5–5). The only independent predictor of late afebrile seizures was the presence of persistent neurologic deficits indicative of cerebral injury.

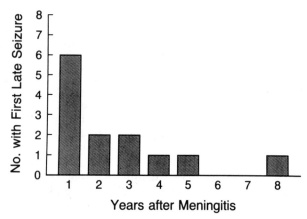

Fig 5–5.—Number of patients with a first late seizure 1 year or more after bacterial meningitis. (Courtesy of Pomeroy SL, Holmes SJ, Dodge PR, et al: *N Engl J Med* 323:1651–1657, 1990.)

Children with persistent neurologic deficits from cerebral injuries sustained during bacterial meningitis are at great risk for epilepsy. A child who has a normal neurologic assessment just after acute meningitis appears to have an excellent chance of escaping serious neurologic sequelae, including epilepsy.

▶ A frequent clinical problem that emerges in treating children with meningitis is the question of therapy for seizures. Thirty percent of children with meningitis will have at least 1 seizure during the acute infection, whereas only 7% will have 1 or more late seizures unassociated with fever. Some clinicians have treated children prophylactically with anticonvulsant medication for weeks to months, or occasionally years, after hospital discharge. Others have treated the seizures only during the period of acute encephalopathy associated with meningitis and have not discharged the patient with prophylactic anticonvulsant therapy. This study supports the latter practice. Those who are neurologically normal have a very low risk of subsequent seizures even if they have had acute seizures during meningitis. On the other hand, those who are neurologically abnormal at the time of discharge are at greater risk for late seizures, whether or not they had acute seizures during meningitis. Early, symptomatic seizures with a variety of encephalopathies do not necessarily result in epilepsy and do not require chronic therapy.—O.B. Evans, M.D.

Subdural Effusion and Its Relationship With Neurologic Sequelae of Bacterial Meningitis in Infancy: A Prospective Study
Snedeker JD, Kaplan SL, Dodge PR, Holmes SJ, Feigin RD (Washington Univ; Baylor College of Medicine, Houston; Duke Univ)
Pediatrics 86:163–170, 1990   5–13

There is controversy over the significance of subdural effusion in bacterial meningitis. Although neurologic deficits, impaired mental status, and other adverse sequelae of bacterial meningitis are commonly attributed to the presence of subdural fluid collections, no studies are available to support this association. A prospective study was performed to determine whether adverse sequelae seen after bacterial meningitis might be related to the occurrence of subdural effusion.

During a 4½-year period, 113 infants aged 1–18 months had bacterial meningitis caused by *Hemophilus influenzae* type b, *Streptococcus pneumoniae*, or *Neisseria meningitidis*. The diagnosis was confirmed by positive CSF culture or positive blood culture with abnormal CSF findings. Neurologic evaluation, transillumination of the skull, and measurement of the head circumference were performed daily until hospital discharge. Subdural paracentesis was performed only in children with symptoms of increased intracranial pressure. Children were reevaluated at 1, 3, 6, and 12 months after hospital discharge, and yearly thereafter. The median follow-up period was 66 months.

During the course of treatment, subdural effusion developed in 43 patients (39%). Young age, rapid onset of illness, low peripheral white blood cell count, high CSF protein levels, and high urinary bacterial antigen excretion were associated with a higher likelihood of effusion developing. Patients with effusion were more likely to have seizures during the course of treatment and to have neurologic abnormalities both at the time of admission and at the end of therapy. However, after long-term follow-up, children with effusion did not have a greater incidence of seizures, hearing loss, neurologic deficits, or developmental delay than children who did not have effusion. When all sequelae were taken together, 14% of the patients with effusion were impaired at follow-up, compared with 16% of the patients in whom effusion did not develop. The difference was not significant.

Subdural effusion is a common event in infants with bacterial meningitis and should be considered part of the meningeal inflammatory process. The findings do not support an association between the occurrence of subdural effusion itself and residual neurologic abnormalities.

▶ The most interesting aspect of this study is that it was conducted more than 15 years ago. The diagnosis was made primarily on examination, transillumination of the skull, and measurement of the head circumference. Subdural paracenteses were performed on children with symptoms of increased intracranial pressure. Although transillumination can detect subdural effusion it is doubtful that all cases can be determined, especially those with small effusions. Thus it is difficult to reach any conclusions based on the data presented here. Of the ones that were identified, however, there were no long-term residual neurologic deficits out of proportion to those that occurred in controls.

The identification and management of subdural effusions have evolved considerably since the early 1950s. At one point there was vigorous therapy for these, including daily tappings, shunts, and other procedures. It was soon discovered that many children were totally asymptomatic from the effusions, and that they resolved spontaneously. For that reason, the interest in attacking these fluid collections waned. At the present time there are few indications for a subdural tap other than suspected empyema or a mass effect.— O.B. Evans, M.D.

Double-Blind, Randomized Trial of Diazepam Versus Placebo for Prevention of Recurrence of Febrile Seizures
Autret E, Billard C, Bertrand P, Motte J, Pouplard F, Jonville AP (Univ of Tours, France)
J Pediatr 117:490–494, 1990   5–14

The recurrence rate of febrile seizure ranges from 30% to 50%. Because the prognosis for most patients with febrile seizures is good, intermittent prophylactic treatment seems a rational approach. Diazepam has been studied extensively, but its efficacy when given orally for preventing recurrence has not been established. The efficacy and tolerance of intermittent oral administration of diazepam during hyperthermia for reducing the recurrence of febrile seizure were assessed in 185 children aged 8 months to 3 years.

The patients were randomly assigned to receive diazepam, .5 mg/kg, orally, followed by .2 mg/kg every 12 hours, or placebo, whenever their rectal temperatures were higher than 38°C. All children had had a first febrile seizure and had normal neurologic development. The children were followed for 3 years. There were a total of 462 febrile episodes and 1,000 days of prophylaxis. The recurrence rates were 16% in the diazepam-treated group and 19.5% in the placebo-treated group, a nonsignificant difference. Children with recurrent seizures were significantly younger at their first seizure than children who did not have recurrences. Among those with recurrent seizures, prophylactic treatment was correctly given to only 1 of 15 children in the treatment group and to 7 of 18 in the control group. The reasons for this poor cooperation included the convulsion being the first manifestation of fever, parental neglect, and refusal to take the medicine. Adverse effects were similar in the 2 groups, although hyperactivity was more frequent in the diazepam-treated group.

Intermittent oral administration of diazepam at the onset of fever offers no advantage over placebo in preventing seizure recurrence in children. This probably reflects a lack of efficacy of the intermittent method, not that of diazepam.

▶ It is not surprising that this study failed to show an effect of oral diazepam in preventing febrile seizures. It is difficult for parents to determine the onset of fever, and often the temperature is 38°C or higher when first taken. Indeed, as the authors and others have found, the febrile convulsion is the first sign of fever in 30% of children. Compliance is always difficult in treating symptoms that occur infrequently in children. This study, like several others, became one of intention to treat rather than one comparing specific therapies.— O.B. Evans, M.D.

Syncope in Childhood: A Case Control Clinical Study of the Familial Tendency to Faint

Camfield PR, Camfield CS (Izaak Walton Killam Hosp for Children, Halifax, NS)
Can J Neurol Sci 17:306–308, 1990   5–15

Little is known about the predisposing characteristics of children who faint. Knowing such factors would help clinicians to establish the differential diagnosis of syncope. It was hypothesized that, although in most individuals fainting can be induced by sufficient stress, the tendency to faint or "the syncope threshold" is influenced by hereditary factors. A controlled study was made of the incidence of syncope among close family members of 30 well children with vasodepressor or vasovagal syncope.

The family history of each child was reviewed. In 24 cases the patient's family history was compared with that of the child's best friend, none of whom had syncope. Twenty-seven of the 30 children and 8 of the 24 friends had at least 1 first-degree relative with syncope. The mothers of 7 of the 8 friends with a parent or sibling with syncope was affected. Four of these 7 mothers had first-degree relatives with syncope. Eleven patients had both a sibling and parent with syncope, compared with 1 control child.

There appears to be an inherited tendency to faint, because most children who faint have a first-degree relative who also faints. This is useful knowledge in the differential diagnosis. This inherited tendency may be multifactorial, requiring an environmental stimulus for expression.

▶ Fainting in children is a difficult diagnosis, particularly in adolescents. Except in children with breath-holding spells, venipuncture seizures, and similar provoked syncope, an etiology is usually not determined. It has been my experience that children with pallid breath-holding spells often have a family history of fainting. Unfortunately, this study excluded young children with pallid syncope. The familial tendency to faint is a real phenomenon and should be kept in mind when evaluating children with spells that resemble fainting.—O.B. Evans, M.D.

Corpus Callosotomy for Intractable Seizures in the Pediatric Age Group

Nordgren RE, Reeves AG, Viguera AC, Roberts DW (Dartmouth-Hitchcock Med Ctr, Hanover, NH)
Arch Neurol 48:364–372, 1991   5–16

Corpus callosotomy is an increasingly popular treatment for intractable epilepsy, but few series have involved only children. The results of callosotomy were assessed in 18 children aged 16 years or younger who were followed for longer than 2 years after operation.

Most patients had a 80% or greater reduction in overall seizure frequency after callosotomy (table). More incapacitating seizures were likely to improve. Eleven of 12 patients who suddenly fell at the onset of seizures no longer had this type of attack after surgery. Simple partial sei-

Results of Callosotomy: Frequency of All Seizures

No. (%)

Postoperative Frequency	Our Patients (N = 18)	Patients Reviewed (N = 50)
Seizure free	1 (6)	6 (12)
>80% reduction	12 (67)	26 (52)
50%-80% reduction	1 (6)	6 (12)
No significant change	3 (17)	12 (24)
Deceased	1 (6)	None reported

(Courtesy of Nordgren RE, Reeves AG, Viguera AC, et al: *Arch Neurol* 48:364–372, 1991.)

zures were the most common type postoperatively. Neuropsychological test scores did not worsen significantly after surgery in any patient, and new language problems have not appeared. No patient has exhibited violent behavior; in many cases, behavior has improved substantially and alertness has increased after callosal sectioning.

Corpus callosotomy should be considered in a young patient who has frequent atonic, tonic, or tonic-clonic seizures. Younger patients appear to tolerate the procedure better than those who are older. Fewer seizures often will promote behavioral and cognitive improvement after callosotomy.

► As a child neurologist, I welcome any new therapy for children with generalized atonic and tonic seizures. Although corpus callosotomy is not new, it is gaining acceptance for treatment of intractable generalized seizures. I believe that it is still underutilized and should be in the treatment algorithm for all children with intractable generalized seizures. Children taking multiple medications for long periods of time with only marginal benefit are probably worse off than they would be after surgery, despite its potential risks and side effects. What is needed, however, is a prospective controlled trial comparing surgery with medical management. Some children with intractable seizures come under control with time. Showing improved seizure control at an earlier age improves outcome and would offset fears of anatomically altering the developing brain.— O.B. Evans, M.D.

Home Use of Rectal Diazepam for Cluster and Prolonged Seizures: Efficacy, Adverse Reactions, Quality of Life, and Cost Analysis

Kriel RL, Cloyd JC, Hadsall RS, Carlson AM, Floren KL, Jones-Saete CM (Univ of Minnesota; Gillette Children's Hosp, St Paul)
Pediatr Neurol 7:13–17, 1991   5–17

About 40% of children with epilepsy have recurrent seizures despite therapeutic serum antiepileptic drug levels. Cluster seizures may be associated with impaired neurologic function, and a large proportion of patients with status epilepticus will have long-term neurologic sequelae.

Rectal diazepam is rapidly absorbed, has a short onset of action, and can end status epilepticus.

Home treatment with rectal diazepam was evaluated in 67 families instructed in this measure from 1982 to 1987. Forty-one families gave their children rectal diazepam in the year after instruction. The indication was prolonged seizures or status epilepticus in 26 instances and cluster seizures in 15 others. The dosage was .3–.5 mg/kg.

A median of 5 doses was given in the year after instruction. In 85% of cases rectal diazepam controlled most or all of the seizures for which it was used. Nearly half of the treated children had unfavorable reactions, e.g., drowsiness, behavioral change, or respiratory difficulty. A possible instance of "respiratory arrest" was noted. Emergency room use declined significantly. Many families felt better able to cope with the seizure disorder, more family activities were possible, and all had greater peace of mind.

Most parents are readily trained to administer rectal diazepam safely and to identify those seizures that are suitable for this treatment. The entire family can enjoy a more normal life-style as a result.

▶ Rectal diazepam is gaining widespread acceptance for the home treatment of prolonged or cluster seizures. Numerous studies cited by the authors support its use. This study should be read with caution, however, as should all retrospective studies. Of the 128 patients identified, only 35 both used rectally administered diazepam and benefited from it. Forty-three did not respond to the questionnaire, thus introducing a sampling bias. The nonuser group had a significant reduction in emergency room visits, as did the user group. There was no significant reduction in seizure severity or frequency. Although I believe that rectal diazepam is effective, it is not without some risks. Five patients had respiratory problems, including 1 with apparent apnea in this series. Prospective studies would be useful in determining the effectiveness of rectal diazepam.— O.B. Evans, M.D.

Rapid Loading of Critically Ill Patients With Carbamazepine Suspension

Miles MV, Lawless ST, Tennison MB, Zaritsky AL, Greenwood RS (Univ of North Carolina)
Pediatrics 86:263–266, 1990   5–18

Carbamazepine is an antiepileptic agent considered the drug of choice for controlling primary generalized tonic-clonic and partial seizures, with and without secondary generalization. It is widely prescribed for children because of its safety and efficacy. Carbamazepine is now available as a suspension. If this suspension is promptly and reliably absorbed in children, it may be useful for rapidly controlling frequent seizures.

The rate and factors affecting carbamazepine absorption were investigated in 6 children in the pediatric intensive care unit. They were given loading doses of carbamazepine suspension, 7.4–10.4 mg/kg, in treatment of frequent seizures. The doses were given by nasogastric or nasoduodenal tube. Drug serum concentrations were assessed by fluorescence polarization immunoassay 15, 30, 60, 120, and 480 minutes after administration.

Therapeutic concentrations of carbamazepine were not attained in 1 patient with an ileus. In the other 5 children, with normal gastrointestinal function, mean serum levels of 4.3 mg/L and 7.3 mg/L were reached at 1 and 2 hours, respectively. Delayed gastric emptying and concurrent enteral feedings apparently slowed down absorption. There were no adverse reactions.

Loading with carbamazepine suspension appears to be a useful alternative for rapidly controlling generalized convulsions and partial seizures in children in acute care settings. Because ileus and coadministration of enteral feedings delay carbamazepine absorption, they should be avoided if rapid onset of antiepileptic effect is necessary.

▶ In most of the subjects in this study, a therapeutic blood level of carbamazepine was achieved within 2 hours after a single enteral dose and, surprisingly, therapeutic concentrations were maintained for up to 8 hours. The dose was only 10 mg/kg in the smaller children, which is a low average daily maintenance dose. Excessive sedation would probably not be a problem in patients in the intensive care setting. Enteral administration of the carbamazepine liquid preparation should be an adjunct in the treatment of seizures that do not respond to initial therapy with intravenous agents. Because highest blood level measured was 9 mg/L, perhaps higher loading doses could be used.—O.B. Evans, M.D.

A Follow-Up Study of Intractable Seizures in Childhood
Huttenlocher PR, Hapke RJ (Univ of Chicago)
Ann Neurol 28:699–705, 1990   5–19

Surgery is being recommended increasingly for children who have refractory seizures, but clear criteria for selecting children for epilepsy surgery are unavailable. Data were reviewed on 145 children with medically refractory seizures who were followed up 5–20 years after onset of seizures. About 60% of the children were mentally retarded, and most of these began having seizures before age 2 years. The mean age at onset of seizures in those with borderline to normal intelligence was 5 years.

Seizure control tended to improve with the length of follow-up (Fig 5–6). Seizures remitted in a significant number of children who had borderline or normal intelligence. The proportion who had persistent seizures declined at a rate of about 4% annually. The rate for retarded children was only 1.5% per year. The type of seizure did not influence the outcome. Children with focal brain atrophy did no worse than those lacking definite pathology on cerebral imaging. No cause was apparent in the majority of children with intractable seizures.

Intractable seizures in childhood frequently are associated with mental retardation, and retarded children have a poorer outlook for seizure

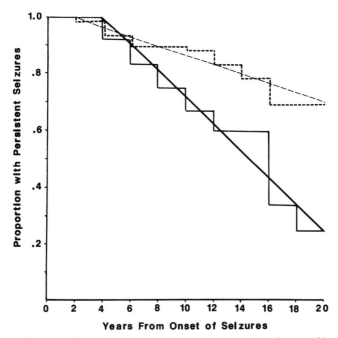

Fig 5–6.—Proportion of patients with persistent seizures (> 1/year) as a function of length of follow-up from onset of seizures (life-table method). *Solid lines* indicate group with IQ ≥ 70; *stippled lines,* group with IQ < 70. (Courtesy of Huttenlocher PR, Hapke RJ: *Ann Neurol* 28:699–705, 1990.)

control. Apart from seizure control itself, decisions regarding surgery should take into account the reactions of children and their families to chronic disease, interference of seizures with normal functioning and school adjustment, and toxic effects of anticonvulsant drugs. The small but definite mortality from uncontrolled seizures also is a consideration.

▶ The prognosis for children with intractable seizures is not good. In children with mental retardation there is a 1.5% remission rate per year. Children with borderline, or near normal, intelligence are not much better off, with a remission rate of 4% per year. In my experience, most families will eagerly consider seizure surgery. Remission rates vary widely in published series, but even a 50% improvement rate would be welcomed by most neurologists and families when faced with years of medications, clinic visits, hospitalizations, and endless determinations of anticonvulsant blood levels. The time for retrospective reviews of surgical and medical treatments for children with poorly controlled epilepsy has passed. Prospective trials are needed to settle issues such as patient selection and risk/benefit outcomes.—O.B. Evans, M.D.

6 Headache

Arterial Responses During Migraine Headache
Iversen HK, Nielsen TH, Olesen J, Tfelt-Hansen P (Gentofte Hosp, Hellerup, Denmark; Bispebjerg Hosp; Univ of Copenhagen)
Lancet 336:837–839, 1990   6–1

Studies on the etiology of migraine have focused on the superficial temporal artery, but one has yet measured its diameter directly. The noninvasive high-resolution ultrasound machine enabled measurement of the luminal diameter of both temporal arteries in 25 patients during unilateral migraine attacks. Diameters of both radial arteries also were measured.

The luminal diameter of the frontal branch of the temporal artery was significantly larger on the symptomatic side than on the nonsymptomatic side during a migraine attack, but both diameters were similar during intervals between attacks (Fig 6–1). The diameters of both radial arteries and the temporal artery on the nonpainful side were smaller during attacks than between attacks.

During unilateral migraine attacks, the generalized vasoconstriction is not shared by the temporal artery on the affected side, suggesting a local

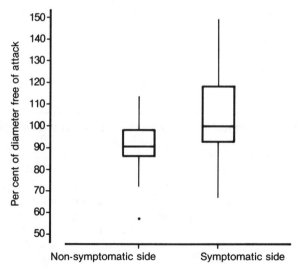

Fig 6–1.—Luminal diameter of the frontal branch of the temporal artery during migraine attack. The *box* covers the middle 50% of the values between the lower and upper quartiles; the *central line* is at the median; the *"whiskers"* extend out to the extremes, but only to those points that are within 1.5 times the interquartiles' range. (Courtesy of Iversen HK, Nielsen TH, Olesen J, et al: *Lancet* 1990; 336:837–839.)

vasodilatory response. Because the adventitia of extracranial and intracranial arteries are richly supplied with sympathetic, parasympathetic, and trigeminal nerves, and contain monoamines and peptide transmitters with vasoactive and inflammatory properties, local vasodilation may sensitize perivascular nociceptors and contribute to the pathogenesis of migraine pain.

▶ This lovely study clearly shows that the temporal artery on the side of the headache dilates while the one on the other side and both radial arteries constrict, leading to the conclusion that, during a migraine headache, there is generalized vasoconstriction with vasodilatation only on the side of the headache. The authors speculate that, because the adventitia of extracranial and intracranial arteries is well supplied with autonomic and trigeminal fibers, and contain monoamine and peptide transmitters with vasoactive and inflammatory properties, the vasodilatation might have something to do with the headaches. Indeed, it might. Speaking personally, my own migraines have been accompanied by a clear-cut peripheral vasoconstriction with coldness of the extremities. Therefore, the long hot tub bath that I take (and also recommend to patients) may work by reversal of the vasoconstriction. It also induces sleep, which is often therapeutic.

The Harvard-Oxford Physicians' Health Study is producing unexpected benefits (1). One aspirin (325 mg) every other day reduces the incidence of migraine by 20%, which is significant. Dalessio, in an editorial (2), says he asks his patients with frequent migraine to take an aspirin every other day.

Another unexpected finding from the same study is the recent note that patients given carotene have fewer heart attacks. It sounds as though we should all take an aspirin and eat a carrot every other day.—R.D. Currier, M.D.

References

1. Buring JE, et al: *JAMA* 264:1711, 1990.
2. Dalessio DJ: *JAMA* 264;1721, 1990.

Temporal Muscle Blood Flow in Chronic Tension-Type Headache
Langemark M, Jensen K, Olesen J (Univ of Copenhagen)
Arch Neurol 47:654–658, 1990   6–2

The pain in chronic muscle-contraction headache is thought to be of ischemic origin. However, blood flow in the pericranial muscles of patients with tension-type headaches has not been measured directly in a large group of patients. To investigate the ischemic theory further, the temporal muscle blood flow was measured using the xenon-133 clearance technique in 40 patients with chronic tension-type headache and in 13 controls. Thirty-five patients had daily headaches, 5 had headaches 15–25 days per month, and 15 had migraine attacks 1–12 days per year. No patients were receiving vasoactive, opioid, or neuroleptic drugs. Pressure-pain thresholds were determined with an algometer in the temporal region the day before blood flow was measured. Temporal blood flow was determined simultaneously on 2 sides at rest and during isometric exercise.

Blood flow parameters did not differ significantly between patients and controls. The resting blood flow was highly correlated between the 2 sides; there were no right/left differences in either patients or controls. During isometric exercise, blood flow increased by approximately fivefold in both patients and controls. Eight patients and 1 control had reactive hyperfusion after isometric exercise. There was no definite correlation between the pressure-pain threshold and corresponding blood flow.

It is unlikely that temporal muscle ischemia is the cause of muscle tenderness and pain in patients with chronic tension-type headaches. Because studies have demonstrated decreased pain perception thresholds in patients with chronic tension headaches, it is possible that pain arises primarily from a disturbance of central pain modulation pathways rather than from a peripheral disturbance of muscle.

▶ This is a careful study by experienced investigators of temporal muscle blood flow in patients with chronic tension-type headache with a negative result. There was no evidence of muscle ischemia in the temporalis muscle. The authors note that, although static low-level muscle contraction can induce headache, ischemia is not the cause.

Goadsby et al. (1) have pulled off a nice trick and found something that may turn out to be an important clue to the understanding of migraine. They discovered an increase during migraine of the calcitonin gene-related peptide in jugular blood. It's one of the vasodilator neuropeptides.—R.D. Currier, M.D.

Reference

1. Goadsby PJ, et al: *Ann Neurol* 28:183, 1990.

Timing and Topography of Cerebral Blood Flow, Aura, and Headache During Migraine Attacks

Olesen J, Friberg L, Skyhøj Olsen T, Iversen HK, Lassen NA, Andersen AR, Karle A (Gentofte Hosp; Rigshospitalet, Univ of Copenhagen; Bispebjerg Hosp, Copenhagen)
Ann Neurol 28:791–798, 1990   6–3

Knowledge of regional cerebral blood flow (rCBF) in migraine with aura is considerable but fragmented. To determine statistically significant sequences of events and spatial relations, studies were made in 63 patients.

The first observable event was a reduction in rCBF posteriorly in 1 cerebral hemisphere. The aura symptoms accompanied further development of this pathologic process. After this, headache occurred. Regional CBF remained decreased. In the headache phase, rCBF gradually changed from abnormally low to abnormally high, with no apparent change in

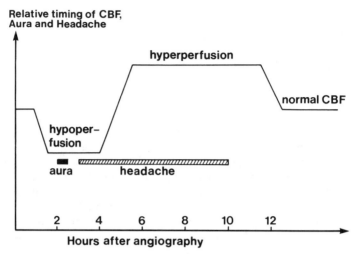

Fig 6–2.—Schematic drawing illustrating the temporal relation between angiography (time 1 hour), hypoperfusion, aura, headach, hyperperfusion, disappearance of headache, and disappearance of hyperperfusion. The time axis is chosen to illustrate what is typical. It does not depict actually recorded times in a single patient or in a group of patients, because the picture only becomes clear by synthesizing information from many patients. It is the sequence of events rather than the exact timing that is important. The angulation of the flow curve is to show that the details about how fast flow changes are unknown. The real course of rCBF is, of course, smooth. (Courtesy of Olesen J, Friberg L, Skyhøj Olsen T, et al: *Ann Neurol* 1990; 28:791–798.)

headache. In some cases, headache disappeared while the rCBF flow was still elevated. In most patients, rCBF reduction and aura symptoms were unilateral, but one third had bilateral headache. Unilateral headache usually localized to the side on which the rCBF was decreased and from which the aura symptoms originated (Fig 6–2).

These findings suggest a simple model for migraine attacks. A pathologic disturbance in 1 cerebral hemisphere first causes the aura symptoms. After a time delay it causes the headache by stimulating local vascular nociceptors. Recent neuroanatomical and neurophysiologic findings may explain bilateral headache caused by a unilateral cerebral disturbance.

▶ This is an article worth reading. These workers are making progress in understanding migraine. They give us some idea as to what happens with CBF during the evolution of migraine, putting to rest the hoary notion of vasoconstriction with the aura and vasodilatation with the headache. It's not that simple, as the fact that a third of their patients with unilateral blood flow changes had bilateral headache shows.

Ferrari et al. (1) found that glutamic and aspartic acid levels are high in migraine patients and go even higher during the headache. They propose a defective cellular reuptake for the 2 amino acids in migraineurs. I can't believe it, having had the top of my head taken off by monosodium glutamate once or twice in the past. But how does it fit in with the blood flow changes?—R.D. Currier, M.D.

Reference

1. Ferrari MD, et al: *Neurology* 40:1582, 1990.

Headache as a Warning Symptom of Impending Aneurysmal Subarachnoid Hemorrhage

Østergaard JR (Univ of Århus, Denmark)
Cephalagia 11:53–55, 1991   6–4

Perhaps half of the patients who sustain an intracranial aneurysm have had previous minor bleeding episodes before a major bleed, the so-called warning leak. Most of those with warning leaks have generalized headache, presumably representing meningeal irritation from blood in the subarachnoid space. In about two thirds of these patients the headache is associated with other features, e.g., nausea-vomiting, meningism or neck pain, visual disorder, and even motor or sensory disturbances. The headache usually is described as unusual in severity and location, and of sudden onset. A missed warning leak is as serious prognostically as a clear sequence of rebleeding episodes.

When a patient without previous severe headaches complains of severe, unremitting pain in the head or face, minor leakage from a saccular aneurysm should be suspected. This is especially the case if the pain is hemicranial or hemifacial, and if vomiting or meningism also occurs. At present, CT is the most satisfactory means of evaluating these patients. Lumbar puncture is indicated once CT has ruled out an intracranial mass lesion or intracranial hypertension. Angiography should be done if xanthochromic CSF is obtained, or if the CSF is bloody after an atraumatic puncture.

▶ The author points out that the warning headache is unusual in both severity and location and is thought by the patient to be unlike any previous headache. He recommends CT followed by lumbar puncture.

It's hard to know what to say about such a recommendation. How can a busy emergency room dealing with all sorts of head pain accurately define those patients who need the CT scan and the lumbar puncture? I suppose one could say, well, if it occurs to you, the physician, then you should do it, like other medical dictums. On the other hand, I can see an emergency room physician who can't get this worry out of his head doing CTs and lumbar punctures on every unusual headache that he encounters. Maybe that is what we will come to.—R.D. Currier, M.D.

Headache Caused by Caffeine Withdrawal Among Moderate Coffee Drinkers Switched From Ordinary to Decaffeinated Coffee: A 12-Week Double-Blind Trial

van Dusseldorp M, Katan MB (Univ of Nijmegen, The Netherlands)
Br Med J 300:1558–1559, 1990   6–5

Although often overlooked, caffeine withdrawal could be an important cause of headache. Information on controlled trials of caffeine withdrawal is limited. The withdrawal effect of caffeine was examined in 45 healthy subjects who regularly consumed 4–6 cups of coffee per day.

Subjects were matched for age, sex, and blood pressure, and then were randomly assigned to receive either 5 cups of coffee each day for 6 weeks followed by 5 cups of decaffeinated coffee for the next 6 weeks, or the protocol in reverse. Both subjects and investigators were blind to the type of coffee consumed. Subjects were prohibited from consuming other products containing caffeine, except for small amounts of chocolate.

Thirty-eight of 45 subjects were unaware that they were drinking decaffeinated coffee. Nineteen subjects had more headache complaints during the first week of drinking decaffeinated coffee in comparison with the mean number of headache complaints during the other 11 weeks (Fig 6–3). Five subjects had fewer complaints during the first week of drinking decaffeinated coffee, and 21 had no change. Subjects also fell asleep more readily when drinking decaffeinated coffee.

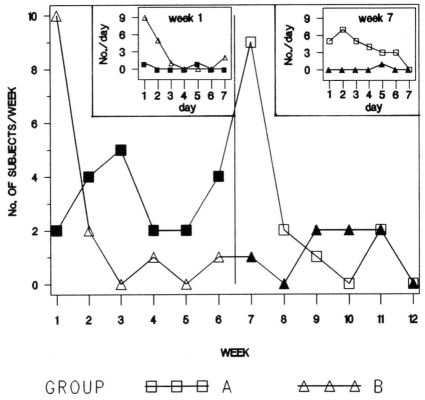

Fig 6–3.—Prevalence of headaches among subjects who habitually consumed 4–6 cups of coffee a day and were switched from ordinary to decaffeinated coffee at the start of study (week 1; *open triangles*) or week 7 *(open squares). Closed triangles* and *closed squares* indicate consumption of ordinary coffee. (Courtesy of van Dusseldorp M, Katan MB: *Br Med J* 300:1558–1559, June 1990.)

Many persons who drink moderate amounts of coffee experience headaches lasting for 2 or 3 days after caffeine withdrawal. This effect is not influenced by subjective expectations. Clinicians should be aware of caffeine withdrawal as a possible cause of headache, particularly when caffeine consumption is sporadic.

▶ Caffeine withdrawal headache has been in the books for many years, but evidently a double-blind crossover study has never before been done. The headaches, after the patients switched to decaffeinated coffee, started on the first or second day (not 16 hours later, as the books say) and lasted for 1–6 days, with a mean duration of 2–3 days. Another cup of decaf, please.—R.D. Currier, M.D.

The Analgesic Effects of Caffeine in Headache
Ward N, Whitney C, Avery D, Dunner D (Univ of Washington)
Pain 44:151–155, 1991   6–6

Although caffeine often is added to preparations of mild analgesics, its effect alone is uncertain. A double-blind, placebo-controlled, multiple crossover study was designed to ascertain the effects of caffeine in 53 patients with nonmigrainous headaches. Subjects received placebo, or caffeine in a dose of 65 mg or 130 mg, or acetaminophen in a dose of 648 mg, alone or combined with either dose of caffeine.

All active treatments reduced headache more than placebo did in the 53 evaluable patients (Fig 6–4). The analgesic effect of caffeine appeared equivalent to that of acetaminophen. It persisted after adjusting for both

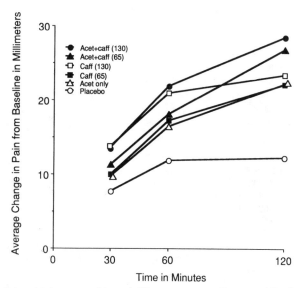

Fig 6–4.—Pain reduction: comparisions of different treatments. (Courtesy of Ward N, Whitney C, Avery D, et al: *Pain* 44:151–155, 1991.)

previous caffeine consumption and the mood effect of caffeine. Caffeine altered ratings of depression and fatigue, but not those of tension, anger, or confusion.

These findings support a direct analgesic effect of caffeine in patients with nonmigrainous headaches. Conceivably, caffeine acts by stimulating D2 or α_2 receptors in the CNS.

▶ This is an unexpected finding, at least to me. The authors postulate possible mechanisms for the analgesic effect of caffeine. Another article by Cameron et al. (1) shows that caffeine given intravenously decreases cerebral blood flow, as observed on positron emission tomography. Is it possible that caffeine works not through any direct analgesic pathway but by decreasing blood flow?—R.D. Currier, M.D.

Reference

1. Cameron, et al: *Life Sciences* 47:1141, 1990.

MSG and Hydrolyzed Vegetable Protein Induced Headache: Review and Case Studies
Scopp AL (Northern California Headache Clinic, Mountain View, Calif)
Headache 31:107–110, 1991   6–7

Up to 50% of patients with migraine report that certain foods can induce headache, among which are monosodium glutamate (MSG), tyramine, and aspartame. The number of foods containing MSG have increased markedly in recent years (Table 1). Chinese restaurants are a relatively minor source of dietary MSG at present. The addition of hydrolyzed vegetable protein, which often contains 20% MSG, to canned or frozen foods may have adverse effects.

Migraine induced by MSG may represent a direct vasospastic effect on peripheral arterial tone. Placebo-controlled studies have shown that about one third of a study group will have symptoms after ingesting MSG. Approved terms indicating the MSG content of foods are listed in

---

TABLE 1.—Partial List of Food Categories That Usually Contain Large Amounts of MSG

```
Frozen food (especially dinner entrees)
Canned and dry soups
Potato chips and prepared snacks
Canned meats, box dinners and prepared meals
International foods
Most diet foods and weight loss powders
Cured and luncheon meats (i.e., salami, bologna, pepperoni)
Most sauces in jars and cans (i.e., tomato and barbecue)
Most salad dressings and mayonnaise
```

(Courtesy of Scopp AL: *Headache* 31:107–110, 1991.)

TABLE 2.—FDA-Approved Food Label Terms Indicating
MSG Content

MSG
Hydrolyzed Vegetable Protein (HVP)
Hydrolyzed Plant Protein (HPP)
Natural Flavor (almost always)
Flavoring (almost always)
Kombu extract

(Courtesy of Scopp AL: *Headache* 31:107–110, 1991.)

Table 2, and the hydrolyzed vegetable protein (HVP) content of commonly prepared foods is shown in Table 3. It remains difficult to identify most dietary sources of MSG through the term "monosodium glutamate" or "MSG" on a label.

Apparently, MSG can trigger migraine headaches, and headache patients should know about the widespread and concealed food sources of MSG. It is helpful to avoid sauces, soups, and salad dressings in restau-

TABLE 3.—Hydrolyzed Vegetable Protein Levels in Common Prepared Foods

Powdered and Dehydrated Soup
Strong meat type-oxtail, kidney, etc.	15–20% of dry soup
Poultry type-chicken, turkey, etc	5–10% of dry soup
Vegetable soups-mixed vegetable, pea	3–10% of dry soup
Gravy powders	20–40% of dry product

Canned Soups and Gravies
Cream soups	0.25–0.6%
Beef broths and consomme	0.5 –2.0%
Vegetable	0.25–0.5%
Poultry soups	0.25–0.6%
Fish soups	0.1 –0.3%
Gravies	0.5 –2.0%

Bouillon and Stock Cubes
Beef type	40–60%
Poultry type	30–50%

Beef stews, hot pot, hashes, etc. steak and kidney pie, beefburgers and other beef products	0.5 –1.0%
Luncheon meat, pasties, pork pie, ham and egg pie and other pork and veal products	0.25–0.5%
English sausage-beef	0.15–0.35%
pork	0.15–0.35%
Liver sausage and pates	0.25–0.35%
Poultry products	0.25–0.5%
Curing brines	0.1 –0.25% on meat weight

(Courtesy of Scopp AL: *Headache* 31:107–110, 1991.)

rants for a 1-month trial period. It also may help for patients to record all foods taken 6 hours before the onset of migraine, or those taken at dinner when migraine occurs at night or shortly after arising.

▶ This author has done us a favor. He has given us lists of things that contain MSG and reports that sometimes MSG, by new Food and Drug Administration (FDA) rule changes, is not identified as such but as hydrolyzed vegetable protein or hydrolyzed plant protein. He has also given us the percentages of these substances in various foods. Talking to the patients in clinic I find that the use of MSG seems to be increasing. Patients use "seasoned salt" routinely (at least here in Mississippi) in their cooking and wonder why they have headaches every day. Perhaps the FDA should rethink their approval of other terms to indicate MSG. How about that, FDA? Possibly they should also require the label, "May cause headaches."

For a comprehensive analysis of dietary influences on migraine see the paper by Seymour Diamond in *Neurology Forum* (1).

Cady et al. (2) record the first American trial of Glaxo's sumatriptan. Given subcutaneously, this serotonin agonist (5-HT$_{1D}$) is a potent vasoconstrictor and is 3 to 4 times more effective than placebo in relieving acute migraine. The sooner it passes the FDA the better.— R.D. Currier, M.D.

References

1. Diamond S: *Neurology Forum* 2:2, 1991.
2. Cady RK, et al: *JAMA* 265:2831, 1991.

Occupational Stress in Migraine: Is Weekend Headache a Myth or Reality?
Morrison DP (Karolinska Inst and Hosp, Stockholm)
Cephalalgia 10:189–193, 1990   6–8

Stress-induced migraine may occur in the relaxation period after stress rather than during its height. With this assumption, there should be an increased number of migraine attacks during the weekend if migraine is associated with job-related stress. To test this hypothesis, 35 women aged 20–59 years prospectively recorded the presence or absence of migraine attacks daily during a 6-week period. Patients also estimated the frequency with which migraine attacks were associated with emotional factors. The diagnosis of common or classic migraine was based on the criteria of the Ad Hoc Committee on the Classification of Headache and the International Headache Society.

Eighteen patients had classic migraine and 17 had common migraine. Patients each completed a mean 37.3 days of records, with a mean 3.5 migraine attacks per patient. Emotional factors were implicated in the migraine attacks by 77% of patients. There was no significant increase in the frequency of migraine attacks during weekends, either in the group as a whole or among those who were employed. There was no association between type of migraine and weekend migraine attacks. This study provided no evidence that delayed onset of migraine during weekends is related to the weekday stress of employment.

▶ This destroys a dearly held myth that migraine headaches more commonly occur on the weekends. Should it be studied further?—R.D. Currier, M.D.

General Practitioners' Detection of Depression and Dementia in Elderly Patients
Bowers J, Jorm AF, Henderson S, Harris P (Australian Natl Univ, Canberra; Woden Valley Hosp, Garran)
Med J Aust 153:192–196, 1990   6–9

The general practitioner is in an advantageous position to detect psychological disturbances in elderly patients. The ability of 11 general practitioners to detect dementia and depression in 101 elderly patients aged 70 or more was evaluated, as was the practitioner's knowledge of these 2 common psychiatric disturbances. Three indices of dementia were used: the Mini-Mental State Examination, the Clifton Assessment Procedures for the Elderly, and the Informant Questionnaire on Cognitive Decline in the Elderly. The 3 indices for depression used were the Diagnostic Interview for Depression, the 12-item General Health Questionnaire, and informant's opinion.

The general practitioners were more accurate in detecting dementia than depression in their elderly patients. Whereas their assessment of dementia corresponded well with the results of dementia tests, the general practitioners failed to identify 12 of 15 patients assessed as depressed by the Diagnostic Interview. The depression recognition rate increased if patients talked about feeling depressed, sad, or irritable. The general practitioners' knowledge of the symptoms and signs of dementia and depression as specified on the *DSM-III-R* diagnostic criteria was limited.

The poor performance in recognizing depression may be attributable to lack of knowledge of depressive symptoms or failure to inquire explicitly about these symptoms. If these findings are confirmed in a larger sample, general practitioners should undertake further training on psychological disturbances, particularly depression, in the elderly.

▶ Unless the patient cries during the interview, I miss the diagnosis of depression routinely. It's nice to see that general practitioners are no better than neurologists. Why the interest in the diagnosis of depression? Read on.—R.D. Currier, M.D.

Headache: A Marker of Depression
Chung MK, Kraybill DE (Montgomery Family Practice Residency Program, Norriston, Pa)
J Fam Pract 31:360–364, 1990   6–10

Several studies suggest a close link between depression and headache and whereas most studies report a high prevalence of headache in patients with depression, the converse has not been well studied. Forty patients aged 15–67 years with a chief complaint of headache were seen in an outpatient family practice setting. All completed a questionnaire that incorporated a 20-item instrument to measure specific characteristics of depression, the Zung Self-Rating Depression Scale index (SDS).

Sixty-three percent of the patients with headache had clinically significant depression, as defined by the Zung SDS score. In fact, 74% of patients who experienced headaches on a daily basis were depressed. The Zung SDS score correlated significantly with the frequency of headache and the length of time that the headache existed. Item analysis of the Zung SDS indicated that 4 questions accounted for 93% of the variance in the Zung SDS score, suggesting that a shorter, more abbreviated screening questionnaire could be developed.

This study demonstrated a strikingly high prevalence of clinically significant depression in patients seen in the primary care setting with the chief complaint of headache. Apparently, headache may be an important marker of depression, suggesting that the clinician may need to focus on treating the entity of depression rather than simply treating the symptoms of headache.

▶ These 2 researchers raise an old problem: How many headache patients are depressed? In their family practice they found 63%, and point out that some of the medications we use in the treatment of headaches, particularly the β blockers, do not help depression. Perhaps we should prescribe propranolol for those patients who have slight or intermittent blood pressure elevations and no trouble with sleep, and antidepressants for those who have trouble with sleep but normal blood pressure.—R.D. Currier, M.D.

Sleep Deprivation Headache
Blau JN (Natl Hosp for Nervous Diseases, London)
Cephalalgia 10:157–160, 1990   6–11

Insufficient sleep as a cause of headache is rarely addressed. A reported 39% incidence of headache as a result of sleep loss in medical and dental students led to an attempt to characterize headaches caused by insufficient or interrupted sleep.

Twenty-five healthy subjects aged 25–27 years who normally required 6–10 hours of sleep per day were studied. In these subjects, sleep loss varying from 1 to 3 hours for 1–3 days caused headaches lasting from 1 hour to all day. The headaches were described as a dull ache or a heaviness or pressure sensation in the forehead and/or at the vertex. Simply over-the-counter analgesics completely or markedly reduced the headache in 20–60 minutes.

Sleep loss is a cause of headache, and this headache differs from a tension headache in site, duration, and response to analgesics. Assuming that pain indicates a regional disturbance, it appears that headaches caused by sleep loss provide support to the notion that sleep has a restorative function.

▶ I agree with the good Dr. Blau. Lack of sleep is one cause of headaches, and it should be on your list of things to ask after you find out the patient has quit smoking, isn't hypertensive, does not take birth control pills, dislikes cheddar cheese and chocolate, and stays away from monosodium glutamate.—R.D. Currier, M.D.

A Comparative Trial of Three Agents in the Treatment of Acute Migraine Headache
Bell R, Montoya D, Shuaib A, Lee MA (Univ of Calgary, Foothills Hosp; Univ of Calgary Gen Hosp, Alta)
Ann Emerg Med 19:1079–1082, 1990   6–12

The management of patients with migraine headache remains a challenge. In a randomized, single-blind study, the relative efficacies of 3 non-narcotic agents—chlorpromazine, lidocaine, and dihydroergotamine—in the treatment of acute migraine headache were compared in 76 patients seen in the emergency department with common or classic migraine. All patients were pretreated with the intravenous administration of 500 mL of normal saline. The patients received either 1 mg of dihydroergotamine, repeated after 30 minutes if the initial response was inadequate; 50 mg of lidocaine at 20-minute intervals to a maximum total dose of 150 mg as required; or chlorpromazine, 12.5 mg repeated at 20-minute intervals to a total maximum dose of 37.5 mg as required; all drugs were administered intravenously. The severity of headache was graded on a 10-point scale before and 1 hour after start of treatment.

Patients treated with chlorpromazine experienced a significantly greater reduction in headache severity compared with those given either of the other 2 drugs. Follow-up at 24 hours by phone determined that 89% of patients treated with chlorpromazine, compared with 53% of patients treated with dihydroergotamine and 29% of patients treated with lidocaine, had persistent relief of headaches. Only minor side effects were reported by patients treated with chlorpromazine, whereas severe gastrointestinal symptoms were reported by those treated with dihydroergotamine. About two thirds of the patients treated with chlorpromazine said that they would use the same treatment for future migraine headaches compared with less than a third of those treated with the other 2 drugs.

▶ Again, chlorpromazine given intravenously turns out to be the winner. Although I don't know, I suspect that it is becoming more commonly used in the emergency room treatment of migraine.—R.D. Currier, M.D.

Recurrent Prolonged Coma Due to Basilar Artery Migraine: A Case Report

Frequin STFM, Linssen WHJP, Pasman JW, Hommes OR, Merx HL (Univ of Nijmegen, The Netherlands)
Headache 31:75–81, 1991   6–13

Basilar artery migraine connotes a functional disturbance of the brain stem, cerebellum, or occipital cortex. Coma is a rare occurrence in basilar artery migraine.

Man, 25, was found stuporous without evidence of seizure activity; he was confused, disoriented, and aggressive when examined. Extensor plantar responses were present bilaterally. The patient deteriorated rapidly, and the limbs became extended and pronated on both sides, with Cheyne-Stokes respiration. Marked

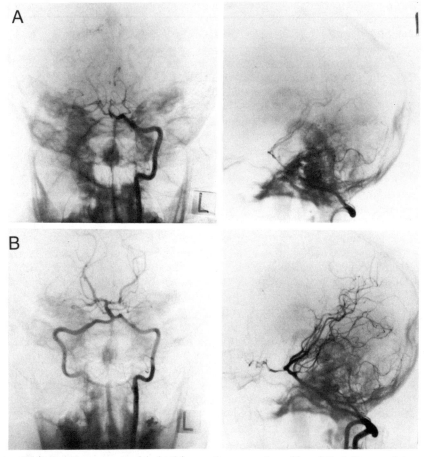

Fig 6–5.—**A,** severe spasm of the basilar artery (anteroposterior and lateral view). **B,** repeated arteriography after 2 weeks shows that the basilar spasm has disappeared. There is no evidence of an arterial aneurysm. (Courtesy of Frequin STFM, Linssen WHJP, Pasman JW, et al: *Headache* 31:75–81, 1991.)

mental slowing resolved in the following weeks, and the patient was able to resume work after 3 months. Cranial CT was negative, but an EEG on the day of admission showed a suppression-burst pattern. Angiography showed severe vasospasm in the basilar artery system (Fig 6–5), which was not evident 2 weeks later. Marked EEG improvement was evident 2 months after the episode. Severe occipital headaches continued, however, and the patient was again unconscious 5 months after his initial presentation, with tonic-clonic seizures and no localizing signs. Consciousness improved slowly, but a third attack occurred in the hospital, resolving after the administration of ergotamine suppositories with phenobarbital. A fourth attack of sudden unconsciousness ensued, followed again by recovery. Phenytoin treatment was instituted; the EEG showed intermittent bilateral synchronous frontotemporal theta-delta activity.

Basilar artery migraine is a diagnosis of exclusion. Attacks can be severe and even life-threatening. The described patient appears to have had upper brain stem dysfunction consequent to basilar artery spasm. Conventional antimigraine agents are of little use in basilar artery migraine, but phenytoin therapy reportedly may be helpful.

▶ Speaking of serious headaches, this sounds like the real thing. It's hard for a migraine sufferer to agree that migraine can cause prolonged coma, but this seems a pretty solid case.—R.D. Currier, M.D.

The Cluster Diathesis
Gawel MJ, Krajewski A, Luo YM, Ichise M (Sunnybrook Health Science Centre, Toronto; Mt Sinai Hosp, Toronto; Univ of Toronto)
Headache 30:652–655, 1990   6–14

Cluster headache has been widely studied and well defined. Vascular reactivity in the anterior cerebral artery on the headache side changes significantly only between the in-cluster and out-of-cluster state. Carbon di-

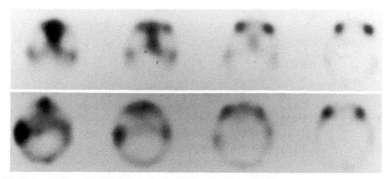

Fig 6–6.—Gallium-SPECT of cluster headache patient shows central area of increased uptake. Below is the scan obtained in the control patient with otitis media showing increased uptake caused by inflammation (nose is at the top; note the 2 areas of increased uptake attributable to the lacrimal glands). (Courtesy of Gawel MJ, Krajewski A, Luo YM, et al: *Headache* 30:652–655, 1990.)

oxide reactivity of the major intracranial vessels in and out of cluster was measured using transcranial Doppler in 119 patients with cluster headache.

Reactivity was significantly reduced during the cluster period, but only in the anterior cerebral artery on the headache side. Nineteen patients were followed sequentially for a full cycle—both in and out of a cluster period. The same changes were seen in these cases. In 3 of 6 patients in an active cluster period, a lesion was seen on gallium single-photon emission CT (SPECT) in the area of the cavernous sinus. This lesion faded as the patient moved out of the cluster state (Fig 6–6).

This study provides additional evidence for a sympathetic defect of vasomotor control of the anterior cerebral artery on the side of the headache during cluster periods. Sequential follow-up is necessary to determine whether the inflammatory changes seen on gallium-SPECT conform to changes in the CO_2 reactivity of the anterior cerebral artery and periods of relapse and remission.

▶ So, now we have a cavernous sinus lesion as shown by SPECT in patients during cluster headache. Can we be sure that it's the cavernous sinus and not simply nasal mucosa that is lighting up? Well, that's the place where those who think about this type of headache have localized it for years, and it shouldn't be too surprising. Now the questions are: What is the nature of the lesion, and what can we do about it? For a thorough review of the mechanisms of pain in cluster headache see Hardebo (1).—R.D. Currier, M.D.

Reference

1. Hardebo JE: *Headache* 31:91, 1991.

7 Epilepsy

Spina Bifida in Infants of Women Treated With Carbamazepine During Pregnancy
Rosa FW (Food and Drug Admin, Rockville, Md)
N Engl J Med 324:674–677, 1991   7–1

Previous studies have reported on the association between exposure in utero to carbamazepine and spina bifida. To investigate further, studies were made in a cohort of pregnant Medicaid recipients who delivered from 1980 to 1988 and who were taking antiepileptic agents during pregnancy. Only infants with spina bifida identified at the time of delivery were considered.

Four infants with spina bifida were born to 1,490 women who were taking antiepileptic drugs during pregnancy, and 3 of these were born to 107 women taking carbamazepine alone (table). The lack of an independent association of phenytoin, barbiturates, or primidone with spina bifida indicates that, unlike valproic acid, these drugs do not confound concurrent maternal exposure to carbamazepine.

Infants With Spina Bifida Born to Women Taking
Antiepileptic Agents During Pregnancy, 1980–1988*

DRUG	CASES OF SPINA BIFIDA/NO. OF PREGNANT WOMEN TAKING DRUG	
	TOTAL[†]	UNCONFOUNDED TOTAL[‡]
Barbiturates	3/1058	1/1018
Phenytoin	1/469	0/444
Carbamazepine	3/107	2/99
Primidone	1/62	0/50
Valproic acid	1/47	0/39
Total	4/1490	—

*The women were all Michigan residents and Medicaid recipients.
†"Total" refers to the total number of infants born to women taking the drugs alone or in combination. Thus, there was a total of 4 infants with spina bifida born to women who had taken the following drugs: carbamazepine and phenobarbital (child born in 1981); carbamazepine, valproic acid, and primidone (child born in 1982); carbamazepine, phenytoin, and mephobarbital (child born in 1985); and phenobarbital (child born in 1985).
‡"Unconfounded total" refers to the totals derived after the removal of the following confounding factors: concurrent use of valproic acid or carbamazepine by women taking barbiturates, phenytoin, or primidone; concurrent use of valproic acid by women taking carbamazepine; and concurrent use of carbamazepine by women taking valproic acid.
(Courtesy of Rosa FW: *N Engl J Med* 324:674–677, 1991.)

In a review of available cohort studies of carbamazepine exposure of fetuses, 9 cases of spina bifida were reported among the 984 exposures in utero to carbamazepine, for a relative risk of about 13.7 (95% confidence limits, 5.6–33.7) times the expected rate. The relative risk of spina bifida associated with exposure in utero to carbamazepine as compared with unconfounded exposure to other antiepileptic drugs was 6.8 (95% confidence limits, 2.4–19.1). The relative risk associated with carbamazepine as compared to valproic acid was .6 (95% confidence limits, .2–1.7). This analysis of all available data indicates that exposure to carbamazepine without concurrent exposure to valproic acid carries a 1% risk of spina bifida.

▶ I wonder how many women at risk for pregnancy have had phenytoin therapy withdrawn and carbamazepine substituted in the past 15 years. Dr Rosa's conclusions is that both carbamazepine and valproic acid may cause spina bifida, although he is not certain because of the small number of cases.

An editorial in *The Lancet* (1) states, "Despite mounting evidence, the case remains to be proven against CBZ (and perhaps also against valproate)," and "treated epilepsy should not preclude a woman from childbearing. More than 90% of such pregnancies will be uneventful and will result in a healthy baby." The editorial notes that carbamazepine is metabolized in the liver partly in the form of a pharmacologically active epoxide, a chemical species that is highly mutagenic. Production of the epoxide is increased by phenytoin and phenobarbital and its breakdown inhibited by valproate—an argument favoring monotherapy in women at risk for pregnancy.

So, what is safe? The lowest possible level of one of the old standbys?—R.D. Currier, M.D.

Reference

1. Editorial: *Lancet* 337:1316, 1991.

Children With Epilepsy as Adults: Outcome After 30 Years of Follow-Up
Sillanpää M (Dept of Public Health, Univ of Turku, Finland)
Acta Paediatr Scand (Suppl 368):1–78, 1990   7–2

A group of 227 patients representative of the epileptic population in southwestern Finland were followed prospectively for 23–39 years. At the last follow-up, 55% of the original group and 63% of the patients seen at the last follow-up evaluation had not had epileptic attacks for at least 3 years (Figs 7–1 and 7–2). This group included more than three fourths of the patients alive at the last follow-up evaluation.

Of the patients who were assessed, 60% were living independently and 21% were living in an institution. The remaining patients were not institutionalized but were receiving a disability pension. The latter, "intermediate" group became progressively smaller as the duration of follow-up

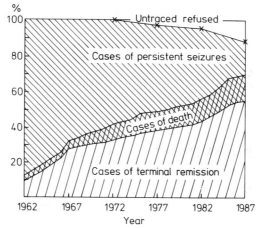

Fig 7–1.—Cumulative annual incidence of cases of terminal remission from seizures of 3 years or more and cases of death during 30-year follow-up period in an epileptic population of 245 patients. (Courtesy of Sillanpää M: *Acta Paediatr Scand* Suppl 368, 1990.)

increased. Mortality was clearly higher for the epileptics as a group than for the general population. Most prominent were respiratory infection, drowning, epileptic attacks, and sudden unexpected deaths. The epileptics exhibited better health behavior than similarly aged persons in the general population, even excluding institutionalized persons. Prominent prognostic factors in this series included the quality of mental development, early response to drug therapy, fine motor status, initial frequency of seizures, and psychotic symptoms.

▶ This remarkable work has been underway for 30 years. It confirms what we often tell patients—that the tendency to be in good control increases with

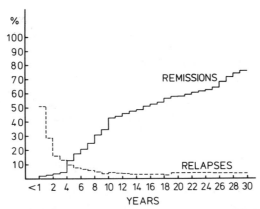

Fig 7–2.—Cumulative annual incidence of terminal remissions from seizures of 3 years or more and that of relapses during 30-year follow-up period in 178 surviving patients. (Courtesy of Sillanpää M: *Acta Paediatr Scand* Suppl 368, 1990.)

age. Congratulations to the author for carrying out this valuable work.— R.D. Currier, M.D.

Idiopathic First Seizure in Adult Life: Who Should Be Treated?
van Donselaar CA, Geerts AT, Schimsheimer R-J (Univ of Rotterdam)
Br Med J 302:620–623, 1991   7–3

Opinions differ on how to manage patients who have a first seizure of unknown origin. Whereas treating all such patients will lower the risk of recurrence, many patients might be treated unnecessarily. A prospective study was made of 165 patients aged 15 and older who had sustained a presumed idiopathic seizure. None had seizures other than febrile seizures in the past, and none had seizures lasting for more than 30 minutes. Electroencephalograms were acquired from 151 patients.

Computed tomography showed a major abnormality in 5% of the patients. The follow-up findings cast doubt on the initial impression in another 6% of patients. The cumulative risk of recurrent seizures within 2 years was 40%, but it was 81% in those in whom an epileptic discharge was observed on a standard or partial sleep deprivation EEG (Fig 7–3). Patients with normal EEGs had a 12% risk of recurrent seizures. More than two thirds of the patients with recurrent seizures were completely controlled by treatment.

Rather than treating all patients who sustain their first seizure in adulthood, it seems reasonable to treat on the basis of the EEG findings. This approach will lessen the number of patients who are treated unnecessarily. A thorough and negative EEG assessment makes the risk of recurrent seizures low.

▶ The EEG, if it was normal, was repeated after sleep deprivation. The EEGs with epileptic discharges (spikes or spike wave complexes) were helpful in predicting who would have a second or more seizures and, therefore, who should be treated after the first seizure. This splendid study should be of clinical use. Perhaps the first EEG should be sleep deprived.

So, now that we know a little more about who should be treated, when can drugs be withdrawn? A recent report of 1,013 patients published in *The Lancet* (1) with editorial comment in the same issue (2) is of help. The patients were all seizure free for 2 years and then were randomized either to continued treatment or to slow drug withdrawal. Five years later, 65% of those still taking medication and 50% of those withdrawn were seizure free. "The most important factors determining outcome were longer seizure-free periods (reducing the risk) and more than one anti-epileptic drug and a history of tonic-clonic seizures (increasing the risk)." The editorial concludes that, in this hawk vs. dove contest, the doves—those physicians who recommend continued drug therapy—have the better of it.— R.D. Currier, M.D.

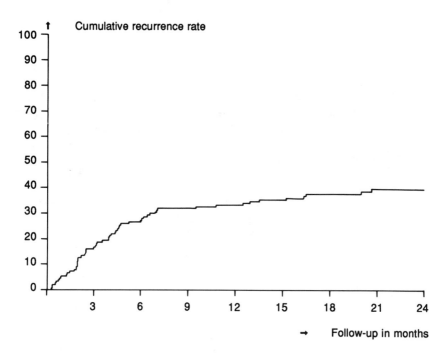

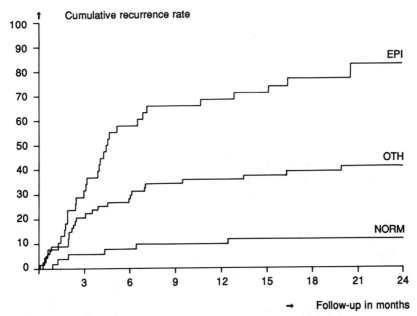

Fig 7–3.—Continuously adjusted recurrence rates in patients with idiopathic first seizures: (top) all patients, (bottom) according to EEG findings. (Courtesy of van Donselaar CA, Geerts AT, Schimscheimer R-J: *Br Med J* 302:620–623, 1991.)

References

1. Chadwick D: *Lancet* 337:1175, 1991.
2. Editorial: *Lancet* 337:1193, 1991.

Seizures of Unknown Origin After the Age of 50: Vascular Risk Factors
Shapiro IM, Neufeld MY, Korczyn AD (Sackler School of Medicine, Tel Aviv Univ, Ramat Aviv, Israel)
Acta Neurol Scand 82:78–80, 1990   7–4

Epilepsy of late onset is not rare, but in a high proportion of these cases the etiology remains unknown. To gain more insight into the etiology of late-onset seizure, 50 consecutive patients whose seizures started after age 50 (range, 55–81; mean, 69 years) and who had a normal CT brain scan were studied.

Most of the patients (72%) had generalized tonic-clonic seizures. The seizures occurred infrequently, with 64% having fewer than 3 seizures yearly. The frequencies of vascular risk factors, including arterial hypertension, ischemic heart disease, peripheral vascular disease, diabetes mellitus, and cigarette smoking, in patients with late-onset seizures were similar to those in the normal age- and sex-matched control group and much lower than those in patients whose seizures followed a stroke or patients with stroke but no seizures.

These data suggest that subclinical cerebrovascular disease is probably an unlikely cause of late-onset seizures of unknown origin. The search for the etiology of these seizures continues.

▶ You and I have long said to patients and their families when the patient's seizures started after age of 50 that, "There was probably a little stroke up in the cortex." Tallis (1), in a recent summary, reinforces that view, saying, Vascular disease is by far the commonest cause" But these Israeli workers find it is not so in most cases. So, what is the cause? The authors conclude it is "still an enigma."

There is a tongue-in-cheek note by Newrick et al. in the *Journal of the Royal Society of Medicine* (2). It's an autopsy study showing a correlation between the palmar life-line length and length of life. The authors suggest that it will require a "properly conducted prospective multicenter study in various populations" to confirm their findings. They do mention, however, that it is possible that palms become more wrinkled as we age.

In the *New England Journal of Medicine* (3), Thompson et al., writing on the Hydergine treatment of Alzheimer's disease, conclude that it is ineffective. Years ago, Wilma Donahue at the University of Michigan, asked me to find something for Alzheimer's disease. I was young and still wet behind the ears and thought I would give Hydergine a whirl. I tried it and couldn't see any effect. However, there have been, over the years, numerous reports in the literature of effective treatment with the drug. This excellent double-blind, placebo-controlled study found "no notable beneficial effect." The authors modestly suggest that their negative results may be because they might have failed to detect a real beneficial effect! However, then they more correctly go on to say that, "We believe that it is more likely that our study improves on previous effects." So it has. But a young friend who is studying Hydergine in the laboratory comments that the recommended dose of 3 mg/day may not be enough to do the job.—R.D. Currier, M.D.

References

1. Tallis R: *Lancet* 336:295, 1990.
2. Newrick PG, et al: *J R Soc Med* 83:449, 1990.
3. Thompson TL II, et al: *N Engl J Med* 323:445, 1990.

A Randomized, Double-Blind Study of Phenytoin for the Prevention of Post-Traumatic Seizures
Temkin NR, Dikmen SS, Wilensky AJ, Keihm J, Chabal S, Winn HR (Univ of Washington)
N Engl J Med 323:497–502, 1990   7–5

Antiepileptic drugs are frequently used to prevent post-traumatic seizures, but previous prospective studies suggest inconclusive evidence for their efficacy. The role of phenytoin in preventing early and late posttraumatic seizures was evaluated in a double-blind, placebo-controlled study involving 404 patients with serious head trauma. An intravenous loading dose (20 mg/kg) was given within 24 hours of injury. The dose of phenytoin was adjusted to maintain serum phenytoin levels in the high therapeutic range, at 3–6 μmol of free phenytoin per liter. In all, 208 patients received phenytoin and 196 received placebo for 12 months. The treat-

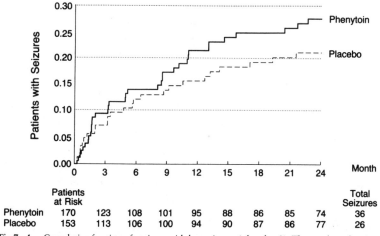

	Patients at Risk								Total Seizures
Phenytoin	170	123	108	101	95	88	86	85	74	36
Placebo	153	113	106	100	94	90	87	86	77	26

Fig 7–4.—Cumulative fraction of patients with late seizures (after day 8). The number of patients at risk for seizures and the total number of seizures are shown at the bottom of the figure. The seizure rates were similar in the phenytoin and placebo groups. (Courtesy of Temkin NR, Dikmen SS, Wilensky AJ, et al: *N Engl J Med* 323:497–502, 1990.)

ment groups were balanced in both demographic variables and severity of head injury. All patients were followed for 24 months.

Between drug loading and day 7, significantly more patients assigned to placebo treatment had seizures (14.2%) compared to patients treated with phenytoin (3.6%), for a reduction of 73% in the risk of seizures for the first week with phenytoin treatment. However, between day 8 and the end of the second year of the study, the frequency of seizures did not differ significantly in the 2 groups (Fig 7–4). Cox regression analysis showed that phenytoin treatment was associated with between a 29% decrease and a 102% increase in late seizures, with a point estimate of a 20% increase. The lack of late protective effect could not be explained by differential mortality, low phenytoin levels, or treatment of some early seizures in patients assigned to placebo.

These data provide convincing evidence on the effectiveness of phenytoin in preventing seizures only during the first week after severe head injury. It appears that phenytoin has an early suppressive effect but not a true prophylactic effect.

▶ This study will probably tend to stop the routine treatment of head-injury patients with phenytoin. There was a clear benefit in the first week, but after that, the phenytoin-treated group had slightly more seizures than the placebo-treated group, although the differences were not significant. As Hauser points out in an editorial in the same issue, the quest should not stop for an agent that will prevent posttraumatic seizures. Hauser also notes that phenobarbital, valproate, and the benzodiazepines theoretically might be more useful for inhibiting the origination of a secondary focus or kindling. Dikmen et al. (1) recently found that phenytoin impaired mental function 1 month after injury in severely injured patients, an effect that had disappeared after 1 year.

Last July, August, and September *The Lancet* published 8 consecutive articles on epilepsy (Epilepsy Octet). The articles are by different authors and are well done. If they had been published separately, the cost would be about equal to a year's subscription to *The Lancet*. Please don't, like me, wait until you are 60 to subscribe to what is arguably the best medical journal in the world. It contains at times more useful clinical neurology than the neurology journals.—R.D. Currier, M.D.

Reference

1. Dikmen SS, et al: *JAMA* 265:1271, 1991.

The Significance of Myoclonic Status Epilepticus in Postanoxic Coma
Young GB, Gilbert JJ, Zochodne DW (Victoria Hosp, London, Ont; Univ of Western Ontario)
Neurology 40:1843–1848, 1990   7–6

Myoclonic status epilepticus (MSE), consisting of generalized, bilateral synchronous myoclonic twitches occurring repetitively for at least half an hour, are common in comatose patients after cardiac arrest. Whether these patients die as a result of the initial anoxic-ischemic insult or from MSE is not clear. To assess the significance of MSE in postanoxic coma, clinical, EEG, and pathologic data were evaluated for 11 unselected patients who died within 2 weeks after the development of MSE following cardiac arrest.

Myoclonic seizures began within .5–48 hours post arrest, lasted from 5–72 hours, and were resistant to antiepileptic drugs. The myoclonic jerks were bilaterally synchronous and always involved the face, particularly the eyelids. Pupillary, oculocephalic-oculovestibular, and corneal reflexes were usually absent. The EEG patterns were not typical of status epilepticus and showed a burst-suppression pattern, periodic complexes, suppression, and an alpha-coma pattern. Pathologically, all patients sustained severe anoxic-ischemic damage to the cerebral cortex and cerebellum, and all had ischemic cell changes involving cerebellar Purkinje cells. In most patients the subcortical gray matter, including the thalamus and basal ganglia, was involved. The spinal cord in 9 of 10 patients showed anoxic myelopathy with similar neuronal ischemic changes in the central gray matter.

These data suggest that the patients died of the initial anoxic-ischemic insult rather than as a result of MSE, and that the seizures are self-limited events that arise from lethal damage to the neurons. When MSE is associated with bilateral loss of pupillary or oculovestibular reflexes and burst-suppression on the EEG, the prognosis is poor and anesthetic barbiturates are unlikely to alter the outcome.

▶ When standing in the intensive care unit watching a decerebrate patient go through this type of seizure, it is not difficult to look on this as the death knell of the cortex, which indeed it seems to be according to these authors. Trying to suppress the seizures may simply speed cell death, although I have never seen such a patient survive, with or without treatment. The syndrome is symptomatic of cortical death, and there is nothing much we can do about it.—R.D. Currier, M.D.

Comprehensive Primary Health Care Antiepileptic Drug Treatment Program in Rural and Semi-Urban Kenya
Feksi AT, Kaamugisha J, Sander JWAS, Gatiti S, Shorvon SD, for the Internal Community-Based Epilepsy Research Group (Provincial Gen Hosp, Nakuru, Kenya; Inst of Neurology, London; Natl Hosp, Gerrards Cross, England; Regional Med Ctr, Ciba-Geigy, Nairobi, Kenya)
Lancet 337:406–409, 1991   7–7

Relatively few patients with active epilepsy who live in developing countries actually receive drug treatment at a given time. A review was made of the results of a comprehensive primary care effort aimed at treating epilepsy in an unselected rural and semiurban population in Kenya, East Africa.

TABLE 1.—Maintenance Dose and Dose Increments for the Different Age Groups

	6–10 yr		11–15 yr		16 and over	
—	CBZ	PB	CBZ	PB	CBZ	PB
1st maintenance dose	400 mg	30 mg	500 mg	45 mg	600 mg	60 mg
Dose increments	100 mg	15 mg	100 mg	30 mg	200 mg	30 mg

Abbreviations: CBZ, carbamazepine; PB, phenobarbital.
First maintenance dose indicates the target dose to which the drugs were first titrated.
(Courtesy Feski AT, Kaamugisha J, Sander JWAS, et al: Lancet 337:406–409, 1991.)

Of 529 patients identified by health workers as having active tonic-clonic seizures, 302 were recruited by a psychiatrist to receive carbamazepine or phenobarbital under supervision by primary health workers (Table 1). Treatment was monitored by a research team. Carbamazepine was given to 152 patients and phenobarbital to 150.

There were 249 patients who completed a 1-year follow-up; 20 patients moved or died, and 33 withdrew because of side effects or for other reasons (Table 2). Fifty-three percent of those completing the trial were free of seizures at 6–12 months (Table 3). One fourth of the patients remained seizure free for the entire follow-up year. The duration of epilepsy and number of seizures did not influence the outcome of treatment. Adverse effects were more frequent with phenobarbital than with carbamazepine.

It appears that health workers can adequately monitor the treatment of newly identified epileptics in developing countries. Although many patients had several years of seizures before receiving treatment, they generally responded well. The view that epilepsy becomes intractable if not treated at an early stage was not supported.

▶ An excellent study. There was essentially no difference between the results after phenobarbital or carbamazepine therapy. The dosage was roughly (in mil-

TABLE 2.—Reasons for Withdrawal

Reason	Carbamazepine	Phenobarbitone
Migrated from the district	8	5
Alcohol or drug abuse	1	3
Non-compliance or refused further treatment	7	10
Side effects*	8	5
Death†	2	4
Total	26	27

Difference in drop-out rates between the 2 drugs was not significant.
*Skin rash (carbamazepine [CBZ] = 4, phenobarbital [PB] = 1); hyperactivity (PB = 3); worsening of seizures—absence and myoclonus (CBZ = 2), psychosis (CBZ = 1, PB = 1), and aggressive behavior (CBZ = 1).
†Because of snake bite (CBZ = 1), paraquat intoxication (PB = 1), lightning (PB = 1), and unknown (CBZ = 1, PB = 2).
(Courtesy of Feski AT, Kaamushiga J, Sander JWAS, et al: Lancet 337:406–409, 1991.)

TABLE 3.—Seizure Frequency During the Second 6 Months
of Trial

Seizure activity during therapy	CBZ (n = 126)	PB (n = 123)
Seizure free	65 *(52%)*	67 *(54%)*
Decreased frequency*	37 *(29%)*	28 *(23%)*
No change in seizure frequency†	17 *(13%)*	18 *(15%)*
Increased frequency‡	7 *(6%)*	10 *(8%)*

There is no significant difference in effect between the 2 drugs.
*Compared with baseline period, >50% reduction in seizure frequency.
†Compared with baseline period, <50% reduction to <50% increase in frequency.
‡Compared with baseline period, >50% increase in frequency.
(Courtesy of Feski AT, Kaamugisha J, Sander JWAS, et al: *Lancet* 337:406–409, 1991.)

ligrams) 10 to 1, carbamazepine to phenobarbital. The side effects were similar, except for a minor difference in skin rash (more with carbamazepine) and hyperactive behavior (more with phenobarbital).

At any rate, these physicians with a minimum of resources have shown us that nearly 89% of epileptics can enjoy substantial seizure reduction or become seizure free with a simple program.

New (and no doubt more expensive) medications are on the way. Vigabatrin (1,2) sounds like it works and should be on this side of the ocean in a few years. Silver et al. have written a nice summary of the way certain drugs act (3). They differ. Valproate markedly inhibits the genesis of epilepsy in the kindling model, whereas carbamazepine does not despite "exhibiting marked anticonvulsant effects." Phenobarbital had some of both actions. Perhaps the day is not too far off when we can legitimately go back to using more than 1 drug at a time.—R.D. Currier, M.D.

References

1. Browne TR, et al: *Neurology* 41:363, 1991.
2. Ring HA, et al: *J Neurol Neurosurg Psychiatry* 53:1051, 1990.
3. Silver JM, et al: *Ann Neurol* 29:356, 1991.

Chloral Hydrate in Intractable Status Epilepticus

Lampl Y, Eshel Y, Gilad R, Sarova-Pinchas I (Edith Wolfson Med Ctr, Holon; Tel Aviv Univ, Israel)
Ann Emerg Med 19:674–676, 1990   7–8

Chloral hydrate was given intrarectally to 5 patients in status epilepticus who had failed to respond to conventional drugs, including intravenous diazepam and diphenylhydantoin (table). Four patients were taking anticonvulsive medication before admission. A dose of chloral hydrate, 30 mg/kg, was given intrarectally every 2 hours, in all cases starting within an hour of onset of seizures.

Three patients ceased having seizures within 5–7 minutes of the start

Clinical Patient Characteristics

Present Medical Treatment	DPH Level In Blood Serum	Result of Chloral Hydrate Treatment
Diazepam, DPH, phenobarbital, chloral hydrate	19.5	Seizure stopped after seven minutes Recurrent focal seizures after eight, 14, and 21 hours
Diazepam, DPH, sodium valporate, chloral hydrate	21	Seizure stopped after five minutes
Diazepam, DPH, sodium valporate	16	Seizure stopped after five minutes
Diazepam, DPH, phenobarbital chloral hydrate	17.5	Seizure stopped after five minutes
Diazepam, DPH, chloral hydrate	17	Seizure stopped after 12 minutes Recurrent seizure after 18 hours

(Courtesy of Lampl Y, Eshel Y, Gilad R, et al: *Ann Emerg Med* 19:674–676, 1990.)

of chloral hydrate therapy, and no new epileptic activity was seen on the EEG. Three patients regained full consciousness and were discharged after several days. One who had recurrent stroke events died without new seizures developing. One patient did not regain consciousness despite resolution of epileptic activity and died 3 weeks later of a massive temporal lobe hemorrhage. No patient had evidence of severe hypoxemia during status epilepticus. None experienced hemodynamic or respiratory side effects from chloral hydrate.

▶ Everyone dealing with this monstrous emergency room problem seeks another medication that might be of some use. Chloral hydrate looks good. All previous treatments had failed in these 5 patients and chloral hydrate was given as a last resort. All of the seizures stopped almost immediately, although in 2 cases there were recurrences hours later. There was no evidence of severe hypoxemia by blood gas analysis, and no endotracheal intubation was needed. In fact, there were no serious side effects from the medication. The authors point out that chloral hydrate and paraldehyde are closely related, but paraldehyde causes more side effects. It sounds like something to keep in mind for that next emergency room patient with status epilepticus who is unresponsive to everything.

The supplement on status in *Neurology* (1990) is worth reading. There is, as one would expect, no mention of chloral hydrate.—R.D. Currier, M.D.

Post-Ictal Recognition Memory Predicts Laterality of Temporal Lobe Seizure Focus: Comparison With Postoperative Data

Andrewes DG, Puce A, Bladin PF (Austin Hosp, Heidelberg, Vic, Australia; Univ of Melbourne, Vic)
Neuropsychologia 28:957–967, 1990   7–9

Verbal memory may be impaired after left temporal lobectomy, whereas visuospatial memory often is deficient after surgery on the right temporal lobe. Selective memory impairment is less evident preoperatively. Standard memory tests were performed in 15 patients with unilateral temporal lobe epilepsy and in 43 reference persons without known neurologic disease. All of the patients had medically resistant focal seizures.

Preoperative scores for interictal difference failed to predict the side of the seizure focus. Subtracting difference scores across postictal and interictal conditions correctly identified the side of the seizure focus in 7 of 8 patients. Patients with a left-sided focus had a relative decrease in verbal memory, whereas those with a right-sided focus had impaired visuospatial memory.

Interictal performance is not a reliable way of predicting the side of a temporal lobe seizure focus, but comparing interictal with postictal performance is more fruitful. The association between side of the seizure focus and selectively impaired postictal memory performance provides a more direct means of making a neuropsychological diagnosis before surgery for temporal lobe epilepsy.

▶ This useful study defines differences between interictal and postictal memory test results to help localize the side of the temporal lobe focus in patients with temporal lobe epilepsy (TLE). Left hemisphere foci are associated with verbal memory deficits in this measure, whereas right hemisphere foci are associated with visuospatial memory loss. These findings are strengthened by the fact that such a dichotomy is expected on the basis of established clinical results. It is often difficult to localize the side of the epileptic focus in patients with TLE, and this is a welcome addition to the clinical armamentarium.—A.M. Galaburda, M.D.

The following review articles are recommended to the reader:

Ring HA, et al: Vigabatrin: Rational treatment for chronic epilepsy. *J Neurol Neurosurg Psychiatry* 53:1051, 1990.
Silver JM, et al: Antiepileptogenic effects of conventional anticonvulsants in the kindling model of epilepsy. *Ann Neurol* 29:356, 1991.

8 Parkinson's Disease

Parkinsonism Due to a Basal Ganglia Lacunar State: Clinicopathologic Correlation
Murrow RW, Schweiger GD, Kepes JJ, Koller WC (Univ of Kansas, Kansas City)
Neurology 40:897–900, 1990   8–1

Parkinson's disease (PD) can result from a variety of insults to the brain. Some authors have proposed a vascular etiology, but others have disagreed, noting the lack of a single pathologically verified case that also had adequate clinical correlation. A clinical syndrome indistinguishable from PD was identified in which a vascular cause for PD was demonstrated on pathologic examination.

Man, 74, died after a 20-year history of PD. The patient initially had problems with walking and in moving his left leg. The next year he had problems moving his left arm. Several years later, when both sides of the body were slow and rigid, PD was diagnosed. The patient initially had a good response to levodopa therapy, but symptoms gradually progressed. A resting tremor developed at 68 years of age that was severe by age 72. Slow, slurred speech developed, and the patient experienced hallucinations, foot dystonia, and motor fluctuations, all of which compromised levodopa therapy. At 70 years of age, the patient entered a nursing home because he could not care for himself. His medical history was significant for hypertension, which was difficult to control. The patient had a family history of hypertension and possibly Alzheimer's disease. A CT examination of the head performed 16 months before his death revealed "generalized atrophy." On a subsequent interpretation, another neuroradiologist noted diffuse bilateral lucencies in the striatum. One month before his death, his condition deteriorated and PD signs were much worse. The patient contracted pneumonia. Respiratory failure developed, leading to death. Postmortem examination revealed widespread atherosclerosis in the thoracic and abdominal aortas and in the coronary arteries. Pathologists noted severe arteriolar nephrosclerosis indicative of hypertensive vascular disease. Microscopically, small arteries and arterioles throughout the kidneys, adrenals, and brain were markedly hyalinized. The coronal section of the brain showed small infarcts and cystic spaces throughout the external capsule and basal ganglia. Branches of the circle of Willis contained eccentrically located atheromatous plaques. Numerous microscopic lacunes were found throughout the basal ganglia and midbrain, including the substantia nigra. There was no evidence of neuronal death or degeneration in routine sections of the substantia nigra.

This case provides pathologic confirmation of the concept of vascular PD. Accurate diagnosis is critical in studies of drug treatment and possible etiologies. Long-standing severe hypertension or vascular abnormalities of the basal ganglia on CT should be exclusion factors for future investigations.

▶ Is this then the answer to the old argument about whether arteriosclerosis can produce parkinsonism? It looks like it. But I'm sure the controversy won't end with this single case report. Some who will try to pick holes in it haven't been heard from yet. It sounds like the real thing, however. There is no reason why small vascular lesions correctly placed shouldn't interrupt the nigrostriatal pathways. The pathology showed very little involvement of the substantia nigra except for multiple small vascular lesions that might be expected to interrupt the pathways. The clinical picture was much like parkinsonism without the extra signs and symptoms supposedly found with arteriosclerotic parkinsonism. Furthermore, the patient responded to dopamine drugs.— R.D. Currier, M.D.

Twin Studies and the Genetics of Parkinson's Disease—a Reappraisal
Johnson WG, Hodge SE, Duvoisin R (Columbia Univ; New York State Psychiatric Inst, New York; Univ of Medicine and Dentistry of New Jersey, New Brunswick)
Mov Disord 5:187–194, 1990   8–2

Although researchers have long believed that Parkinson's disease (PD) has a hereditary component, 3 recent twin studies failed to find any significant genetic component in the etiology of this disease. Three twin studies were examined to determine whether such a conclusion might not be premature.

Investigators reviewed statistical tests of twin concordance rates and calculated G, the coefficient of genetic determination that is a measure of the contribution of heredity to a multifactorial trait. These questions were considered when evaluating the twin concordance data: (1) Are monozygotic (MZ) twins concordant more often than expected by chance alone? (2) Are MZ twins concordant more often than dizygotic (DZ) twins? Four levels of diagnostic criteria were used. At level 1, only typical PD was included; at level 2, both typical and possible PD were included; at level 3, atypical PD was added; and at level 4, isolated dementia was added.

At the first diagnostic level, concordance among MZ twins was no more frequent than that anticipated by chance; however, at the other 3 levels, the difference was statistically significant at the .01 level or better. When MZ and DZ concordance rates were compared, MZ rates were slightly higher than DZ rates at all 4 diagnostic levels, but the differences were not significant. At all 4 diagnostic levels, the estimate of G was nonzero, but the 95% confidence interval was sufficiently broad that, when using the formula G = 1 (i.e., variation in a trait results entirely from genetic factors) and G = 0 (i.e., variation in a trait results entirely from nondiagnostic factors), neither possibility could be excluded. The one exception was that at the third level, G = 1 was excluded. In other words.

the variation in the trait could be attributable either entirely to nongenetic factors or—except at the third diagnostic level—entirely to genetic factors.

Low MZ concordance rates can be compatible with substantial genetic contributions to the etiology of PD. The very broad 95% confidence limits for G made it impossible for twin-study data to either verify or disprove a substantial genetic component to PD. Furthermore, changing clinical concepts of PD have cast doubt on the assumptions underlying the methodology of the PD twin studies.

▶ This is another paper that made me happy. Studies of the heredity of PD have been more or less negative, and yet you and I once in a while see patients with a history of familial parkinsonism. The authors analyzed the data of previous studies and concluded that there is a good possibility of a substantial genetic contribution to the causation of the disease. One expects that studies of that other common supposedly nongenetic cellular neurodegenerative disease, amyotrophic lateral sclerosis, would produce the same result. Every disease has a genetic component.

In the same issue of *Movement Disorders,* there is a comprehensive analysis of Rett syndrome by FitzGerald et al. (1) that is of interest in that it provides some information on how patients appear when they reach adulthood and the pathologic findings. Have a look.

Also in the same issue are 2 further interesting notes. The first, by Waters et al. (2), found, at autopsy, surviving adrenal tissue but no cellular outgrowth in the caudate of a transplanted Parkinson's patient who died 6 weeks after operation. The second, by Friedman and Ambler (3), found only a reduction of small neurons and fibrillary gliosis in the putamen of a woman who died with senile chorea at 99 years of age with onset at 70 years of age. So, senile chorea exists as a separate entity.—R.D. Currier, M.D.

References

1. FitzGerald PM, et al: *Mov Disord* 5:195, 1990.
2. Waters C, et al: *Mov Disord* 5:248, 1990.
3. Friedman JH, Ambler M: *Mov Disord* 5:251, 1990.

Promotion of Central Cholinergic and Dopaminergic Neuron Differentiation by Brain-Derived Neurotrophic Factor But Not Neurotrophin 3

Knüsel B, Winslow JW, Rosenthal A, Burton LE, Seid DP, Nikolics K, Hefti F (Univ of Southern California; Genetech Inc, South San Francisco, Calif)
Proc Natl Acad Sci 88:961–965, 1991   8–3

Brain-derived neurotrophic factor (BDNF) and neurotrophin 3 (NT-3) and 2 recently cloned molecules closely related to nerve growth factor (NGF). To assess the role of BDNF and NT-3 in the CNS, recombinant human BDNF (rhBDNF) and NT-3 (rhNT-3) produced from human cDNA expressed in human embryonic kidney cells were tested in cultures of dissociated fetal rat brain cells containing basal forebrain cholinergic neurons.

Choline acetyltransferase activity increased significantly in a dose-dependent manner after the addition of rhBDNF to basal forebrain cultures, but not with rhNT-3. The stimulatory action of rhBDNF was similar to NGF, which is well established as a neutrophic factor for these cells. When added to basal forebrain cultures at either 2 days or 9 days in vitro, rhBDNF was particularly effective during early development in vitro, whereas the stimulatory action of NGF was more pronounced later in the development of cultures. Further studies on the selectivity of the rhBDNF-mediated trophic action showed that rhBDNF increased dopamine uptake activity in cultures of ventral mesencephalon containing dopaminergic cells as well as γ-aminobutyrate uptake in basal forebrain cultures, whereas rhNGF appeared to act rather selectively on cholinergic neurons and not on central dopaminergic neurons.

These findings suggest that BDNF stimulates the development of cholinergic neurons, similar to NGF. However, unlike NGF, BDNF exerts its most pronounced action during early development of basal forebrain cholinergic neurons in vitro, and also stimulates the survival of cells other than the cholinergic neurons.

▶ The original studies of the first well-described neurotrophic factor, NGF, have now led to a description of a family of related neurotrophic polypeptides. The most prominent members of this family are now recognized to be BDNF and NT-3. Whereas NGF is well known to enhance the survival, maintenance, and cholinergic function of basal forebrain cholinergic neurons, it has little effect on dopaminergic neurons. Similarly, BDNF was found to enhance cholinergic function. However, BDNF was also found to enhance dopamine uptake in ventral mesencephalic neurons, but NGF and NT-3 had no such effects. If similar effects can be documented in animal models in vivo, the neurotrophic factor BDNF may well represent a trophic molecule of potential relevance to nigrostriatal degeneration in Parkinson's disease.—S.H. Appel, M.D.

Reversal of Experimental Parkinsonism by Lesions of the Subthalamic Nucleus
Bergman H, Wichmann T, DeLong MR (Johns Hopkins Hosp)
Science 249:1436–1438, 1990   8–4

In Parkinson's disease (PD), loss of dopamine results in an increased inhibitory output from the basal ganglia to the thalamus. Increased activity in the subthalamic nucleus (STN) stimulates neurons in the internal part of the globus pallidus, leading in turn to increased inhibition of the thalamus and thalamocortical neurons. The role of excessive output from the STN was examined in monkeys treated with 1-methyl-4-phenyl-1,2,3,6-tetrahydropyridine (MPTP), a model resembling human parkinsonism.

Lesions of the STN lessened all major motor disorders in the contralateral limbs of MPTP-treated monkeys, including akinesia, rigidity, and tremor. Tremor was abolished almost completely. Histologic study several weeks after lesioning confirmed that lesions were confined to the STN.

These findings support a role for excessive STN activity in the development of motor abnormalities in PD. They also suggest a potential role for surgically or pharmacologically inactivating the STN as a treatment for PD, but further knowledge of the long-term effects of STN lesions is needed.

▶ The loss of dopamine in PD appears ultimately to result in increased transmission from the basal ganglia to the thalamus and decreased output from the thalamus to the cortex. The most cogent hypothesis explaining the physiologic events suggests that in PD there is excessive output from the subthalamic nucleus that activates globus pallidus neurons and, in turn, thalamic neurons. The present study documents that monkeys rendered parkinsonian by treatment with MPTP demonstrated improvement in all major motor disturbances after lesions of the subthalamic nucleus. This important physiologic information should pave the way for developing unique approaches to parkinsonism other than through the current dopamine-receptor interactions.—S.H. Appel, M.D.

Effects of Tobacco Smoke Constituents on MPTP-Induced Toxicity and Monoamine Oxidase Activity in the Mouse Brain
Carr LA, Basham JK (Univ of Louisville)
Life Sci 48:1173–1177, 1991   8–5

Epidemiologic studies have suggested an inverse relationship between smoking and Parkinson's disease. Exposure to cigarette smoke reportedly lessens the reduction in striatal dopamine produced by 1-methyl-4-phenyl-1,2,3,6-tetrahydropyridine (MPTP) in mice. Exposure also inhibits monoamine oxidase (MAO) activity in brain tissue. Whether specific constituents of smoke can be identified as causing these effects was investigated.

Mice were treated chronically with nicotine, 5-phenylpyridine, and hydrazine. All 3 compounds prevented the MPTP-induced fall in dopamine metabolites, but dopamine levels did not change significantly. None of the agents inhibited cerebral tissue MAO activity after exposure in vivo. An extract of particulate matter from tobacco smoke, however, markedly inhibited both MAO A and MAO B activities. Unidentified components of tobacco smoke may inhibit the formation of an active neurotoxin through oxidative mechanisms.

▶ The reason for the protective effect of smoking on parkinsonism remains in limbo. This basic science article (for which you can thank the Mosby-Year Book people who send everything under the sun to their editors) points out some interesting facts. Mice were treated with nicotine, 4-phenylpyridine, and hydrazine. None inhibited MAO activity in MPTP-treated mice. However, an extract of tobacco smoke particulate matter caused marked inhibition of MAO A and MAO B activity in vitro. The authors conclude that there is something in tobacco smoke, but not in the above 3 drugs, that inhibits brain MAO and perhaps alters the formation of the active metabolite of MPTP, MPP^+, thus preventing parkinsonism. Something good is coming out of the tobacco research institute after all. Maybe we should all just simply swallow a little tobacco juice every day, that is, without smoking or chewing it. Pass the spittoon.

Neurology published 2 good supplements on parkinsonism recently (1,2) entitled *On Emerging Strategies in Parkinson's Disease* and the *Preclinical Detection of Parkinsonism.* Both are fascinating and worth an hour or 2 of an evening. And my favoriate neurology journal *The Lancet* has 2 neat articles, 1 on the pathophysiology (3) and the other on management of the disease (4). Copies to the residents.—R.D. Currier, M.D.

References

1. *Neurology* (Suppl 3), 1990.
2. *Neurology* (Suppl 2), 1991.
3. Agid Y: *Lancet* 337:1321, 1991.
4. Clough CG: *Lancet* 337:1324, 1991.

9 Neuromuscular Disease

Exacerbation of Isoniazid Induced Peripheral Neuropathy by Pyridoxine
Nisar M, Watkin SW, Bucknall RC, Agnew RAL (Fazakerley Hosp, Liverpool; Broadgreen Hosp, Liverpool, England)
Thorax 45:419–420, 1990   9–1

Isoniazid is commonly used in the treatment of pulmonary tuberculosis. In some patients peripheral neuropathy develops, usually when the drug's half-life is prolonged or higher doses are used. The *British National Formulary* recommends doses of 100–200 mg of pyridoxine in patients with established peripheral neuropathy. At doses of more than 50 mg/day, pyridoxine may contribute to neuropathy.

Man, 51, with rheumatoid arthritis had a 2-month history of dry cough and weight loss. Chest radiographs at admission revealed right upper lobe consolidation with cavitation suggestive of active pulmonary tuberculosis. Therapy with rifampicin, isoniazid, and pyrazinamide was begun. Although the patient improved clinically and radiographically, a classic glove-and-stocking peripheral sensory deficit developed. On the assumption that the neuropathy was caused by isoniazid, chemotherapy was withdrawn and treatment with pyridoxine, 150 mg daily, started. The patient was later confirmed to be a slow acetylator of isoniazid. He continued to deteriorate, and electromyography revealed predominantly sensory axonal peripheral neuropathy consistent with isoniazid neuropathy. Symptomatic deterioration continued until pyridoxine was withdrawn after 10 weeks. Acid-alcohol-fast bacilli were identified in culture as *Mycobacterium kansasii*, sensitive to rifampicin and ethambutol. The patient improved clinically and radiographically with this treatment and slow but appreciable improvement occurred in the peripheral neuropathy.

Pyridoxine may cause peripheral neuropathy. This case illustrates the need for caution in the use of pyridoxine in the prevention and treatment of isoniazid-induced peripheral neuropathy. The lower dose of 10 mg/day, recommended as prophylaxis against isoniazid-induced neuropathy, should not cause peripheral neuropathy, and may be recommended.

▶ This is another instance of pyridoxine being harmful to patients with peripheral neuropathy. If you have wondered where the idea originated that neuropathy should be treated with pyridoxine, the authors note that the *British National Formulary* recommends it at a dose of 10 mg as prophylaxis for patients taking isoniazid, and at a dose of 100–200 mg daily for the treatment of established peripheral neuropathy. The authors hope that their formulary will reconsider its recommendation. We note that moderate doses of pyridoxine (100–200 mg/ day) are still being used in the treatment of undiagnosed neuropathy in the United States. The vitamin is easily available in "health" food stores. One wonders if our Food and Drug Administration ought not to look into the labeling of this particular vitamin.—R.D. Currier, M.D.

Blood Thiamine and Thiamine Phosphate Concentrations in Excessive Drinkers With or Without Peripheral Neuropathy
Poupon RE, Gervaise G, Riant P, Houin G, Tillement JP (INSERM, Villejuif, France; Centre Hosp Gén Louis Doumergue, Martinique; Hôp Intercommunal, Creteil; CHU Purpan, Toulouse, France)
Alcohol Alcoholism 25:605–611, 1990   9–2

Several syndromes ascribed to thiamine deficiency, including peripheral neuropathy and Wernicke-Korsakoff encephalopathy, are associated with excessive alcohol consumption in industrialized countries. Widely varying estimates are given for the prevalence of subclinical thiamine deficiency in alcoholics. Apart from insufficient dietary intake, intestinal malabsorption and a toxic effect of alcohol could dispose to thiamine deficiency in heavy drinkers.

Blood levels of free thiamine and thiamine phosphate were estimated in 251 patients seen at an alcoholic-oriented medicine service or an ophthalmic department. Daily alcohol intake did not relate to the presence of neuropathy in excessive drinkers, but those with neuropathy had taken excessive alcohol for a longer time. Although free thiamine levels did not differ significantly, thiamine phosphate levels were significantly lower in excessive drinkers than in controls. Liver enzymes were elevated in some drinkers regardless of whether or not neuropathy was present.

The minor thiamine phosphate deficiency present in excessive drinkers could reflect reduced availability of free thiamine or, more likely, defective phosphorylation at the hepatic level. Thiamine deficiency probably does not have a determining role in the development of peripheral neuropathy in this setting.

▶ The authors studied thiamine levels in alcoholics with peripheral neuropathy by direct analysis and found no thiamine deficiency except for a mild decrease of thiamine phosphate, probably the result of liver disease. Several questions come to mind: What about the Wernicke-Korsakoff syndrome? If thiamine deficiency is not the cause of alcoholic peripheral neuropathy, is it the alcohol itself, or something else?

Further on the possibility of alcohol as a toxin, Tözün et al. (1) have courageously given alcohol to persons recovering from hepatitis A, B, or C. A mean of 26 grams of alcohol daily made no difference in liver function tests or recovery as compared to a control hepatitis group not given alcohol. These authors believe that previous reports of alcoholic relapse of hepatitis may have included some persons with earlier and heavier alcohol consumption.—R.D. Currier, M.D.

Reference

1. Tözün N, et al: *Lancet* 337:1079, 1991.

Polyneuropathy Syndromes Associated With Serum Antibodies to Sulfatide and Myelin-Associated Glycoprotein

Pestronk A, Li F, Griffin J, Feldman EL, Cornblath D, Trotter J, Zhu S, Yee WC, Phillips D, Peeples DM, Winslow B (Washington Univ; John Hopkins School of Medicine; Univ of Michigan)
Neurology 41:357–362, 1991   9–3

Antimyelin-associated glycoprotein (MAG) antibodies in patients with demyelinating sensorimotor neuropathy syndromes are cross-reactive with compounds that contain sulfate-3-glucuronate epitopes, which include myelin components. To determine which sensory neuropathy syndromes are associated with serum antibody reactivity to the glycolipid sulfatide, an enzyme-linked immunosorbent assay (ELISA) was used to test sera from 64 patients with peripheral nerve disorders and prominent sensory involvement. Also tested were 35 normal individuals and blood bank donors, 21 patients with chronic inflammatory polyneuropathies, and 20 patients with amyotrophic lateral sclerosis. The ELISA used purified glycolipids and glycoproteins as antigens. High-performance thin-layer chromatography and Western blotting were done to test the specificity of the results.

In 12 patients with sensorimotor polyneuropathies with physiologic evidence of demyelination, high titers of IgM antibodies directed against MAG were seen. Another 8 patients, most of whom had predominantly sensory neuropathies, had high titers of antibody reactivity to sulfatide but not of IgM to MAG. An associated IgM paraprotein was present in 2 of these patients. Physiologic tests showed no predominantly demyelinating features in any patients with selective serum antisulfatide activity.

In patients with chronic demyelinating sensorimotor neuropathies, high ELISA titers of antibodies to MAG may be more common than was previously suspected. High serum titers of antisulfatide antibodies may give clues to the pathogenesis of idiopathic, axonal, predominantly sensory neuropathies. Clinical trials are necessary to test this conclusion.

▶ In an ideal sense, detection of different antibodies would set apart distinct diseases, indicate pathogenesis, and point toward the appropriate treatment. Although anti-MAG antibodies have been linked to demyelinating neuropathies, anti-GM_1 to neuropathy with multifocal conduction blocks and lower motor neuron syndromes and, now, antisulfatide antibodies to sensory neuropathies, such correlations remain imperfect. Eleven of 18 patients in this study with antisulfatide antibodies also had anti-MAG antibodies. Among the 7 patients with isolated antisulfatide antibody, only 3 had a pure sensory neuropathy.—S.H. Subramony, M.D.

Phenotypic Heterogeneity of Spinal Muscular Atrophy Mapping to Chromosome 5q11.2-13.3 (SMA 5q)

Munsat TL, Skerry L, Korf B, Pober, B, Schapira Y, Gascon GG, Al-Rajeh SM, Dubowitz V, Davies K, Brzustowicz LM, Penchaszadeh GK, Gilliam TC (Tufts-New England Med Ctr; Children's Hosp Med Ctr, Boston; Hadassah Hosp, Jerusalem; King Faisal Specialist Hosp and Research Ctr, Riyadh, Saudi Arabia; Hammersmith Hosp, London; et al)
Neurology 40:1831–1836, 1990   9–4

Both the chronic and acute forms of spinal muscular atrophy apparently map to the q11.2-13.3 region of chromosome 5 (SMA 5q). The phenotypic features of 14 SMA 5q families and of 2 other families not clearly mapping to this region were analyzed. In most families it was possible to discern linkage to DNA markers on chromosome 5q.

Mutations at the 5q locus had a broad range of clinical abnormalities. Tongue fasciculations were present in most patients with early-onset disease. About one fourth of the patients (especially those with a later onset) had trunk and limb fasciculations. Common findings also included areflexia and prominent polyminimyoclonus. In the single family that clearly lacked linkage with 5q, disease began relatively late and there were early deaths.

The severity of SMA 5q correlates closely with the age at onset, and an early onset is associated with early death. There are exceptions, however. Phenotypic variation in SMA 5q ranges from acute disease leading to death within the first months of life to a late-onset indolent disorder causing only modest functional impairment. It remains uncertain whether a significant minority of true SMA results from nonallelic mutations (as in neurofibromatosis and polycystic kidney disease).

▶ The number of different genes that could give rise to the clinical syndrome of spinal muscular atrophy is an extremely important concern currently being addressed by several laboratories. This paper by Munsat et al. provides important new information that most of the lower motoneuron syndromes that usually develop in childhood may map to a relatively limited region on chromosome 5. Thus whether the disease occurs before 6 months of age and proceeds rapidly to death by 4 years or the onset is after age 6 months and a more benign course follows, mapping is still to the chromosome 5q11.2-13.3 region. Clinical heterogeneity may well depend on modifying factors or the variable involvement of the gene as described in the clinical variants of the Duchenne locus on the X chromosome. A definition of the specific gene and the gene product involved in the spinal muscular atrophies should have a major impact on motoneuron biology as well as on therapy. This paper is an important step in this process.—S.H. Appel, M.D.

Type 1 Neurofibromatosis Gene: Identification of a Large Transcript Disrupted in Three NF1 Patients

Wallace MR, Marchuk DA, Andersen LB, Letcher R, Odeh HM, Saulino AM, Fountain JW, Brereton A, Nicholson J, Mitchell AL, Brownstein BH, Collins FS
(Univ of Michigan; Washington Univ)
Science 249:181–186, 1990   9–5

von Recklinghausen neurofibromatosis (NF1) is a common autosomal dominant disorder characterized by abnormalities in multiple tissues emanating from the neural crest. An inability to identify a reliable cellular phenotype marker has made it difficult to identify the gene. Earlier studies mapped the NF1 gene to chromosome 17q11.2. Subsequent cloning efforts, focused on the region between the breakpoints, determined that there is more than 1 gene in the interval. Researchers used chromosome jumping and yeast artificial chromosome technology to identify a large, ubiquitously expressed and highly conserved gene, NF1LT, that is definitely interrupted by 1—and probably both—translocutions, contains the previous candidate genes within it, and is altered in a new mutation NF1 patient. This most likely represents the true NF1 gene.

To survey the pattern of expression of NF1LT in different normal and pathologic tissues, the RNA polymerase chain reaction with primers from the translated region was used to analyze a number of tissues. The NF1LT gene was expressed in many human tissues, including those providing signals on Northern RNA blots, immortalized B lymphoblasts (both NF1 and non-NF1), NF1 skin fibroblasts, spleen, lung, muscle, thymoma, neuroblastoma, an NF1 neurofibrosarcoma cell line, a colon carcinoma cell line, and breast cancer. Other experiments detected expression in other tissues, suggesting that NF1LT is widely expressed.

Previously identified candidate genes that failed to show abnormalities in NF1 patients are apparently found within introns of NF1LT, on the antisense strand. A new mutation patient with NF1 was identified by a de novo .5-kb insertion in the NF1LT gene.

These findings, together with the high spontaneous mutation rate of NF1, which is indicative of a large locus, suggest that NF1LT is representative of the NF1 gene. Homozygous loss of NF1LT expression might lead to increased expression of EV12 and NF1-c2. These gene products might ultimately be responsible for some NF1 phenotypic features; however, it is more likely that NF1LT alterations alone lead to the NF1 phenotype.

▶ Advances in molecular genetics have begun to yield important payoffs in our understanding of the genetic defects in neurologic disease. Several years ago the gene for Duchenne muscular dystrophy was discovered and the protein product dystrophin identified. This present paper is a landmark contribution by Collins et al. to reverse genetics, i.e., discovery of the gene without knowledge of the abnormal protein. Neurofibromatosis (NF) is a relatively common autosomal dominant disorder with abnormalities in multiple tissues. The key to recognition of the NF gene was the identification of mutations in NF patients, in whom the mutation rate is known to be high. Now the challenge is to determine what the function of the gene might be. Most investigators believe that the normal NF gene probably plays a role in restraining cell growth and thus may be involved in growths other than those occurring in von Recklinghausen's disease. If the gene really is a tumor suppressor gene, the variable manifestations of the disease may be explained: Some patients have only a few tumors, whereas others are covered with them. One third of these patients have major problems such as malignant tumors, seizures, and sometimes severe disfigurement. Two thirds of NF patients can lead relatively normal lives. Further understanding of the function of the NF gene not only will shed light on the pathogenesis of the disease, but also should offer important insights into carcinogenesis in man.— S.H. Appel, M.D.

Flunarizine Protects Neurons From Death After Axotomy or NGF Deprivation
Rich KM, Hollowell JP (Washington Univ)
Science 248:1419–1421, 1990   9–6

Exogenous nerve growth factor (NGF) can prevent neuronal death after axotomy of dorsal root ganglion neurons in the newborn or adult rat, but the mechanism is not clear. The ability of the calcium channel blocker flunarizine to prevent neuronal death after withdrawal of trophic support was examined in vitro and in vivo in neonatal rats. Experimentally, flunarizine had a cerebral protective effect in ischemic-hypoxic rats.

Flunarizine at a concentration of 30–40 µM prevented the death of embryonic sensory and sympathetic neurons after the abrupt withdrawal of NGF in cell culture. Control neurons consistently died within 72 hours of NGF deprivation. In studies of sciatic nerve axotomy in neonatal rats, flunarizine treatment resulted in a loss of 71% fewer than treatment without flunarizine. The protective effect of flunarizine did not appear to be related to decreased protein synthesis.

Flunarizine may protect against neuronal death by an action at an intracellular site, apart from its effect in blocking voltage-dependent calcium channels. This type of drug may have clinical value.

▶ It is well known that neurotrophic factors such as NGF are important for neuronal survival during development and possibly for neuronal maintenance thereafter. The specific mechanism by which NGF withdrawal results in cell death is becoming increasingly clear. Recent data (1,2) suggest that trophic factor withdrawal results in the synthesis of specific proteins leading to neuronal death. The present paper suggests another important mechanism whereby the entry of calcium into the cell, possibly through L-type calcium channels, may contribute to the process of cell death. These observations are of great interest, because they suggest that cell death after neurotrophic factor deprivation, or even after axotomy, may be prevented by calcium channel blockers. If similar mechanisms are operative in neurodegenerative disease, the present findings would be of great importance. As the authors point out, "Such pharmacologic agents have promise in future clinical approaches." I couldn't agree more.—S.H. Appel, M.D.

References

1. Oppenheim RW, Prevette DM: *Soc Neurosci Abstr* 14:368, 1988.
2. Martin DP, et al: *J Cell Biol* 106:829, 1988.

Control of Embryonic Motoneuron Survival In Vivo by Ciliary Neurotrophic Factor
Oppenheim RW, Prevette D, Qin-Wei Y, Collins F, MacDonald J (Bowman Gray School of Medicine, Wake Forest Univ; Synergen, Inc, Boulder, Colo)
Science 251:1616–1618, 1991   9–7

With the neurotrophic hypothesis, it is believed that survival of only a proportion of neurons during normal development is regulated by the limited availability of neurotrophic agents. Ciliary neurotrophic factor (CNTF) is a putative neurotrophic agent that promotes the survival of ciliary, sensory, and sympathetic neurons in vitro. To test the role of CNTF in neuronal survival in vivo, purified human recombinant CNTF was administered daily at various doses to chick embryos in ovo from embryonic day 6 (E6) to E9 and E9 to E14, which is a period of naturally occurring ciliary neuronal death.

Daily treatment of chick embryos in vivo with CNTF had no significant effect on the survival of sensory, sympathetic, nodose, or sympathetic preganglionic neurons from E6 to E9 and E9 to E14, compared with control embryos. In fact, CNTF at high concentrations appeared to reduce survival. However, CNTF did promote the in vivo survival of spinal motoneurons in a dose-response relationship. The number of pyknotic motoneurons in the lumbar spinal cord on E8, the peak time of cell death, was significantly reduced by CNTR, indicating that CNTF prevented the degeneration of cells.

These findings suggest that CNTF may not act as a neurotrophic agent in vivo for those embryonic neurons, particularly the ciliary neurons, on which it acts in vitro. However, CNTF may be involved in regulating the in vivo survival of motoneurons.

▶ The demonstration of neurotrophic activity in tissue culture is only the first step in documenting the potential efficacy of the trophic factor in enhancing neuron survival. With respect to motoneurons only, cholinergic development factor (CDF) has been documented to work in vitro and in vivo. Now a second neurotrophic factor, CNTF, known to influence motoneurons as well as ciliary, sensory, and sympathetic neurons in vitro, has been tested in an in vivo chick embryo system. Surprisingly, no effect was noted on sensory or sympathetic neurons in vivo even though definite effects have been documented in vitro. However, spinal motoneurons were noted to survive in a dose-dependent fashion, which suggests that CNTF may act as a neurotrophic agent regulating the survival of motoneurons. Thus, at least from a theoretical point of view, CDF as well as CNTF may be of value in motoneuron diseases in man.—S.H. Appel, M.D.

Manganese, Selenium and Other Trace Elements in Spinal Cord, Liver and Bone in Motor Neurone Disease
Mitchell JD, East BW, Harris IA, Pentland B (Royal Preston Hosp, Preston; Scottish Universities Research and Reactor Ctr, Glasgow; Astley Ainslie Hosp, Edinburgh)
Eur Neurol 31:7–11, 1991   9–8

Trace elements long have been linked with neurologic disorders, including motor system degeneration, but few studies of essential and nonessential trace elements have been carried out and many of these have involved only small numbers of patients and controls. Trace element levels were measured by neutron activation analysis in specimens of spinal cord, liver, and bone from 15 patients dying of motor neuron disease (MND) and 7 dying of non-neurologic disorders.

Cord manganese levels were significantly increased in MND cases, but the liver manganese concentration was significantly reduced in this group. Spinal cord selenium was significantly increased in MND cases at the cervical level only. The study patients also had increased selenium levels in liver and bone. There were no significant group differences in mangesium, chromium, iron, cobalt, zinc, rubiditum, cesium, or antimony.

Spinal cord levels of selenium and manganese are increased in MND, possibly reflecting abnormal free radical activity. High selenium levels may be a protective response to an environmental factor underlying MND, or may potentiate the adverse effects of a causative substance.

▶ This study of MND from Scotland shows clearly that the selenium level was significantly elevated in the patients with MND, not just in the CNS but also in the more tenacious liver and bone. The authors nicely review the possible causes for such a condition and point the way for further research. As they indicate, if manganese can cause parkinsonism, why wouldn't selenium cause MND? They don't mention the work history of their patients.—R.D. Currier, M.D.

Clinical Features and Associations of 560 Cases of Motor Neuron Disease
Li T-M, Alberman E, Swash M (Royal London Hosp, London)
J Neurol Neurosurg Psychiatry 53:1043–1045, 1990   9–9

Data were reviewed on 560 patients with motor neuron disease diagnosed at 3 centers between 1965 and 1984. The mean age at onset of disease was 56 years, and the mean duration of illness was 2½ years.

Most patients initially complained of muscle weakness. The upper limbs were first affected in 44% of the patients, the lower limbs in 37%, and the bulbar muscles in 19%. A bulbar presentation was relatively frequent in older women. Dysarthria was a feature in half of the patients and dysphagia in 41%. Only 2.5% of patients had sensory abnormalities. Nearly 40% had surgery previously, although not appreciably more than a control group had. Smoking habits also were similar in the patient and control groups, and there were no unusual occupational associations. More patients than controls had never drunk alcohol.

▶ This negative retrospective study is interesting because it tends to quiet some of the excitement about previously reported associations.

The authors don't mention how many of their patients had familial motor neuron disease, a point of importance because of the recent finding of the 21st chromosomal locus of the familial type of amyotrophic lateral sclerosis (ALS) by Siddique et al. (1). Our own twin study (2) tended to show that the twin with ALS was more likely to have a history of influenza and to be the more physically active of the pair. It is hoped that future prospective studies will ask specific questions to check our findings.— R.D. Currier, M.D.

References

1. Siddique T, et al: *N Engl J Med* 324:1381, 1991.
2. Currier RD, Conwill DE: In Rose & Norris (eds): *Amyotrophic Lateral Sclerosis.* London, Smith-Gordon-Nishimura, 1990, pp 23–28.

Lymphoma, Motor Neuron Diseases, and Amyotrophic Lateral Sclerosis
Younger DS, Rowland LP, Latov N, Hays AP, Lange DJ, Sherman W, Inghirami G, Pesce MA, Knowles DM, Powers J, Miller JR, Fetell MR, Lovelace RE (Columbia-Presbyterian Med Ctr, New York)
Ann Neurol 29:78–86, 1991   9–10

The syndrome of motor neuron disease (MND) in patients with lymphoma was first reported in 1963. Since that time, 23 additional patients with this syndrome have been described. The cause of the syndrome is still unknown.

Nine patients were studied, and several new observations were made. Motor neuron syndromes were associated with either Hodgkin's disease or non-Hodgkin's lymphoma. The syndromes were not limited to lower motor neuron disorders. Eight patients had definite or probable upper motor neuron signs as well, qualifying for the diagnosis of amyotrophic lateral sclerosis. In 2 postmortem examinations, corticospinal tracts were seen to be affected. The combination of MND and lymphoma was frequently associated with paraproteinemia, increased CSF protein content, and CSF oligoclonal bands. In 2 cases asymptomatic non-Hodgkin's lymphoma was discovered only because the finding of paraproteinemia prompted a bone marrow examination. Some patients with both upper and lower motor neuron signs had physiologic signs of conduction block in peripheral nerves or autopsy abnormalities in peripheral nerves.

Lymphoma and MND may have a common cause, possibly a retroviral infection. The frequency of paraproteinemia seen in patients with both lymphoma and MND suggests that an immunologic disorder may also have a role in the pathogenesis of the neurologic disorder.

▶ The understanding of this peculiar type of amyotrophic lateral sclerosis is becoming clearer. The authors suggest that if your patient has a high CSF protein content, evaluation for a lymphoma would be worthwhile.—R.D. Currier, M.D.

A Mutation in the tRNA$^{Leu(UUR)}$ Gene Associated With the MELAS Subgroup of Mitochondrial Encephalomyopathies

Goto Y, Nonaka I, Horai S (Natl Inst of Neuroscience, Tokyo; Hokkaido Univ School of Medicine, Sapporo; Natl Inst of Genetics, Shizuoka, Japan)
Nature 348:651–653, 1990   9–11

The acronym MELAS denotes a subgroup of mitochondrial myopathy associated with encephalopathy, lactic acidosis, and strokelike episodes. Other groups are myoclonus epilepsy associated with ragged-red fibers (MERRF), related to a transition mutation at the mitochondrial transfer (RNA^{Lys}) gene; and chronic progressive external ophthalmoplegia (CPEO), associated with large deletions of mitochondrial DNA.

An A-to-G transition mutation was identified at nucleotide pair 3,243 in the dihydrouridine loop of mitochondrial tRNA$^{Leu(UUR)}$, which is specific to patients having MELAS. The mutation creates an *Apa*I restriction site, permitting a simple molecular diagnostic test for the disease. The mutation was found in 26 of 31 patients with independent MELAS and in 1 of 29 patients with CPEO. It was absent in 5 patients with MERRF and 50 controls. Southern blot studies confirmed that the mutant DNA invariably coexists with wild-type DNA (heteroplasmy).

It remains unclear how abnormalities of tRNAs lead to defects in respiratory-chain enzymes and produce functional and morphological changes in mitochondria. Nuclear factors conceivably could also contribute to the pathogenesis of mitochondrial disorders.

▶ Mitochondrial encephalomyopathies are often not diagnosed early in the course of disease because weakness may not be a prominent symptom or sign. When strokelike episodes, nausea, and vomiting associated with lactic acidosis or cognitive deterioration are present in young individuals, examination of a muscle biopsy specimen can be of significant value in calling attention to a maternally inherited mitochondrial defect. Now this study by Goto et al. describes a diagnostic test that can define the specific mutation. It should help to shed light on the way in which the metabolic defect results in the clinical picture.—S.H. Appel, M.D.

Prednisone in Duchenne Dystrophy: A Randomized, Controlled Trial Defining the Time Course and Dose Response
Griggs RC, Moxley RT III, Mendell JR, Fenichel GM, Brooke MH, Pestronk A, Miller JP, and the Clinical Investigation of Duchenne Dystrophy Group (Univ of Rochester, NY; Vanderbilt Univ; Washington Univ; Ohio State Univ; Walter C McKenzie Ctr for Health Sciences, Edmonton, Alta)
Arch Neurol 48:383–388, 1991   9–12

The only treatment shown to alter the course of Duchenne muscular dystrophy is prednisone at a dosage of .75 or 1.5 mg/kg/day. A study was done to define the time course of improvement and the dose response to treatment in 99 boys aged 5 to 15 years.

Thirty-two patients received placebo, 33 received prednisone at a dose of .3 mg/kg, and 34 received prednisone at a dose of .75 mg/kg/day for 6 months. Manual muscle and myometry testing, timed functional testing, and laboratory measurements were done at 10 days and after 1, 2, 3, and

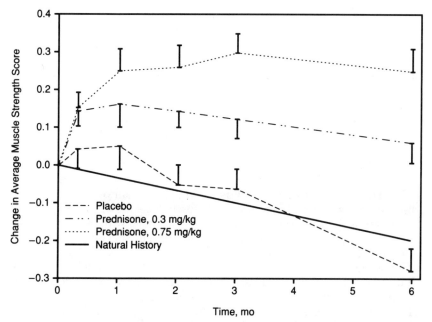

Fig 9–1.—Change (mean ± SEM) in the score for average muscle strength in the placebo and prednisone groups after the initiation of their regimens. *Dashed line* indicates placebo; *dashed-dotted* line indicates prednisone, .3 mg/kg; *dotted line* indicates prednisone, .75 mg/kg. *Solid line* ("natural history") represents the values for change observed in 177 patients with Duchenne dystrophy who received no treatment. (Courtesy of Griggs RC, Moxley RT III, Mendell JR, et al: *Arch Neurol* 48:383–388, 1991.)

6 months of treatment. Side effects were also assessed through examination of the patients and interviews with the parents.

Beginning at 10 days after the start of therapy, boys in the 2 prednisone-treated groups had higher average muscle strength scores than boys given placebo. A dose response was indicated by the significantly greater strength of boys in the higher-dose group compared with boys in the lower-dose group at 3 months (Fig 9–1). However, patients given the higher dose experienced significant side effects by 6 months, including weight gain, cushingoid appearance, and excessive weight gain. Patients given the lower dose had only weight gain. No side effects were seen at 10 days or 1 month despite the improvements in muscle strength and function.

In boys with Duchenne dystrophy, prednisone produces a rapid increase in muscle strength and function. Strength gain is maximal at a dose of .75 mg/kg or less. Treatment may have to be reduced or ceased in some patients because of side effects.

▶ In this follow-up study, the occurrence of improvement very early during the treatment tends to exclude the possible role of unblinding of the observers as a result of prenisone-induced side effects. The minimum dose required appears to be between .3 and .75 mg/kg, because the previous study did not document differences between doses of .75 mg/kg and 1.5 mg/kg. Prednisone's mechanism of action is unknown, but it may be related to its immunosuppressant action.— S.H. Subramony, M.D.

Hyperkalemic Periodic Paralysis and the Adult Muscle Sodium Channel α-Subunit Gene
Fontaine B, Khurana TS, Hoffman EP, Bruns GAP, Haines JL, Trofatter JA, Hanson MP, Rich J, McFarlane H, Yasek DM, Romano D, Gusella JF, Brown RH Jr (Massachusetts Gen Hosp, Charlestown, Mass; Harvard Med School; The Children's Hosp, Boston)
Science 250:1000–1002, 1990   9–13

Hyperkalemic periodic paralysis (HYPP) is an autosomal dominant disorder characterized by episodes of muscle weakness as a result of depolarization of the muscle cell membrane associated with an increased serum level of potassium. Electrophysiologic studies suggest a role for the adult muscle sodium channel in HYPP.

Using the rat sodium model, 2 regions of the human adult muscle sodium channel α-subunit, Na2 and Na3, were amplified by the polymerase chain reaction with normal adult human skeletal muscle single-stranded cDNA as the template. The plasmids h-Na2 and h-Na3 were cloned and sequenced, and were localized by somatic cell hybrids to the long arm of chromosome 17. Restriction fragment length polymorphism (RFLP) analysis showed a single Bgl II RFLP that was mapped near the human growth hormone locus on chromosome 17.

In a large pedigree affected by HYPP with myotonia, these 2 loci showed tight linkage to the genetic defect with no recombinants detected. These data suggest that the sodium channel α-subunit gene contains the HYPP mutation.

▶ Electrophysiologic studies have suggested that slow inactivation of the voltage-gated sodium channel may explain the abnormalities noted in HYPP. Since the α-subunit of the adult muscle sodium channel has been cloned, it was possible to test for genetic linkage between HYPP and the locus for the α-subunit. In a large pedigree affected by the clinical variant of HYPP that expresses myotonia, tight linkage to the genetic defect was documented with no recombinants detected. Thus the genetic data support the fact that abnormalities in the sodium channel α-subunit gene may be responsible for this variant of HYPP.— S.H. Appel, M.D.

10 Multiple Sclerosis

Multiple Sclerosis Among United Kingdom-Born Children of Immigrants From the Indian Subcontinent, Africa, and West Indies
Elian M, Nightingale S, Dean G (Oldchurch Hosp, Romford; Queen Elizabeth Hosp, Birmingham, England)
J Neurol Neurosurg Psychiatry 53:906–911, 1990   10–1

Multiple sclerosis (MS) is uncommon in Asia, Africa, and West Indies, as well as the ethnic Asian and African immigrants in England, suggesting that these immigrants maintain their low risk for MS when they migrate to high prevalence areas. To determine whether the British-born children of these immigrants have the same low risk for MS developing, the point prevalence of probable or possible MS among British-born children of Asian, African, and West Indian immigrants was determined using birthplace data of their parents obtained from the 1971 census.

In the age groups available for study, British-born children of Asian, West Indian, and African immigrants showed a high prevalence of MS on an order similar to the age and specific prevalence rates from the study in the London borough of Sutton. There were 26 observed patients with probable MS among British-born West Indians compared with the expected number of 34.74 patients in the Sutton study. Among British-born Asians there were 12 observed patients with MS compared with the expected number of 10.95 patients in the Sutton study. The calculated standard prevalence ratio for British-born West Indians in greater London and the West Midlands was .75 and for Asians, 1.10. Multiple sclerosis in British-born West Indians took a particularly severe course, and MS in British-born Asians had an unusually early onset.

This study found that British-born children of Asian, African, and West Indian immigrants have a high prevalence of MS in contrast to the very low MS risk of their immigrant parents. These data suggest that place of birth and residence in early life may be of great importance in the development of MS.

▶ This study shows that when one moves to places with a high prevalence of MS, one's hereditary background is not very protective. What is it in the new environment that sets off this disease?

Miller et al. (1), who studied MS in Australia and New Zealand, found a marked variation between the northern part of Australia and the southernmost point of New Zealand—a variation of 7 times between the 2 and conclude that it is the environment that does it—a mystery that has been going on for my practice lifetime.

Dean and Gray in the same journal have studied the risk of multiple sclerosis in nurses and doctors and find out that it is no higher than the general population, to my surprise.— R.D. Currier, M.D.

References

1. Miller DH, et al: *J Neurol Neurosurg Psychiatry* 53:903, 1990.
2. Dean G, Gray R: *J Neurol Neurosurg Psychiatry* 53:899, 1990.

Cauda Equina Syndrome After Continuous Spinal Anesthesia
Rigler ML, Drasner K, Krejcie TC, Yelich SJ, Scholnick FT, DeFontes J, Bohner D (Univ of California, San Francisco; Northwestern Univ; Suburban Gen Hosp, Norristown, Pa; Kaiser Permanente, Orange City, Calif)
Anesth Analg 72:275–281, 1991   10–2

There are no clear guidelines for safely administering local anesthetics via an indwelling subarachnoid catheter. Four patients from 3 centers had a persistent neurologic deficit after continuous spinal anesthesia.

Man, 68, scheduled for transurethral prostatic resection, had a 22-gauge spinal needle placed at L3–L4 while seated. A 28-gauge catheter was advanced 3 cm into the subarachnoid space and, with the patient supine, 150 mg of 5% lidocaine with 7.5% glucose was injected over 15 minutes. Another 25 mg of lidocaine with .25 mg of morphine was injected an hour later. A left S1–S4 radiculopathy was present the next day and improved only slightly. Computed tomography was not helpful. After 7 months the patient had no spontaneous bowel movements and had to strain to urinate. Numbness was present in the penis, left testicle, anus, and left posterior thigh and buttock.

All 4 patients remained hemodynamically stable, and there was no evidence of localized ischemia. A direct neurotoxic effect of local anesthetic is a possible cause of cauda equina syndrome in these cases. A relatively high dose of anesthetic and maldistribution may be factors. The catheter should be inserted just far enough into the subarachnoid space to maintain placement and the lowest effective dose of anesthetic should be used after a test dose.

▶ Having a long-held prejudice that spinal anesthetics might be a factor in the causation of multiple sclerosis (MS) and of worsening in established MS, I was interested to see that the cauda equina syndrome can be induced after spinal anesthesia. Previous studies of tens of thousands of patients after spinal anesthesia have not shown such an association and thus weakened my belief and caused hedging on advice to MS patients to stay away from spinal and dental local anesthesia. Years ago the dental anesthesia connection with MS was strengthened when Wallace Tourtellotte explained that it represents an injection of a possibly injurious substance in or near one of the most highly myelinated nerves in the body, the trigeminal nerve, which itself is connected directly through a very short stem to a part of the CNS commonly involved in the lesions of MS, the pons. Neither of these possibilities has been proven by me or anyone else. They are difficult to prove, but I hope that some of you in the future will consider these as ideas for clinical and laboratory research. Can MS be produced in the experimental animal by repeated exposure to local anesthesia?—R.D. Currier, M.D.

Autoreactive T Lymphocytes in Multiple Sclerosis Determined by Antigen-Induced Secretion of Interferon-γ
Olsson T, Wei Zhi W, Höjeberg B, Kostulas V, Yu-Ping J, Anderson G, Ekre H-P, Link H (Huddinge Univ Hosp, Huddinge; Karolinska Inst, Huddinge; Kabi Biopharma, Stockholm)
J Clin Invest 86:981–985, 1990   10–3

An autoimmune pathogenesis has been proposed for multiple sclerosis (MS), but there have been no conclusive data on the number of T cells autoreactive with myelin antigens in MS patients compared with controls. Because T cells may secrete interferon-gamma (IFN-γ) in response to a presented antigen, it is possible to estimate the number of T cells reactive with different myelin antigens by applying an immunospot assay. Mononuclear cells from the peripheral blood and CSF were examined in 39 untreated patients with clinically definite MS. Sixteen patients had acute aseptic meningitis and 25 had tension headache.

On average, T cells reactive with myelin basic protein (MBP), 2 different MBP peptides, and proteolipid protein were about 7- to 10-fold more common in the peripheral blood of MS patients than in those with aseptic meningitis or tension headache. In the CSF, the MBP reactive T cells were about 30-fold more common in MS CSF mononuclear cells than in patients with meningitis or headache. In MS patients the frequency of MBP reactive T cells was about 70-fold higher in the CSF than in the peripheral blood.

This study demonstrates that T cells reactive with MBP are increased in the peripheral blood and strongly enriched in CSF of patients with MS. The use of peptide antigens to detect autoreactive T cells may allow definition of immunodominant T cell epitopes in individual MS patients for development of specific immunotherapy.

▶ I venture into research papers that I only partially understand with real fear, but it looks as though this does provide a missing link in MS research. The T cells both in blood and spinal fluid do react with myelin autoantigens in MS. This has been difficult to prove until now. What else is going on in MS basic research?

Workers in Amsterdam (1) have shown that if you eliminate the macrophage before the clinical signs of experimental allergic encelphalomyelitis (EAE) appear, the EAE is markedly suppressed. In my innocence, I did not know that the macrophage played an active role in production of the disease, but I see in a leaflet of the National MS Society macrophages apparently busy chewing up myelin.

And workers at Yale (2) have found that treating the recipient mouse with antibodies that neutralize lymphotoxin and tumor necrosis factor prevents the transfer of EAE.

Losy et al. (3) note that human IgG, the antigens of which have been something of mystery, can be subclassified into 4 subtypes. Those most commonly found in MS, IgG_1 and IgG_3, are those usually reported in patients with chronic viral infections and autoimmune diseases.

And from Finland (4) comes a report of antibody levels in twins, showing that when comparing the affected and unaffected twin, 3 viral antibodies are found more often in the MS patient—those to the measles, mumps, and the Epstein-Barr viruses.

Finally, from London and Yugoslavia (5) is a note that the oligoclonal IgG from tears in MS patients is not abnormal, as was found previously. That is satisfying, because it was hard to understand previous reports of abnormal IgG in tears. But perhaps we haven't heard the end of it.—R.D. Currier, M.D.

References

1. Huitinga I, et al: *J Exp Med* 172:1025, 1990.
2. Ruddle NH, et al: *J Exp Med* 172:1193, 1990.
3. Losy J, et al: *Acta Neurol Scand* 82:4, 1990.
4. Kinunnen E, et al: *Arch Neurol* 47:743, 1990.
5. Mavra M, et al: *Neurology* 40:1259, 1990.

Occurrence of MRI Abnormalities in Patients With Isolated Optic Neuritis
Städt D, Kappos L, Rohrbach E, Heun R, Ratzka M (Univ of Würzburg, Germany)
Eur Neurol 30:305–309, 1990   10–4

Optic neuritis is a manifestation of a number of diseases, but it occurs most frequently in patients with multiple sclerosis (MS). Because the diagnosis of MS depends on both dissemination in space and time, 24 patients with clinically isolated optic neuritis were examined with MRI to determine whether this procedure may detect other cerebral lesions as evidence for dissemination in space in defining the risk for and perhaps the diagnosis of MS. The median age of the patients was 26 years.

All patients had pathologic visual evoked potentials (VEP) of the affected eye; 4 patients also had pathologic VEP of the contralateral eye. Only 5 patients (21%) had a normal MRI scan. The other 19 patients (79%) had clinically silent lesions detected on MRI. The number of lesions ranged from none to 38 (median, 2) and were located predominantly in the frontal and parietal white matter. All patients with more than 2 lesions on MRI had pathologic CSF findings. The number and locations of lesions did not correlate with age at onset of optic neuritis.

These data suggest that isolated optic neuritis does not really exist as a clinical entity because of the rather high rate of clinically silent lesions detected on cerebral MRI. Further studies are warranted to define the predictive value of MRI in isolated optic neuritis.

▶ Is MS, then, always multifocal in origin? It has been commonly said that about half of the patients with optic neuritis will progress to MS. Does it follow that some optic neuritis is benign and will never lead to MS? It would be helpful if the authors could follow their group for 20 more years and give us another report. Other questions are raised by such a finding. Should one say that these patients have MS? If so, should the patient be told that he has MS? Because immune suppressive treatments are now coming on line for MS, should treatment be started at this early stage? Questions, questions.—R.D. Currier, M.D.

Breakdown of the Blood-Brain Barrier Precedes Symptoms and Other MRI Signs of New Lesions in Multiple Sclerosis: Pathogenetic and Clinical Implications

Kermode AG, Thompson AJ, Tofts P, MacManus DG, Kendall BE, Kingsley DPE, Moseley IF, Rudge P, McDonald WI (Inst of Neurology, London; Natl Hosp for Nervous Diseases, London)

Brain 113:1477–1489, 1990   10–5

The use of MRI has facilitated the study of acute lesions in patients with multiple sclerosis (MS). A consistent finding in new lesions in relapsing/remitting and secondary progressive MS is gadolinium-DTPA (Gd-DTPA) enhancement, signifying breakdown of the blood-brain barrier. How early the blood-brain barrier breakdown occurs was investigated.

From an extensive serial MRI study in MS patients, researchers identified 4 cases in which disruption of the blood-brain barrier, as detected by Gd-DTPA enhancement, preceded other MRI abnormalities. All 4 patients were studied during an acute relapse. The group included 3 men and 1 woman aged 25–54 years.

Serial scans of 3 patients showed that blood-brain barrier breakdown can precede the appearance of new lesions on T2-weighted MRI. In a patient in the relapsing/remitting phase, blood-brain barrier breakdown preceded clinical expression of the new lesion. In the 3 patients with relapsing/progressive MS, there was a clear discrepancy between MRI abnormalities and clinical symptoms.

Inflammation appears to occur very early in the evolution of a new lesion. This finding is in agreement with the growing evidence that inflammation is possibly the primary event in the development of new white matter changes in MSI. Lesions observed on MRI may be associated with clinical deficit in some instances. Similarly, substantial functional deterioration may occur in the absence of relevant new lesions observed on MRI. Such disparity is to be expected given the early occurrence of inflammation.

▶ Well, some have long said that MS involves the breakdown of the blood-brain barrier, and these workers, using MRI scanning of early lesions, have shown it. One wonders whether a severe demyelinating syndrome such as Schilder's disease (1) is caused by a marked change in the immune response of

the individual, or by a difference in blood-brain barrier breakdown characteristics—or are they one and the same?—R.D. Currier, M.D.

Reference

1. Eblen F, et al: *Neurology* 41:589, 1991.

Effect of Low Saturated Fat Diet in Early and Late Cases of Multiple Scle-rosis
Swank RL, Dugan BB (Oregon Health Sciences Univ, Portland)
Lancet 336:37–39, 1990   10–6

In 1950 researchers suggested that the frequency of multiple sclerosis
(MS) was related to fat consumption. Accordingly, 144 MS patients were
put on a low-fat diet. The effects of the 34-year consumption of low-fat
diets in relation to severity of MS were evaluated.

Neurologic status was graded on a 7-point scale and neurologic disability categorized as minimum, moderate, or severe. Patients eliminated
butter fats and hydrogenated oils, and saturated animal fats were limited
to 15 g/day. Five grams of cod liver oil and 10–40 g/day of vegetable oils
were added. Coconut and palm oils were not permitted. The daily diet
included 60–90 g of protein from fish, seafood, white meat of chicken,
and turkey cooked without skin, as well as skimmed milk, small amounts
of lean meat, 1 egg a day, vegetables, cereals, and nuts. Results in those
who followed the diet were compared with those who did not.

Patients who followed the diet had significantly less deterioration and
much lower death rates than did those who consumed more than 20 g of
fat per day. This was true regardless of the initial neurologic classification of disability; however, those who had minimum disability at the
beginning of the trial had the greatest benefit. At the end of the trial,
good dieters with an initial neurologic grade of 1 had a mean neurologic grade of 1.9, whereas poor dieters with the same initial neurologic
grade had a mean neurologic grade of 5.3. One good dieter with initial minimal disability died of MS or its complications, as did 4 poor
dieters.

When the diet was begun before the patients' normal activities became
restricted, about 95% of MS patients remained only mildly disabled for
approximately 30 years. Even those good dieters with moderate and severe disabilities initially had significantly less deterioration and lower
death rates, however.

▶ Over the years, I have recommended a low-fat diet to many MS patients, so
I was glad to see this. An accompanying editorial correctly points out that the
control group, which consists of those who did not follow the diet, may well be
those who did not respond to it. Perhaps they had exacerbations while on the
diet and then eliminated themselves from the treatment group. Those who
stayed on the diet may be those who did not have exacerbations. If this is true,

the value of the study is negated. Does this mean that the low–saturated-fat diet therapy for MS will have to be tested again over another 35 years?

In the meantime, I can't see that it will do harm. Certainly, one would expect it to increase longevity in MS patients (and in all of us) simply by decreasing the effects of fat on the vascular system, so I for one am going to continue to recommend it, albeit as an unproven therapy.— R.D. Currier, M.D.

Efficacy and Toxicity of Cyclosporine in Chronic Progressive Multiple Sclerosis: A Randomized, Double-Blinded, Placebo-Controlled Clinical Trial
Wolinsky JS, for the Multiple Sclerosis Study Group (Univ of Texas, Houston)
Ann Neurol 27:591–605, 1990   10–7

Cyclosporine A is a cyclic undecapeptide with potent immunosuppressive activity exhibited by a relatively selective inhibitory effect on the helper population of T lymphocytes. The efficacy and safety of cyclosporine in the treatment of chronic progressive multiple sclerosis (MS) were evaluated in a double-blind, placebo-controlled, 2-year, multicenter parallel study involving 547 patients. These patients had clinically definite MS, mild to moderately severe neurologic disability as evidenced by an entry score of between 3 and 7 on the Expanded Disability Status Scale (EDSS), and a progressive course defined by an increase in the EDSS of between 1 and 3 grades in the year before entry. The cyclosporine dosage was adjusted for toxicity, and a median trough whole-blood level was maintained between 310 and 430 ng/mL.

In all, 273 patients received cyclosporine and 274, placebo; the 2 groups were similar in age, gender, duration of illness, and neurologic disability. Only 56% of those given cyclosporine and 68% of those given placebo completed the 2-year study. More placebo-treated patients were withdrawn prematurely from the study because of treatment failure. Upon completion of or withdrawal from the study, cyclosporine-treated patients had a mean deterioration in neurologic function, as measured by the EDSS, of .39, compared with an EDSS of .65 in their placebo-treated counterparts.

Of the 3 primary efficacy criteria, cyclosporine delayed the time to become wheelchair bound (Fig 10–1), but significant differences were not observed for time to sustained progression or on a composite score of activities of daily living. Mean physician and patient global assessments of improvement favored cyclosporine. Multivariate analysis showed substantial effects of baseline neurologic disability on the outcome. Most common adverse effects were nephrotoxicity and hypertension, which accounted for most of patient withdrawal in the cyclosporine arm of the study.

These data show that continuous oral therapy with cyclosporine is associated with a significant but clinically modest delay of progression of disability in patients with moderately severe and progressive multiple sclerosis. Adverse effects of cyclosporine are common, particularly

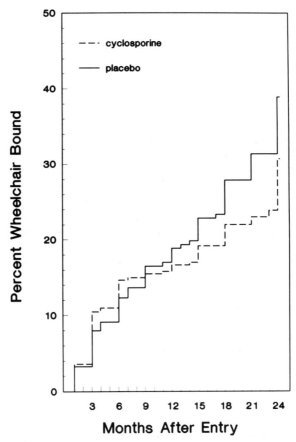

Fig 10–1.—The probability of becoming wheelchair bound is displayed as the cumulative percentage of all patients at risk who have reached this end point over time. Wheelchair bound status was defined as reaching an extended disability status scale (EDSS) score of 7 or an Ambulation Index rating of 7. Of the 547 evaluable patients, 248 cyclosporine- and 250 placebo-randomized patients were at risk from entry to reach this milestone. Of these, only 13 cyclosporine-treated and 6 placebo-treated patients who were prematurely withdrawn from this study failed to reach this milestone. The survival curves differ at the *P* level of .038. (Courtesy of Wolinsky JS, for the Multiple Sclerosis Study Group: *Ann Neurol* 1990; 27:591–605.)

nephrotoxicity, and may temper consideration of its use to treat this disease.

▶ Cyclosporine held great hope for the treatment of MS, but the results have been disappointing. Apparently, it is partially effective, delaying the time to become wheelchair bound but otherwise is not useful. Forty-four percent of the cyclosporine-treated patients in this placebo-controlled, double-blind study withdrew from treatment, usually because of nephrotoxity and hypertension. It appears we must look elsewhere for safe and effective treatment.

Hoogstraaten and Minderhoud in Groningen (1) found that ACTH produced a short-term improvement in MS, but the benefit was gone 6 months later. In the ACTH group, the side effects were greater and the relapse rate higher, although that did not reach significance. As one who has used ACTH for 35 years in various ways to treat MS, I can only agree. It too does not seem to be the answer.

A Swiss group (2) compared cyclosporine with azathioprine in a 12-month study and found the azathioprine-treated patients had not improved, but the cyclosporine-treated group showed mild improvement. This is not too surprising, because azathioprine takes 2–3 years to become effective.

There is an interesting note by Birk et al. (3) on the clinical course of MS during and after pregnancy, which is contrary to some of the recent comments that pregnancy does not seem to increase the overall exacerbation rate. Six of 8 women studied prospectively had a relapse within 7 weeks after delivery. Why?—R.D. Currier, M.D.

References

1. Hoogstraaten MC, Minderhoud JM: *Acta Neurol Scand* 82:74, 1990.
2. Steck, et al: *Eur Neurol* 30:224, 1990.
3. Birk K, et al: *Arch Neurol* 47:738, 1990.

A Placebo-Controlled, Double-Blind, Randomized, Two-Center, Pilot Trial of Cop 1 in Chronic Progressive Multiple Sclerosis
Bornstein MB, Miller A, Slagle S, Weitzman M, Drexler E, Keilson M, Spada V, Weiss W, Appel S, Rolak L, Harati Y, Brown S, Arnon R, Jacobsohn I, Teitelbaum D, Sela M (Albert Einstein College of Medicine, Bronx; Baylor College of Medicine, Houston; Weizmann Inst of Science, Rehovot, Israel; Maimonides Med Ctr, Brooklyn)
Neurology 41:533–539, 1991   10–8

Cop 1 is one of a series of basic copolymers of L-alanine, L-glutamic acid, L-lysine, and L-tyrosine. It is immunologically cross-reactive with myelin basic protein at the cellular level. Cop 1 has suppressed experimental allergic encephalomyelitis in rabbits, mice, and nonhuman primates without producing toxicity.

Patients with definite multiple sclerosis (MS) and evidence of a chronic-progressive course for 18 months or longer participated in the trial. They had experienced no more than 2 exacerbations in the preceding 2 years. The age range was 20–60 years. The 106 patients were evaluated using the Kurtzke Expanded Disability Scale.

After 9 months, placebo recipients exhibited more progression than did patients given Cop 1 (Fig 10–2). Significant progression was recorded in 18% of treated patients and 25% of placebo recipients. The overall survival curves did not differ significantly. The risk of progression after 2 years was significant at 1 center but not at the other. Transient vasomotor responses were more frequent in treated patients.

This study failed to demonstrate significant arrest or reversal of MS by Cop 1 treatment. A pilot finding of more definite benefit in exacerbating-

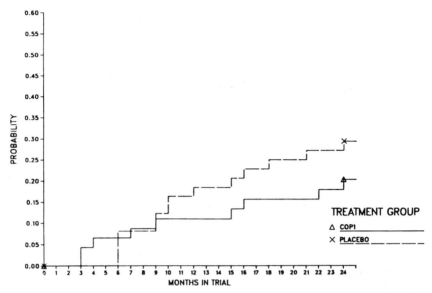

Fig 10–2.—Curve demonstrates the probability of progressing at each time point along the 24-month continuum. Confirmed progression is defined as an increase in EDSS of 1 or 1.5 units maintained for an additional 3 months. Includes patients from both centers. (Courtesy of Bornstein MB, Miller A, Slagle S, et al: *Neurology* 41:533–539, 1991.)

remitting cases suggests that treatment be considered early in the course of disease.

▶ This stuff looks good, at least fairly good, in patients with chronic progressive MS. If something works on them, the chances are it really does work. Why the drug showed benefit at 1 center and not at the other is curious. I suppose studies will have to be continued. Another problem is that Cop 1 is given in 2 daily injections and must be kept frozen.

Recently, reports have been published on the treatment of MS with cyclophosphamide, levamisole, azathioprine, and hyperbaric oxygen. There is something imperfect about all of them. Joining in, we recently completed a small study of low-dose oral methotrexate, which was reported at the ANA meeting in Seattle in 1991. A note on the suppressive effect of bromocriptine on the immune system of rats led to a look in the Clinical Trials compendium of the National MS Society (April 1991) to see if anyone is using it in the treatment of MS. Yes, those energetic fellows up in London, Ontario, are—their study finishes late next year. And now comes a letter from Paul Richter pointing out that the elevated prolactin level after delivery could have something to do with the frequent worsening of MS post partum. He has started bromocriptine treatment in some of his patients who have chronic progressive MS.

Hang on, folks, happier days are coming in the treatment of this brain-mangling disease.—R.D. Currier, M.D.

Reference

1. Riskind PN, et al: *Ann Neurol* 29:542, 1991.

11 Infections of the Nervous System

Frequency of Adverse Reactions to Influenza Vaccine in the Elderly: A Randomized, Placebo-Controlled Trial
Margolis KL, Nichol KL, Poland GA, Pluhar RE (Hennepin County Med Ctr, Minneapolis; Veterans Affairs Med Ctr, Minneapolis; Mayo Clinic and Found, Rochester, Minn)
JAMA 264:1139–1141, 1990   11–1

Concern about adverse effects is a major deterrent to patient compliance with influenza vaccination. However, there is little information about the occurrence of side effects in the population targeted for immunization. A randomized, double-blind, crossover trial was done to compare the frequency of side effects after administration between 1988 and 1989 of trivalent split-antigen influenza vaccine with those of saline placebo in 336 outpatient veterans aged 65 years or older. The participants were randomly assigned to receive vaccine followed by placebo injection 2 weeks later or placebo followed by vaccination 2 weeks later.

Similar proportions of patients in the 2 groups reported disability or systemic symptoms, including fever, cough, coryza, fatigue, malaise, myalgia, headache, nausea, sore arms, and disability. Influenza vaccine produced no increase in systemic adverse effects or disability in the elderly. Symptoms attributed by patients to a recent influenza vaccination are probably the result of a coincidental illness coupled with heightened somatic awareness after the injection. These findings should help physicians and other health professionals to address patient concerns about side effects associated with influenza vaccination.

▶ This solves a problem in dealing with those to whom you have just recommended a flu vaccination. The placebo and the modern flu vaccination were nearly identical with regard to reported symptoms except for a sore arm found in 20% of the flu vaccinees and 5% of the placebo vaccinees. The chances of "any symptoms" occurring was 27.7% in the flu group and 23% in the placebo group, an insignificant difference. There might have been some uncovering of the double-blind component because of the common occurrence of sore arm with the flu vaccination.—R.D. Currier, M.D.

Rapid Diagnosis of Herpes Simplex Encephalitis by Nested Polymerase Chain Reaction Assay of Cerebrospinal Fluid

Aurelius E, Johansson B, Sköldenberg B, Staland Å, Forsgren M (Central Microbiological Lab, Stockholm; Karolinska Inst, Danderyd Hosp, Sweden)

Lancet 337:189–192, 1991   11–2

Early and specific detection of herpes simplex virus encephalitis or demonstration of viral antigen previously necessitated invasive and potentially risky brain biopsy. The polymerase chain reaction (PCR) technique with nested primers has made amplification of virus-specific target DNA sequences possible with increased specificity and sensitivity.

The assay was applied to 151 CSF samples obtained from 43 patients with herpes simplex encephalitis and compared to 87 CSF samples obtained from 60 patients with acute febrile focal encephalopathy. The PCR procedure detected herpes simplex virus (HSV) DNA in 42 of 43 patients with proven herpes simplex encephalitis. The method was negative in 1 patient treated with acyclovir within 20 hours of onset of symptoms. The 87 control samples and all contamination controls were PCR negative. The PCR results remained positive in samples drawn up to 27 days after onset of neurologic symptoms.

The PCR technique may be difficult to master, but its reproducibility is high. It may be useful to include a weak positive sample in each run and to analyze duplicate samples. The specificity and sensitivity of the PCR assay are enhanced through the nested approach. This is a rapid, noninvasive diagnostic method for herpes simplex encephalitis.

▶ Diagnostic testing for herpes simplex encephalitis using the PCR in this series seems to be 100% correct unless the patient had previously received acyclovir. So, get the CSF specimen before treatment begins. There is a fine accompanying editorial in the same issue of *The Lancet* (1), which predicts that "specific PCR methods should lead to accurate diagnosis of the 60–70% of cases of acute encephalitis of presumed viral origin." How long before this test becomes available in the United States?—R.D. Currier, M.D.

Reference

1. Editorial: *Lancet* 337:205, 1991.

Pre-Mortem Diagnosis of Creutzfeldt-Jakob Disease by Detection of Abnormal Cerebrospinal Fluid Proteins

Blisard KS, Davis LE, Harrington MG, Lovell JK, Kornfeld M, Berger ML (VA Med Ctr, Albuquerque; Natl Inst of Mental Health, Bethesda, Md; Univ of New Mexico, Albuquerque)

J Neurol Sci 99:75–81, 1990   11–3

The triad of rapid progressive dementia, startle myoclonus, and periodic EEG complexes for the diagnosis of Creutzfeldt-Jakob disease (CJD) occurs only in 62% of patients and may develop relatively late in the course of disease. Prompted by previous reports of the presence of abnormal proteins in the CSF of patients with CJD, protein separation by 2-dimensional electrophoresis and detection by silver staining was performed premortem on CSF specimens obtained from 2 patients with progressive dementia. The initial diagnosis of CJD was confirmed on autopsy.

The 2 patients, aged 61 and 66 years, had progressive dementia. Findings on brain biopsy, performed in the early course of the disease, were not characteristic of CJD in 1 patient and were normal in the second. Spinal fluid analysis with 2-dimensional electrophoresis and silver staining confirmed the presence of 2 abnormal proteins, numbers 130 and 131, with relative molecular masses of 26,000 and 29,000 daltons, respectively, and isoelectric points of 5.2 and 5.1, respectively. In both patients, autopsy confirmed the diagnosis of CJD.

These 2 abnormal CSF proteins have been reported previously in patients with CJD, although their presence in the CSF is not specific for CJD. The detection of these 2 proteins appears to be a valuable adjunct in the evaluation of patients with unexplained progressive dementia.

▶ This technique, I hope, will hold up and become useful. Certainly, at the present time it is a difficult diagnosis, especially in the early stages.

For a method of eliminating the virus from formalin-fixed tissues in the neuropathology laboratory see the note by Brown et al. (1). To be safe, include a formic acid step.

And see a nice concise editorial in *The Lancet* (2) on prion disease—spongiform encephalopathies. It notes that with the broadening of the neuropathologic spectrum, the number of cases diagnosed annually in the United Kingdom could be as many as 9,000! Copy to the residents.—R.D. Currier, M.D.

References

1. Brown P, et al: *Neurology* 40:887, 1990.
2. Editorial: *Lancet* 336:21, 1990.

Spontaneous Neurodegeneration in Transgenic Mice With Mutant Prion Protein

Hsiao KK, Scott M, Foster D, Growth DF, DeArmond SJ, Prusiner SB (Univ of California, San Francisco)
Science 250:1587–1590, 1990   11–4

Gerstmann-Sträussler-Scheinker syndrome (GSS) is a rare neurodegenerative disorder that is vertically transmitted as an autosomal dominant trait. It has been transmitted horizontally to primates and rodents through intracerebral inoculation of brain homogenate. Ataxia and dementia develop in the third to seventh decades of life, and death occurs within 10 years. The protease-resistant isoform of prion protein (PrP) is implicated in the pathogenesis and transmission of GSS, as well as scrapie, a similar disease affecting animals.

A leucine substitution at codon 102 of the human PrP gene, on the short arm of chromosome 20, is linked genetically with GSS. Transgenic mice were created to assess genetic linkage between GSS and this substitution in mice. Neurologic disease developed spontaneously in mice expressing PrP with the leucine substitution, and spongiform degeneration and gliosis were observed resembling what is seen in mouse scrapie. Disease appeared at a mean age of 166 days. It is hoped that studies of neurodegeneration in these mice will help to elucidate the pathogenesis of more common genetic and sporadic CNS disorders such as Huntington's disease and Alzheimer's disease.

▶ The role of prions as proteinacious transmissible agents responsible for spongiform encephalopathies in man has reached a new level of significance with this publication. Skeptics were always concerned that agents copurifying with prions and contaminating preparations were responsible for infectivity. The fact that spongiform degeneration can develop in transgenic mice with a single AA substitution of the human PrP gene should quiet the critics and provide support for one of the most innovative concepts in human neurobiology that is possibly applicable to a range of neurodegenerative diseases.—S.H. Appel, M.D.

Nationwide Survey of HTLV-I–Associated Myelopathy in Japan: Association With Blood Transfusion
Osame M, Janssen R, Kubota H, Nishitani H, Igata A, Nagataki S, Mori M, Goto I, Shimabukuro H, Khabbaz R, Kaplan J (Kagoshima Univ; Ctrs for Disease Control, Atlanta; Utano Natl Hosp, Kyoto; Nagasaki Univ; Nagasaki-Chuo Natl Hosp; et al)
Ann Neurol 28:50–56, 1990   11–5

Tropical spastic paraparesis (TSP) is associated with human T cell lymphotropic virus type I (HTLV-I). A similar HTLV-1–associated spastic paraparesis reported in Japan has been termed HTLV-I–associated myelopathy (HAM). The latter disease and HTLV-1–associated TSP are now thought to be the same disorder (HAM/TSP). The relationship between HAM/TSP and transmission by blood transfusion is not clear. Two surveys were conducted to study the epidemiology of HAM/TSP in Japan.

Between October 1986 and March 1989, there were 589 cases of definite HAM and 121 cases of probable HAM reported. Most of the patients (69%) with definite HAM lived in areas having the highest prevalence of HTLV-I. To determine the role of blood transfusion in the pathogenesis of HAM, a case-control study was performed in the Kagoshima district (Fig 11–1).

The frequency of a history of blood transfusion among patients with HAM in the Kagoshima district (20%) was significantly higher than the frequency of blood transfusion among residents responding to a random

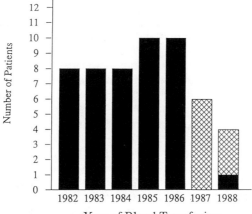

Year of Blood Transfusion

Fig 11-1.—Number of patients reported with transfusion-associated HTLV-I-associated myelopathy (HAM) by year of blood transfusion, 1982–1988, Japan. *Filled bars* represent patients reported to the surveillance system (observed); *cross-hatched bars* represent expected patients with transfusion-associated HAM had blood donors not been screened for HTLV-I. (Courtesy of Osame M, Janssen R, Kubota H, et al: *Ann Neurol* 28:50–56, 1990.)

health survey (3%) or among hospitalized neurologic patients (5%). Cumulative percentages of the intervals between blood transfusion and onset of symptoms of HAM fit a log normal curve, suggesting transfusion as an important common exposure.

After the screening of blood donors began in 1986, the number of patients with transfusion-associated HAM decreased significantly. The number of patients with no history of blood transfusion remained relatively stable. The median latent period between blood transfusion and disease onset was 3.3 years.

▶ This study throws some light on the mystery of how this disease is transmitted. Those with the myelopathy were more likely to have had blood transfusion. Starting in 1986, donors have been screened, and the number of cases has decreased. It can't be the whole answer, however; the drop in cases has been only 16%.

What else is new in infectious disease? Halperin et al. (1) report on the peripheral nervous system manifestations of Lyme neuroborreliosis. Most patients had some type of peripheral abnormality. The authors reason there must be widespread axonal damage because the pattern of electrophysiologic abnormalities was the same in all; reversible abnormalities of distal conductions were common, and demyelinating neuropathy was rare.

Gustafson et al. from Sweden (2) report that antibodies to Lyme borreliosis are found, for the most part, in persons living in Liso, an area south of Stockholm, as are antibodies to tickborne encephalitis. A further study by Holmgren and Forsgren (3) confirms that the tickborne encephalitis is concentrated in the islands around the coastline areas of the Baltic and Lake Malar near Stockholm. They are trying to decide whether vaccination for encephalitis is to be recommended.

Workers from Würzburg, Germany (4), in an interesting retrospective study of the outcome in untreated acute monophasic neuroborreliosis from old records, found no significant difference compared to the follow-up of 66 patients recently treated. They believe that this may support the notion that the neurologic manifestations of Lyme disease are of an allergic nature, more easily treated with prednisone than with antibiotics. Nevertheless, they recommend that it be treated with high-dose intravenous antibiotics because there is no way to predict who will have a chronic course.

English workers (5) studied more than 1,000 patients with acute shingles and found definite seasonal variation, with the peak occurring in the summer and the fewest cases in the spring. They conclude that shingles is not contagious, and that reexposure to the virus of chickenpox is not the cause. The highest incidence of chickenpox in England and Wales is in the spring and summer, rather than in the summer and fall as is found with shingles. They also could find no evidence that patients who attended the physiotherapy department for other reasons were likely to contract shingles from infected patients also being treated there.

Finally, Collinge et al. from London (6) report a case of Gerstmann-Sträussler-Scheinker syndrome studied with prion protein gene analysis. Neuropathologically, there was no spongiform encephalopathy, which raises the question of possible transmission of the disease from the brain that ultimately does not show the classic pathologic picture.— R.D. Currier, M.D.

References

1. Halperin J, et al: *Brain* 113:1207, 1990.
2. Gustafson R, et al: *Scand J Infect Dis* 22:297, 1990.
3. Holmgren EB, Forsgren M: *Scand J Infect Dis* 22:287, 1990.
4. Krüger H, et al: *Acta Neurol Scand* 82:59, 1990.
5. Glynn C, et al: *J R Soc Med* 83:617, 1990.
6. Collinge J, et al: *Lancet* 336:7, 1990.

12 Other Things of Interest

The Aetiology of Transient Global Amnesia: A Case-Control Study of 114 Cases With Prospective Follow-Up
Hodges JR, Warlow CP (Oxford Univ; Western Gen Hosp, Edinburgh)
Brain 113:639–657, 1990   12–1

Although transient global amnesia (TGA) is a well-recognized syndrome, its etiology remains unknown. The most widely held theory is that TGA is caused by thromboembolic cerebrovascular disease; however, evidence is conflicting. The prevalence of various putative risk factors was determined in a TGA population and the findings compared with control populations drawn from the community and those with transient ischemic attacks (TIAs).

In all, 114 cases were collected by 2 methods: 51 cases (designated the retrospective group) were taken from the files; 63 cases comprised the prospective group and were considered potential cases of TGA. Prospective cases were interviewed for demographic data; details of attacks, including duration, potential precipitating factors, and accompanying neurologic features; medical history; smoking and alcohol consumption histories; and family history. All patients underwent a standard clinical examination including evaluation for vascular disease. If possible, patients were investigated after attacks by blood count, fasting blood lipids and glucose, ECG, chest radiogram, EEG, and CT scan of the head. Prospectively ascertained patients were reviewed 6 months after the attack and followed by questionnaire at 6-month intervals thereafter. Retrospective cases were reviewed by 6-month questionnaire. There were 109 community-based controls and 212 controls who had experienced transient ischemic attacks (TIAs).

Eighty-five percent of TGA cases were seen after a single attack. The mean duration of amnesia was 4.2 hours. There was no evidence of an increased risk of TGA associated with any conventional risk factors for cerebrovascular disease. However, migraine headache was significantly more common in TGA patients than in either control group. Actuarial life-table analysis found that the prognosis of TGA patients was significantly better than that of TIA controls. Seven percent of TGA cases became epileptic, generally within 1 year of presentation with TGA.

In most cases there is no thromboembolic etiology for TGA. There is reason to link migraine and TGA causally and, in a few cases, epilepsy may mimic TGA. In the remaining cases, the cause of TGA cannot yet be determined.

▶ This contribution may be a landmark in the understanding of this fascinating problem. As have previous smaller studies, this confirms the lack of association of TGA with the conventional risk factors for cerebrovascular disease. Migraine was more common in the TGA group and epilepsy developed in a minority within 1 year of the first episode.

If TGA is not thromboembolic in origin, what is it? The connection of migraine or an equivalent in the middle-aged and elderly is supported by a short report by Stillhard et al. (1) from Zurich, who performed single-photon emission CT scanning on a 71-year-old woman who had a history of migraine since adolescence and episodes of TGA in the preceding 9 years. During an episode, severe bitemporal hypoperfusion was seen that cleared as memory improved. Is TGA a migraine equivalent in the elderly that, for some reason, affects the temporal lobes bilaterally and is painless?—R.D. Currier, M.D.

Reference

1. Stillhard G, et al: *J Neurol Neurosurg Psychiatry* 52:339, 1990.

Syndromes of Transient Amnesia: Towards a Classification. A Study of 153 Cases
Hodges JR, Warlow CP (Radcliffe Infirmary, Oxford, England; Western Gen Hosp, Edinburgh)
J Neurol Neurosurg Psychiatry 53:834–843, 1990   12–2

Transient global amnesia (TGA), a heterogenous clinical syndrome of unknown etiology, may be caused by cerebrovascular disease, but epilepsy and migraine have also been proposed as causes of the syndrome. Studies were made in 153 patients who had acute transient amnesia, 114 of whom fulfilled proposed strict diagnostic criteria for TGA. The 2 groups of patients, TGA and non-TGA, were compared for demographic data, clinical details, and prognosis.

Seven characteristics are required for definite TGA. The attacks must be witnessed by a capable observer; there must be clear-cut anterograde amnesia during the attack; loss of personal identity must be absent; there should be no accompanying focal neurologic symptoms during the attack and no significant neurologic signs afterward; epileptic features must be absent; the attacks must resolve within 24 hours; and patients must not have had a recent head injury or active epilepsy. The 2 groups did not differ significantly in age, prevalence of migraine, alcohol intake, vascular risk factors, or in the behavior manifestations observed during the attack. Two TGA patients had a family history of the syndrome.

The outcome differed significantly for the 2 groups. Patients with TGA had a .6% annual rate of major vascular events, compared with 7.7% in non-TGA patients (Fig 12–1). There were 2 deaths in the TGA group,

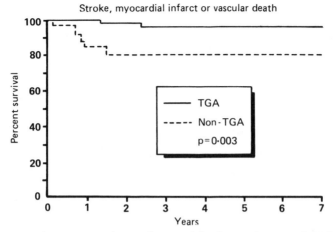

Fig 12–1.—Kaplan-Meier survival curves for survival free from stroke, myocardial infarction, or sudden death (excluding nonvascular deaths) comparing the TGA and non-TGA cases. (Courtesy of Hodges JR, Warlow CP: *J Neurol Neurosurg Psychiatry* 53:834–843, 1990.)

both attributable to nonvascular causes, whereas 4 of 5 deaths in the non-TGA group resulted from vascular causes. The mortality rate in the non-TGA group, standardized for length of follow-up, was about 9 times that in the TGA group.

Fourteen patients became overtly epileptic during the study, 8 in the definite TGA group and 6 in the non-TGA group. The development of epilepsy was associated with the number of previous transient amnesia attacks at presentation. Whereas 50% of TGA patients whose attack lasted for less than 1 hour became epileptic, only 2.9% of patients with longer attacks were similarly affected. The duration of the attack was a better predictor than multiplicity. The recurrence rate of amnesia was low in both groups, excluding cases with subsequent epilepsy.

Findings suggest that there are several distinct causes of transient amnesia, and patients experiencing pure TGA attacks have a good prognosis. Patients experiencing probable epileptic amnesia, attacks of less than 1 hour or rapidly recurrent attacks, and probable transient ischemic amnesia or additional focal neurologic deficits during the attack have a more guarded prognosis and require further investigation.

▶ Not all TGA is benign. However, the subgroup fulfilling the diagnostic criteria did have a benign prognosis, whereas the smaller group who did not have "pure" TGA had a prognosis similar to that associated with vascular disease and epilepsy.

Hodges and Oxbury (1) found that patients tested 6 months after attacks of TGA were defective in verbal memory and facial and famous event recognition, indicating persistent hippocampal diencephalic dysfunction. They couldn't say whether the deficit antedated or was a result of the TGA. It's still a mystery.— R.D. Currier, M.D.

Reference

1. Hodges JR, Oxbury SM: *J Clin Exp Neuropsychology* 12:904, 1990.

Effects of Anesthesia on Superior Brain Functions in Elderly Subjects

Forster A, Altenburger H, Gamulin Z (Hôp Cantonal Universitaire, Geneva, Switzerland)
Presse Med 19:1577–1581, 1990   12–3

Postoperative cognitive impairment is often attributed to general anesthesia, whereas local/regional anesthesia (LRA) is thought to have no effect on CNA function. The effects of GA and LRA on superior brain function were compared among patients older than age 60 undergoing identical surgical procedures.

Of 64 patients undergoing elective operations of the lower limbs, 32 (median age, 72 years) were randomly allocated to undergo general anesthesia and 32 (median age, 74 years) to undergo LRA. Among the patients who had LRA, 8 received epidural anesthesia, 16 were given continuous spinal anesthesia, and 8 had simple spinal anesthesia. The groups were matched for gender, anesthetic risk factors, number and type of preexisting disorders, and preoperative medication histories. Cognitive function was evaluated 24 hours before operation and 24 hours and 7 days after operation by the Mini-Mental State (MMS) test. The highest possible MMS score is 30 points; a score of 20 points or less is considered abnormal.

The mean preoperative MMS scores were 26.3 in the LRA group and 27.3 in the general anesthesia group. The mean MMS scores did not change significantly throughout the study. None of the patients in the general anesthesia group had scores below 20 at any time. In contrast, 4 patients in the LRA group briefly had MMS scores below 20 after operation, but all CNS disturbances were attributable to perioperative and postoperative hypoxemia resulting from hemorrhage, cardiorespiratory arrest, confusion after receiving pethidine, or cardiac decompensation.

The occurrence of such CNS disturbances as confusion and amnesia after operation is not usually related to the type of anesthesia administered. The disturbances are probably the result of hypoxemia associated with perioperative and postoperative incidents.

▶ I have often wondered if general anesthesia didn't eliminate some of the memory neurons. This study directly assesses that possibility and comes to a negative conclusion, somewhat to my surprise. Perhaps it will be restudied with a larger group somewhere, some time.—R.D. Currier, M.D.

Correlation Between Essential Tremor and Migraine Headache

Biary N, Koller W, Langenberg P (Univ of Illinois, Chicago; Kansas Univ Med Ctr)
J Neurol Neurosurg Psychiatry 53:1060–1062, 1990   12–4

Clinical observations suggest that there may be a correlation between essential tremor and migraine. A cross-sectional study of this possible relationship was made in which 74 patients with essential tremor and 102 controls with tremor were enrolled.

In the control group, 18% had migraine, compared with 36.5% of the patients with essential tremor. In a third group of 58 patients with migraine, 17.2% were found to have essential tremor. Of 85 controls without migraine, only 1.2% had essential tremor. The prevalence of essential tremor in controls with migraine was greater than that in controls without migraine, occurring in 22% and 1%, respectively. Younger patients with essential tremor seem more likely to have migraine.

Although essential tremor and migraine are both common neurologic disorders, these data indicate that the 2 occur together more often than can be explained by chance alone. The reason for this association is difficult to explain. A greater understanding of the pathophysiology of both disorders is needed.

▶ I suppose we should have suspected this association because propranolol is useful in the treatment of both essential tremor and migraine. Does that thought mean that both will be found to be associated with hypertension? I have all 3.

Lou and Jancovic (1) do not mention migraine as a correlate of essential tremor in their study of 350 patients but do note that in 20% parkinsonism developed subsequently, a belief that is dear to my heart.

And neither mentions Critchley's 3 essential tremor associations that I have long preferred: longevity, fecundity, and higher intelligence. Now that's talking.—R.D. Currier, M.D.

Reference

1. Lou JS, Jancovic J: *Neurology* 41:234, 1991.

Symptomatic and Essential Rhythmic Palatal Myoclonus
Deuschl G, Mischke G, Schenck E, Schulte-Mönting J, Lücking CH (Neurologische Klinik and Poliklinik, Breisgau, Germany; Universität Freiburg, Breisgau)
Brain 113:1645–1672, 1990   12–5

Rhythmic palatal myoclonus (RPM) is a rare movement disorder characterized by continuous synchronous jerks of the soft palate and other muscles innervated by the cranial nerves, and, occasionally, trunk and limb muscles. Most patients with RPM have cerebellar or brain stem disease (symptomatic RPM), but some have no known structural lesion (essential RPM). To define criteria that may distinguish these 2 conditions, data on 287 patients with RPM previously reported in the literature were reviewed.

There were 210 patients with symptomatic RPM and 77 with essential RPM. Forty percent of the patients had cerebrovascular disease, whereas

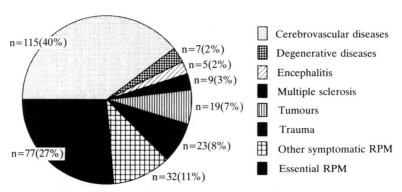

n=115(40%)

n=7(2%)
n=5(2%)
n=9(3%)

n=19(7%)

n=23(8%)

n=77(27%)

n=32(11%)

☐ Cerebrovascular diseases
▦ Degenerative diseases
▨ Encephalitis
■ Multiple sclerosis
▥ Tumours
■ Trauma
⊞ Other symptomatic RPM
■ Essential RPM

Fig 12–2.—Etiology of 287 cases with RPM. Note that more than a quarter belong to essential RPM. (Courtesy of Deuschl G, Mischke G, Schenck E, et al: *Brain* 113:1645–1672, 1990.)

27% had no known cause for RPM (Fig 12–2). Patients with essential RPM were relatively young (mean, 30.4 years) with an equal sex distribution. Objective ear clicks, which are rare in the symptomatic form, are the most common symptom in essential RPM patients. Eye and extremity muscles are rarely involved and, despite the long course of the disease, patients do not have further signs or symptoms of neurologic disease other than the palatal myoclonus. The hyperkinesia is mostly persistent and remissions may occur. The rhythmicity of RPM is more profoundly affected by sleep, coma, and general anesthesia in essential than in symptomatic RPM.

Patients with symptomatic RPM were older (mean age, 49.2 years) with a male predominance. The majority (82%) were seen for complaints related to the neurologic disease underlying the RPM. Extrapalatal involvement is frequent. The jerk frequency is higher than in essential RPM, the duration of kyperkinesia is lifelong, and the prognosis is related to the underlying disease. The pathology in symptomatic RPM is hypertrophic degeneration of the inferior olive.

These data suggest that symptomatic and essential RPM should be separated as distinct clinical entities. The pathogenesis of symptomatic RPM is well established, with cells of the hypertrophied inferior olives representing the oscillator. Essential RPM may represent its functional analogue, based only on transmitter changes.

▶ The authors divide palatal myoclonus into symptomatic and essential, a new thought to me, having always believed that those with a nondemonstrable lesion in truth had lesions in other parts of the nervous system. But they may be right.

They believe that the hypertrophied inferior olives provide the oscillator for the movement, an interesting concept, because it had always been my feeling that the hypertrophied inferior olive was a nonfunctional organ with dead olivary cells, a notion shared with Arnulf Koeppen. Nor do the authors subscribe to the idea that the palatal movement is a release of ancient gill breathing, another quaint idea that has always pleased me. It certainly is a fascinating subject.—R.D. Currier, M.D.

Autoantibodies to GABA-ergic Neurons and Pancreatic Beta Cells in Stiff-Man Syndrome

Solimena M, Folli F, Aparisi R, Pozza G, De Camilli P (Yale Univ; Univ of Milan, Italy)
N Engl J Med 322:1555–1560, 1990   12–6

Stiff-man syndrome, a rare disease of the CNS, is characterized by progressive rigidity and painful muscle spasms. Its cause is unknown. Investigators previously reported finding autoantibodies against glutamic acid decarboxylase (GAD) in a patient with stiff-man syndrome, insulin-dependent diabetes mellitus, and epilepsy. The enzyme GAD is selectively concentrated in neurons secreting the neurotransmitter gamma-aminobutyric acid (GABA) and in pancreatic beta cells.

Investigators collected serum samples from 11 men and 21 women who had stiff-man syndrome; CSF samples were available from 24 patients. Control serum samples were obtained from 16 healthy subjects and 202 patients with a variety of neurologic disorders. Tissue samples were available from some patients. Laboratory studies were performed to detect autoantibodies against GABA-ergic neurons and other organ-specific antibodies.

Investigators found autoantibodies to GABA-ergic neurons in 20 of 33 patients with stiff-man syndrome. The principal autoantigen was GAD. In those patients positive for autoantibodies against GABA-ergic neurons, there was a marked association with organ-specific autoimmune diseases, principally insulin-dependent diabetes mellitus. Four patients without stiff-man syndrome were also positive for autoantibodies against GABA-ergic neurons. Three of these patients had insulin-dependent diabetes mellitus. The fourth had other organ-specific diseases and was at risk for insulin-dependent diabetes mellitus.

Stiff-man syndrome is apparently an autoimmune disease in which GAD is the primary autoantigen. The possibility that the same autoimmune mechanism might cause stiff-man syndrome, insulin-dependent diabetes mellitus, or both cannot be excluded.

▶ It's a shame that the original describers of the stiff-man syndrome, Drs. Moersch and Woltman, are not alive to read this article. Who in the neurologic community would have guessed that it would turn out to be an autoimmune disorder? The authors suggest that immunotherapy might work, but so far only 1 of 3 patients has responded.—R.D. Currier, M.D.

Idiopathic Intracranial Hypertension Without Papilledema

Marcelis J, Silberstein SD (Temple Univ Hosp; Germantown Hosp and Med Ctr, Philadelphia)
Arch Neurol 48:392–399, 1991   12–7

TABLE 1.—Ophthalmoscopic Examination

		No. of Patients
Fundi	WNL	9/10 (drusen, 1)
	Papilledema	0/10
	Venous pulsations	8/9
Visual fields	WNL	9/10
	Bilateral superior temporal field cut	1/10
Visual acuity	WNL	19/20 eyes
	Light perception	1/20 eyes
Fluorescein angiogram	WNL	7/7

Abbreviation: WNL, within normal limits.
(Courtesy of Marcelis J, Silberstein SD: *Arch Neurol* 48:392–399, 1991.)

The first patient with idiopathic intracranial hypertension (IIH) without papilledema was reported in 1972, since which time there have been several reports of IIH with unilateral, asymmetric, or no papilledema.

Ten patients were referred for investigation of headache during a 13-year period. All had complete general, neurologic, and ophthalmoscopic examination, as well as CT and/or MRI and 1 or more lumbar punctures. Endocrinologic examination was done in 7 patients.

The patients' historic and demographic features were no different from those of IIH patients with papilledema. None of the patients had papilledema, exudates, hemorrhages, enlarged blind spot, elevated intraocular pressure, or abnormal pupillary responses (Table 1). Visual field studies were normal in all but 2 patients. Lumbar puncture was within normal limits in 7 patients. Imaging studies showed an empty sella in 2 patients (Table 2). Standard headache therapy was given in all cases. Surgical intervention was eventually required in 3 patients. During 2 months to 10 years of follow-up, 1 of the 7 medically treated patients died and the other 6 required periodic lumbar puncture to relieve symptoms. In no patient did papilledema develop.

This disease may occur without papilledema. Initially, possible inciting agents should be removed, with weight loss if applicable and standard

TABLE 2.—Investigations

Study		No. of Patients
LP		
Elevated Opening pressure, mm H₂O	Range, 230-450; average, 322	10/10
Composition	WNL	7/10
	Low protein content	3/10
MRI/CT	WNL	6/10
	Empty sella	2/10
	Small ventricles	1/10
	Cortical atrophy	1/10

Abbreviations: LP, lumbar puncture; *WNL*, within normal limits.
(Courtesy of Marcelis J, Silberstein SD: *Arch Neurol* 48:392–399, 1991.)

headache therapy. Lumbar puncture and diuretic treatment should be tried before corticosteroids. Patients with prolonged incapacitating headache that does not respond to medical management or lumbar puncture may be candidates for surgery.

▶ It should not be a surprise that some patients with IIH do not have papilledema. What is interesting is the frequency with which patients with chronic recurrent headaches are evaluated without ever having a diagnostic spinal tap. These authors show us that IIH without headache occurs in the same group of obese women of childbearing age. Diagnosis and treatment depend on lumbar puncture with pressure measurement.—J.J. Corbett, M.D., Professor and Chairman of Neurology, University of Mississippi Medical Center

---

Idiopathic Intracranial Hypertension: A Prospective Study of 50 Patients
Wall M, George D (Tulane Univ)
Brain 114:155–180, 1991   12–8

The presence and progression of visual loss should be the basis of management for patients with idiopathic intracranial hypertension (IIH). Clinical status was monitored, with special attention to visual status, in 50 patients with newly diagnosed IIH to better characterize the clinical course of the disease. Follow-up averaged 12.4 months.

At each follow-up visit, patients underwent a neuro-ophthalmologic examination, color vision testing, and Goldmann perimetry. Forty-six of the 50 patients were women, and the average age at onset of symptoms was 31 years. Also, 94% were obese (mean weight, 90 kg). Symptoms included headache in 92% of patients, transient visual obscurations in

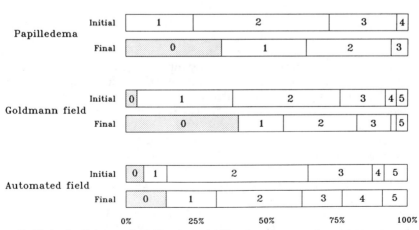

Fig 12–3.—Papilledema grade, Goldmann visual field grade, and automated visual field grade at the initial and final visits by percentage [grade in worst eye used; normal findings are represented by grade zero *(stippled area)*]. (Courtesy of Wall M, George D: *Brain* 114:155–180, 1991.)

72%, and intracranial noises in 60%. The initial complaint in 26% was sustained visual loss.

Visual loss was disclosed by Goldmann perimetry in 96% of patients and by automated perimetry in 92%. Whereas 50% had abnormal contrast sensitivity, 22% had abnormal Snellen acuity. Bilateral blindness occurred in 2 patients. Most patients (60%) had improvement of the Goldmann visual field grade, but 10% had deterioration (Fig 12–3). The only factor that was significantly associated with deterioration of visual field grade was weight gain in the year before diagnosis.

Patients with IIH commonly experience visual loss, which is often reversible. Appropriate perimetric and contrast sensitivity testing should be done in these patients, along with careful optic disk examination. Both papilledema and perimetry grades improve with treatment, but these 2 grades were not correlated.

▶ With only 1 exception, all other studies of IIH have been retrospective. This study confirms and amplifies earlier observations of frequent and severe visual loss in these patients. Once the diagnosis of IIH is established, follow-up must include frequent visual field tests and the services of an ophthalmologist. Visual acuity testing alone (what most neurologists would do) is inadequate, and the appearance of the disk correlates poorly with overall visual outcome.—J.J. Corbett, M.D.

Symptoms of Low Blood Pressure: A Population Study
Wessely S, Nickson J, Cox B (Inst of Psychiatry, London; Univ of Cambridge)
Br Med J 301:362–365, 1990   12–9

Systolic blood pressures in the "low normal" range are regarded as desirable in English and American medical practice but are considered pathologic by French and German medical practice in which "neurasthenic" symptoms (e.g., tiredness, weakness, fainting, and dizziness) are attributed to low blood pressure. A cross-sectional, population-based survey was conducted to ascertain the relationship between blood pressure measurements and self-reported common symptoms. A total of 7,383 adults aged 18 and older, chosen randomly from the electoral register in England, Wales, and Scotland, participated in a population-based health and life-style survey. All had satisfactory physiologic measurements.

Potential confounders, as determined by the general health questionnaire, were elevated in relation to systolic pressure. True confounders were age, sex, taking of drugs, physical illness, exercise, and body mass index. There was a negative association between systolic blood pressure and self-reported tiredness and feeling faint, even after adjusting for confounders. This association was most pronounced for women younger than age 50. There was also a negative association between systolic blood pressure and headache and a positive association between systolic blood pressure and palpitation. Both associations disappeared after adjusting for age.

These data show that systemic hypotension is associated with persistent tiredness. However, there is no clear pathophysiology to explain this relationship, and it is possible that both tiredness and low blood pressure may be linked to a third unidentified factor, e.g., anemia. Therefore, it would be difficult to justify recommending treatment of low blood pressure. Rather, low blood pressure may be associated with opposite effects on mortality, in contrast with morbidity.

▶ This nice study does show a relationship between complaints of tiredness and low blood pressure, to my surprise. It does not show a relationship to other neurasthenic symptoms, such as weakness, fainting, dizziness, and headache. The authors point out that although the continental practice is to treat low blood pressure, the English and Americans regard it as a healthy bonus conducive to a long life and do not treat it.—R.D. Currier, M.D.

Muscle Performance, Voluntary Activation, Twitch Properties and Perceived Effort in Normal Subjects and Patients With the Chronic Fatigue Syndrome
Lloyd AR, Gandevia SC,. Hales JP (Prince Henry Hosp, Sydney; Univ of New South Wales, Sydney, Australia)
Brain 114:85–98, 1991   12–10

Disabling fatigue sometimes persists after a viral or other infection. Many studies have focused on epidemics of this disorder, but most cases occur sporadically in the community. The hallmark of "chronic fatigue syndrome" is marked tiredness after minor physical activity and an inability to perform tasks that formerly were achieved readily.

Performance during prolonged submaximal isometric (elbow flexor) activity was assessed in 12 men with this syndrome and 13 healthy men (controls). Maximal voluntary isometric muscle torque was measured at 5-minute intervals during 45 minutes of repetitive isometric contractions lasting for 6 seconds, with 4-second rest intervals. Contractions produced 30% of initial peak voluntary torque. In addition, electrical stimuli were delivered to the elbow flexors to measure the contractile force between voluntary contractions. Central motor activation during peak contraction was estimated using a method of twitch interpolation. Perceived effort was recorded on a self-report scale.

Both patients and controls achieved a high degree of central activation in maximal contractions during the endurance sequence. There was no significant difference in relative torque produced by either voluntary or stimulated contractions, and no difference in perceived exertion.

Apparently neither muscle contractile failure nor inadequate motivation can explain the chronic fatigue syndrome. Any pathophysiologic abnormality must lie in the CNS above the level of the motor cortex.

▶ So, by actual measurement, the muscular effort and endurance of the patients and the controls were the same. The authors' conclusion that muscle contractile failure is not part of the chronic fatigue syndrome seems acceptable.—R.D. Currier, M.D.

Is Chronic Fatigue Syndrome Synonymous With Effort Syndrome?
Rosen SD, King JC, Wilkinson JB, Nicon PGF (Charing Cross Hosp, London)
J R Soc Med 83:761–764, 1990   12–11

Chronic fatigue syndrome is characterized by the inability to make and sustain effort. It has included myalgic encephalomyelitis and postviral syndrome. The prevalence of chronic hyperventilation was determined in 100 consecutive patients given a diagnosis of chronic fatigue syndrome and in 40 asymptomatic controls. The respective mean ages were 36.5 years and 40 years. Forced hyperventilation testing was done to assess the tendency to continue overbreathing after breathing deeply and rapidly for 3 minutes to lower the $PetCO_2$ to 20 mm Hg or less.

Performance declined to a mean of 40% of the self-perceived "normal" levels during hyperventilation. The mean time between presumed viral infection and referral was 3½ years, but the mean time for which the patient had felt incapable of normal performance was nearly 6 years.

The labels chronic fatigue syndrome, myalgic encephalitis, and postviral syndrome should not be used until chronic habitual hyperventilation is definitively ruled out. The latter is a disorder for which effective rehabilitative measures are available.

▶ Another interesting study on the chronic fatigue syndrome. Ninety-three of 100 patients were found to be hyperventilating by respiratory studies. So, it looks like we may be getting somewhere. Before we throw the syndrome out completely, read the comment by Thomas English in the *JAMA* (1). Dr. English details in 1 brief page his problems with the chronic fatigue syndrome, which sound very real.

And 2 researchers from Bonn (2) give a nice review of the situation for those of you who are German literate. Their conclusion that "current knowledge does not allow specific therapeutic recommendations" is certainly correct.—R.D. Currier, M.D.

References

1. English TL: *JAMA* 265:964, 1991.
2. Ewig S, Dengler HJ: *Klin Wochenschr* 68:789, 1990.

The following review article is recommended to the reader:

Lloyd AR, Gandevia SC, Hales JP: Muscle performance, voluntary activation, twitch properties and perceived effort in normal subjects and patients with the chronic fatigue syndrome. *Brain* 114:85–98, 1991.

13 Treatment

Neurological Deterioration in Young Adults With Phenylketonuria
Thompson AJ, Smith I, Brenton D, Youl BD, Rylance G, Davidson DC, Kendall
B, Lees AJ (Natl Hosp for Nervous Diseases, London; Inst of Child Health, Lon-
don; Univ College and Middlesex School of Medicine, London; Alder Hey Chil-
dren's Hosp, Liverpool, England; Children's Hosp, Birmingham, England)
Lancet 336:602–605, 1990   13–1

There have been reports of late-onset neurologic disability in patients
with phenylketonuria. Seven patients with phenylketonuria were seen in
whom neurologic disability developed in adolescence or early adult life.

In 4 patients the diagnosis was made by routine neonatal screening and
they were started on a low phenylalanine diet in infancy. These 4 patients
represented a frequency of .4% among those with phenylketonuria detected at infancy who later experienced neurologic deterioration in adolescence or early adulthood. In the other 3 patients the diagnosis was
made in early childhood because of developmental delay; dietary treatment was then started. In all patients, dietary control deteriorated in later
years and was withdrawn in middle to late childhood.

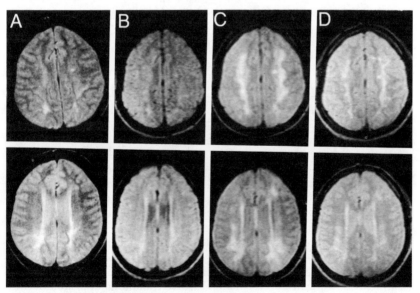

Fig 13–1 —Axial T2-weighted MRI scans (SE 2,000/60) of patient at 2 levels through the brain.
Abnormal high-signal (light) areas, mainly periventricular and posterior, but with some discrete lesions.
Scan taken at 23 (A), 24 (B), and 25 (C) years of age, and at 2 months after resumption of strict diet (D).
(Courtesy of Thompson AJ, Smith I, Brenton D, et al: *Lancet* 336:602–605, 1990.)

All had signs of upper motor neuron damage; 4 patients had spastic paraparesis or quadriparesis, 1 had epilepsy, and another had pronounced intention tremor. When strict diet was resumed after the onset of neurologic deterioration in 4 patients, 1 made as low but almost complete recovery, 2 had reduced behavioral problems, and 1 had reduced tremor during follow-up for 3–10 years (mean, 6 years). Six patients underwent MRI and abnormal high-signal areas were observed in the cerebral white matter in all 6. One of these 6 had serial MRI scans demonstrating clinical deterioration that resolved within 2 months of resumption of dietary control (Fig 13–1).

This study confirms previous reports on the development of late neurologic deterioration in patients with phenylketonuria despite varying periods of dietary treatment during childhood. If these findings are confirmed, it seems prudent to continue strict dietary control into adulthood in some patients with phenylketonuria.

▶ These investigators followed their phenylketonurics into adult life and found that when the diet was discontinued, some deteriorated neurologically. How long should the diet be continued? Forever? The apparent improvement after diet was restarted in the 25-year-old patient is striking. The similarity of the white matter changes on MRI scan to that of other demyelinating diseases is noted.

Pearsen et al. (1), who reviewed the MRI changes of phenylketonuria in 15 patients, described rather symmetrical periventricular white matter lesions on T2 that tend to cluster around the posterior horns of the lateral ventricles and are not found in the brain stem.—R.D. Currier, M.D.

Reference

1. Pearsen KD, et al: *Radiology* 177:437, 1990.

Sulpiride in Tardive Dyskinesia
Schwartz M, Moguillansky L, Lanyi G, Sharf B (Bnai-Zion Med Ctr, Haifa, Israel; Fluegelman Psychiatric Hosp, Acre, Israel)
J Neurol Neurosurg Psychiatry 53:800–802, 1990   13–2

The abnormal involuntary movements of tardive dyskinesia are caused by the long-term use of neuroleptic drugs. Although postsynaptic dopaminergic receptor blockers can suppress tardive dyskinesia, most induce parkinsonian signs. Sulpiride, a benzamide derivative and a selective antagonist of D2 receptors, was evaluated for its clinical benefit in a group of 15 psychiatric inpatients.

The patient's mean age was 67 years; they had undergone neuroleptic treatment for a mean of 28.3 years. Tardive dyskinesia appeared in these patients at least several months before the start of sulpiride treatment. The agent or placebo was administered orally at 50 mg twice a day, with weekly increases of 100 mg/day until marked clinical improvement with-

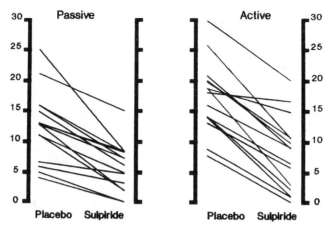

Fig 13–2 —Tardive dyskinesia scores: body movements. (Courtesy of Schwartz M, Moguillansky L, Lanyi G, et al: *J Neurol Neurosurg Psychiatry* 53:800–802, 1990.)

out side effects was noted. Two weeks after patients reached their optimal dosage, the sulpiride and placebo groups were switched. After completion of the first phase of the study, sulpiride was reintroduced to all patients at the optimal dosage for 3 months and then discontinued.

The patients had significantly lower tardive dyskinesia scores with sulpiride treatment than with placebo (Fig 13–2). Improvement was marked in 6 patients, and only 3 patients had no real benefit from the drug. Women generally responded to sulpiride better than men. Nine to 12 months later the patients were reassessed for signs of tardive dyskinesia and neurologic side effects. After completing the 3-month course of sulpiride, involuntary movements reappeared in only 4 patients.

The side effects of sulpiride in most of the patients were insignificant. Most patients reached their optimal dosage at 200–400 mg daily. The mechanism by which sulpiride brought about improvement is not fully understood. The drug may effect a loss of hypersensitivity in the dopamine receptors of the striatum, or it may reinstate the normal function of the receptors.

▶ Well, the world needs a drug to treat tardive dyskinesia and it looks like we may be getting one. I do not know its status in the United States, but the hope is that it will get here sooner rather than later, because it appears effective.— R.D. Currier, M.D.

Predictors of Improvement in Tardive Dyskinesia Following Discontinuation of Neuroleptic Medication
Glazer WM, Morgenstern H, Schooler N, Berkman CS, Moore DC (Yale Univ; Univ of California, Los Angeles; Univ of Pittsburgh; Columbia Univ)
Br J Psychiatry 157:585–592, 1990   13–3

It has been difficult to study the natural course of tardive dyskinesia after discontinuation of neuroleptic drugs because many patients relapse and must resume their medication before an adequate follow-up period is completed. An extended follow-up, which included some nonschizophrenic patients, was possible in 1 series that allowed conclusions to be reached on the demographic and clinical variables predictive of the outcome of tardive dyskinesia after discontinuation of neuroleptics.

The course of involuntary movements was studied prospectively in 49 chronic psychiatric outpatients with tardive dyskinesia. The mean follow-up after discontinuation of neuroleptic medication was 40 weeks. Ten patients were schizophrenic; other diagnoses included major depressive disorder and lifetime bipolar disorder. There were 3 outcome measures: first improvement, overall improvement, and mean improvement.

By completion of the study, 24 patients had relapsed, 20 had left treatment, 1 had died, and 4 were being actively followed. If a patient could be without neuroleptic medication for 24 weeks, the estimated probability of achieving a 50% reduction in the total Abnormal Involuntary Movement Scale (AIMS) score was 42.5%. The probability of such a reduction was 93% at 1 year. Variables predicting time until first improvement were a baseline dose of neuroleptic medication higher than 100 mg of chlorpromazine equivalents, being employed, and having a psychiatric diagnosis of schizoaffective or affective disorder.

Predictors of greater mean improvement were a baseline AIMS score of 6 or more and a psychiatric diagnosis other than schizophrenia. Patients younger than age of 55 and those with a history of psychiatric illness of 20 years or more experienced greater overall improvement. Although complete and persistent reversibility of tardive dyskinesia occurred in only 2% of patients, many had noticeable improvement. Both the type and the history of psychiatric illness appear to affect the course of tardive dyskinesia after discontinuation of neuroleptic therapy.

▶ Who should get the sulpiride? It looks as though these investigators are able to predict which patients will persist with tardive dyskinesia after the neuroleptic drug has been discontinued. The problem, of course, is that it should not be discontinued in many patients, otherwise the schizophrenia returns. The drug noted in the above article may turn out to be quite useful because it can be given with the neuroleptic.—R.D. Currier, M.D.

A Controlled Trial of Transcutaneous Electrical Nerve Stimulation (TENS) and Exercise for Chronic Low Back Pain
Deyo RA, Walsh NE, Martin DC, Schoenfeld LS, Ramamurthy S (Seattle Veterans Affairs Med Ctr; Univ of Washington; Univ of Texas, San Antonio)
N Engl J Med 322:1627–1634, 1990   13–4

Although numerous treatments are widely prescribed for chronic low back pain, few have been assessed rigorously. The efficacy of transcutaneous electrical nerve stimulation (TENS), a program of stretching exercises, and a combination of both was evaluated in 145 patients who had experienced low back pain for a median of 4.1 years. Thirty-six received daily treatment with TENS, 36 with sham TENS, 37 with TENS plus exercises, and 36 with sham TENS plus exercises.

After 1 month there were no clinically or statistically significant treatment effects of TENS on any of 11 indicators of outcome. Nor was there an interactive effect between TENS and exercise. Overall, pain indicators improved by 47% with TENS and by 42% with sham TENS, which was not a significant difference. By contrast, patients in the exercise groups had significant improvement in self-rated pain scores, a decrease in the frequency of pain, and higher levels of activity compared with patients in the nonexercise groups. The mean reported improvement in the exercise groups' pain scores was 52%, compared with 37% in the nonexercise groups. Two months later, however, most patients had stopped exercising, and the initial improvements were lost.

For patients with chronic low back pain, treatment with TENS is no more effective than treatment with a placebo. Further, TENS adds no apparent benefit to that achieved with exercise alone.

▶ After 2 decades and the sale of countless thousands of expensive TENS units, someone has evaluated their effectiveness for relief of chronic low back pain. As a matter of fact, it looks as though the exercise groups had better results than did the TENS-treated groups, although the benefit of neither lasted.

Meade et al. (1) analyzed the treatment of low back pain by chiropractic vs. hospital outpatient physical therapy in a careful, large, 11-center, 2-year trial. Chiropractic won, although it was given more frequently and for a longer time, and the trial, although randomized, was not blinded in any way.— R.D. Currier, M.D.

Reference

1. Meade TW, Frank AO: *Br Med J* 300:1431, 1990.

Spinal Cord Stimulation in 60 Cases of Intractable Pain
Simpson BA (London Hosp, London)
J Neurol Neurosurg Psychiatry 54:196–199, 1991   13–5

Analgesic effects of electrical stimulation have been recognized since Roman times when an electric fish was used to relieve gouty pain. The results of implanting a spinal cord stimulator were examined in 60 patients who had experienced pain for a median of 7–8 years and who were followed for a median of 29 months. Electrodes were inserted by laminectomy and usually sutured to the dura. Bipolar plate electrodes were most frequently used.

Four patients were made worse by cord stimulation, and 2 others worsened after initially benefitting. Twelve patients noted no change in their pain. Twenty-eight patients (47%) reported significant improvement

Results Related to Diagnosis

	Total	SB	MB	NE	MW
Traumatic and unplanned surgical peripheral denervation	6	5	—	1	—
Painful paraparesis, paraplegia and hemiparesis					
— trauma	2	2	1	1	1
— chronic disease	5	2	1	1	1
— CVA	1	1	—	—	—
— idiopathic	1	1	—	—	—
Painful conus lesion (trauma)	7	4	1	2	—
"Failed back" syndrome	4	1	2	1	—
Phantom pain (leg)	4	1	—	1	—
Stump pain—arm	3	1	1	—	—
—leg	10	3	3	2	2
*Anaesthesia dolorosa (face)	1	—	—	1	1
†Thalamic syndrome	2	2	—	—	—
Post thalamotomy pain	4	2	1	2	—
Ischaemic leg	6	3	3	—	1
Nociceptive (eg carcinoma, spondylosis)	1	—	1	—	—
Idiopathic chronic focal pain (loin, groin etc)	1	—	1	1	—
Syrinx	3	—	1	—	—
Tabes dorsalis	1	—	1	—	—
Post herpetic neuralgia	3	1	—	2	—

The total exceeds 60 as some had more than one pain, e.g., stump and phantom, which are noted separately.
*One patient was made worse but first enjoyed significant benefit for 3 years and 6 months and is therefore recorded as SB in the table.
†One patient was made worse after initial modest benefit; the overriding result was MW. (Courtesy of Simpson BA: *J Neurol Neurosurg Psychiatry* 54:196–199, 1991.)

and 10 were totally relieved of pain. The outcome is related to diagnosis in the table (SB, significant benefit; MB, modest benefit; NE, no effect; MW, made worse). Effective frequencies most often were in the range of 50–120 cycles per second. No neurologic deterioration resulted from stimulation. Nearly half of the patients required only 1 implant procedure.

Spinal cord stimulation is a reversible nondestructive procedure causing little morbidity and does not itself produce deafferentation pain. It can be effective in selected patients with chronic pain for whom little else is available.

▶ This is a summary of 1 hospital's use of this technique for intractable pain. I have always had the feeling that eventually this form of therapy would fail in every case, but that does not seem to have happened in this series, most of the patients benefitting. The majority of electrodes did not require removal, although infection and lead breakage were significant problems.—R.D. Currier, M.D.

Risk of Anginia Pectoris and Plasma Concentrations of Vitamins A, C, and E and Carotene
Riemersma RA, Wood DA, MacIntyre CCA, Elton RA, Gey KF, Oliver MF (Univ of Edinburgh; Univ of Berne, Switzerland)
Lancet 337:1–5, 1991   13–6

Interest in the possible role of free radicals in atheroma is growing. Oxidative modification of low-density lipoprotein (LDL) particles in the arterial subendothelium leads to structural changes, which may make them more atherogenic than native LDL. Vitamins E and C are the most readily available naturally occurring antioxidants in food. To test the hypothesis that plasma concentrations of vitamins with antioxidant properties may be associated with the risk of angina, and to assess the extent to which such risk is independent of class risk factors for coronary heart disease (CHD), a case-control study was carried out. The series included 110 patients with angina, identified by the Chest Pain Questionnaire, and 394 controls. The group was selected from 6,000 men aged 35–54 years.

Plasma levels of vitamins C and E and carotene and the risk of angina were significantly inversely correlated. Vitamin A levels were not significantly related to angina risk. After adjustment for smoking, the inverse relationship between angina and low plasma carotene disappeared, and that with plasma vitamin C was greatly reduced. However, vitamin E remained independently inversely related to the risk of angina after adjustment for smoking, age, blood pressure, lipids, and relative weight. The adjusted odds ratio for angina between the lowest and highest quintiles of vitamin E levels was 2.68.

Some populations with a high incidence of CMD may benefit from eating diets rich in natural antioxidants, especially vitamin E. The mechanism by which low plasma vitamin E and C predisposes a person to CHD has yet to be determined.

▶ After reading this article, I looked up vitamin E and find it is in most everything. A little extra can do no harm, so I swallow the vitamin my wife shoves across the breakfast table every morning. What prevents angina should prevent stroke.—R.D. Currier, M.D.

Regression of Coronary Artery Disease as a Result of Intensive, Lipid-Lowering Therapy in Men With High Levels of Apolipoprotein B
Brown G, Albers JJ, Fisher LD, Schaefer SM, Lin J-T, Kaplan C, Zhao X-Q, Bisson BD, Fitzpatrick VF, Dodge HT (Univ of Washington)
N Engl J Med 323:1289–1298, 1990   13–7

With the advent of more effective therapies for hyperlipidemia, new arteriographic methods for assessing atherogenesis, and new insights into atherogenesis, the question of whether the progression of atherosclerosis can be retarded or reversed with treatment of hyperlipidemia can be addressed. In a randomized, double-blind, placebo-controlled study, the effect on coronary artherosclerosis of intensive lipid-lowering therapy in men at high risk for cardiovascular events was assessed by quantitative arteriography.

A series of 146 men 62 years or younger with elevated apolipoprotein B levels (≥125 mg/dL), documented coronary artery disease, and a family history of vascular disease participated in the 2-year study. Patients were given dietary counseling and assigned to 1 of 3 treatment groups: lovastatin, 20 mg twice a day, and colestipol, 10 g 3 times a day; niacin, 1 g 4 times a day, and colestipol, 10 g 3 times a day; or conventional therapy with placebo [or colestipol if the low-density lipoprotein (LDL) cholesterol level was elevated]. The primary end point was the average change between the initial and follow-up (after treatment) coronary arteriography in the percent stenosis of the worst lesion in each of 9 proximal segments.

Among the 120 men who completed the study, the levels of LDL and high-density lipoprotein (HDL) cholesterol changed only slightly in the conventionally treated group but more substantially in patients treated with levostatin and colestipol and those treated with niacin and colestipol. Definite lesion progression as the only change occurred more frequently in conventionally treated patients (46%) than in those who received lovastatin and colestipol (21%) or niacin and colestipol (25%). Regression as the only change was uncommon in conventionally treated patients (11%), whereas it was 3 times more common in the intensively treated patients (32% and 39%, respectively).

Intensive lipid-lowering therapy reduced the frequency of cardiovascular events, e.g., death, myocardial infarction, or revascularization for worsening symptoms. Clinical events occurred in 3 of 46 men treated with lovastatin and colestipol and in 2 of 48 given niacin and colestipol, compared to 10 of 52 men assigned to conventional therapy. Multivariate analysis showed that reduction in apolipoprotein B levels (or LDL cholesterol) and systolic blood pressure, and increases in HDL cholesterol correlated independently with regression of coronary lesions.

These data show that intensive lipid-lowering therapy in men with coronary artery disease who are at high risk for cardiovascular events reduces the frequency of progression of coronary lesions, increases the frequency of regression, and reduces the incidence of cardiovascular events.

▶ Those who have argued that you can't reverse coronary artery disease and therefore also other atherosclerosis are wrong. This looks to be proof that you can. Get on that diet, ladies and gentlemen.—R.D. Currier, M.D.

Ubidecarenone in the Treatment of Mitochondrial Myopathies: A Multi-Center Double-Blind Trial

Bresolin N, Doriguzzi C, Ponzetto C, Angelini C, Moroni I, Castelli E, Cossutta E, Binda A, Gallanti A, Gabellini S, Piccolo G, Martinuzzi A, Ciafaloni E, Arnaudo E, Liciardello L, Carenzi A, Scarlato G (Univ of Milan; Univ of Torino; Univ of Padua; Univ of Bologna; Univ of Pavia, Italy; et al)

J Neurol Sci 100:70–78, 1990   13–8

Earlier trials involving small numbers of patients suggest that Ubidecarenone (CoQ10) may be beneficial in some patients with mitochondrial myopathy, as evidenced by the partially corrected elevated levels of serum lactate and improved cardiac function. To further evaluate the usefulness of CoQ10 therapy and identify features that may delineate patients who respond to therapy, an open, multicenter trial was undertaken involving 44 patients with mitochondrial myopathies.

Patients received CoQ10, 2 mg/kg/day, for 6 months to identify those who would respond to therapy. The CoQ10 therapy was associated with a significant reduction in 5-minute postexercise serum lactate levels and significant increases in mitochondrial activity of platelet succinate dehydrogenase and succinate cytochrome c reductase and reduction of citrate synthetase, as well as significant strength improvement in the global, axial, and upper and lower distal muscles. In 16 patients at least a 25% reduction of postexercise lactate was achieved; these 16 were considered responders. There was no significant correlation between response to CoQ10 therapy and serum and platelet CoQ10 levels or the presence or absence of mtDNA deletions.

In the double-blind phase of the trial, the 16 responders were treated for another 3 months with either CoQ10 or placebo. Serum lactate levels after exercise did not decrease further and platelet mitochondrial enzyme activities did not increase significantly. In contrast, the group given placebo showed worsening of postexercise lactate levels relative to previous levels and a reversed nonsignificant trend for platelet mitochondrial enzyme activities. The differences between these 2 groups were not significant.

It is not clear why CoQ10 has therapeutic effects in some patients but not in others with the same clinical symptoms and biochemical defect. It appears that a dose of 2 mg/kg/day, CoQ10 therapy requires a long administration time before a response is evident.

▶ A trial of CoQ10 needed to be done, and these workers have carried it out. It seems fairly clear, but not certain, that CoQ10—something that can be obtained in the local health food store—is not effective in the mitochondrial myopathies.—R.D. Currier, M.D.

Reversal of Early Neurologic and Neuroradiologic Manifestations of X-Linked Adrenoleukodystrophy of Bone Marrow Transplantation

Aubourg P, Blanche S, Jambaqué I, Rocchiccioli F, Kalifa G, Naud-Saudreau C, Rolland M-O, Debré M, Chaussain J-L, Griscelli C, Fischer A, Bougnères P-F (Hôp Saint Vincent de Paul, Paris; Hôp des Enfants Malades, Paris; Centre Hospitalier, Lorient, France; Hôp Debrousse, Lyon, France)
N Engl J Med 322:1860–1866, 1990   13–9

X-linked adrenoleukodystrophy is an inherited peroxisomal disease caused by a defective gene within the Xq28 region of the X chromosome. Initial attempts to treat the disease with bone marrow transplantation were unsuccessful, and some thought that treatment might have accelerated neurologic deterioration. However, transplantation may have been performed too late. Bone transplantation must be performed after the demonstration of CNS involvement but early enough for some effects to be reversed.

Boy, 8 years, a dizygotic twin, had normal motor and cognitive development throughout early childhood. Like his unaffected twin brother, he had scores below the middle range in school. At aged $6\frac{1}{2}$ years he contracted a mild viral infection that triggered vomiting and coma. Adrenal insufficiency was diagnosed after 2 additional episodes within the year. Six months later, dystonia developed, as well as pyramidal signs and corresponding lesions of the internal capsules, pallidum, and caudate nuclei. He also had marked behavioral and cognitive changes. Symptoms rapidly worsened, and an MRI examination 1 month before transplantation showed that lesions of the pyramidal tracts now extended to the pons (Fig 13–3). The patient's mother was heterozygous for adrenoleukodystrophy; 2 of her brothers had died in childhood of acute adrenal insufficiency, and her grandfather may have had an adult form of adrenoleukodystrophy. The patient underwent bone transplantation and dietary therapy. At 79 days after transplantation, the oxidation of very-long-chain fatty acids by peripheral blood leukocytes derived from the donor was normal, and it remained so at 12 months after transplantation. Eighteen months after transplantation the plasma $C_{26:0}$ concentration and $C_{26:0}/C_{22:0}$ ratio were completely normal. Six months after transplantation, results of neurologic examination were similar to those before transplantation; however, verbal fluency was better, and the patient could participate normally in school. Within 12 months, dystonia and pyramidal signs disappeared, and the neurologic examination was normal. By 18 months, neurodiagnostic studies were normal.

In adrenoleukodystrophy, functional bone marrow cells from a donor may cross the blood-brain barrier and produce favorable effects in mechanisms leading to demyelination. Studies suggest that perivascular microglial cells—a subset of CNS cells—are derived from bone marrow. This finding may be particularly relevant in adrenoleukodystrophy. The results here support further evaluation of bone marrow transplantation for treatment of adrenoleukodystrophy.

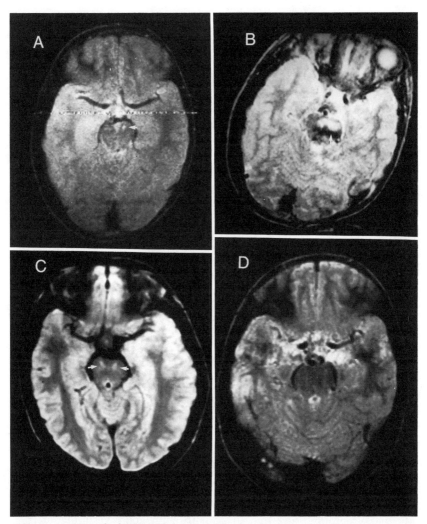

Fig 13–3 —T2-weighted MRI scans show evolution of the lesions (*arrows*) located within the pons and cerebral peduncles, **A**, before bone marrow transplantation, and **B**, 6 months, **C**, 12 months, and **D**, 18 months thereafter. (Courtesy of Aubourg P, Blanche S, Jambaqué I, et al: *N Engl J Med* 322:1860–1866, 1990.)

▶ My ignorance in this particular situation is nearly complete. It strains belief to be told that a form of CNS demyelination may be treated by bone marrow transplantation. One can only congratulate these scientists on not only inventing this therapy, but carrying on further trials when the first efforts did not succeed. Adrenoleukodystrophy is no laughing matter, and if this treatment, when examined further, continues to be effective, it would seem that neurologists and neuroradiologists will be obligated to extend every effort to diagnose it early and to make friends with their nearest bone marrow transplantation team.

Here is an example of one of the chief reasons for the continuing rise of medical costs. Bone marrow transplantation is expensive, but who would deny it to a young boy with early signs of this disorder.— R.D. Currier, M.D.

The Beneficial Effect of Methylprednisolone in Acute Vestibular Vertigo
Ariyasu L, Byl FM, Sprague MS, Adour KK (Kaiser Permanente Med Ctr, Oakland, Calif)
Arch Otolaryngol Head Neck Surg 116:700–703, 1990   13–10

There are no previous published reports of clinical trials showing the benefit of short-term corticosteroid therapy to treat patients with acute vestibular vertigo. Twenty patients were randomized to receive either placebo or a single 32-mg dose of methylprednisolone orally on the first day followed by divided doses of 16 mg twice daily for 3 days. Dosage was tapered to 0 after 8 days. If patients had relief from vertigo, nausea, and vomiting, they continued treatment. If no significant relief of symptoms was obtained after 24 hours, they were switched to the other treatment. Investigators performed electronystagmography before treatment and at 1 week and 1 month afterward.

Patients given methylprednisolone tended to have more severe vertigo. Initial vestibular signs were similar in the 2 groups, and most patients in both groups had nausea. Nine of 20 patients had signs of cranial polyneuritis. Of the 10 patients receiving methylprednisolone, 9 had a marked reduction in symptoms of vertigo; the tenth patient switched to placebo. Of the 10 patients given placebo, 3 had relief of vertiginous symptoms. Seven patients with persistent symptoms switched to methylprednisolone and experienced relief of vertigo symptoms within 24 hours. In all 16 patients who took methylprednisolone, electronystagmograms returned to normal within 1 month. However, electronystagmograms remained abnormal in 2 of 4 patients who took placebo only. One patient receiving methylprednisolone had renewed symptoms when the dose was tapered; however, these resolved when the dosage was increased to 32 mg/day.

Methylprednisolone is much more effective than placebo in reducing the symptoms of vertigo in patients with acute vestibular vertigo. The variability of symptoms associated with vestibular vertigo may be caused by the randomness of the clinical presentation of polyneuritis.

▶ I was unaware of the effect of corticosteroids on this disorder. This double-blind study demonstrated rapid relief of symptoms in those who took the oral steroid as compared to those who took a placebo. The treatment was gradually reduced to 0 over 8 days. The authors comment that "The division of acute vestibular vertigo into such entities as vestibular neuritis, epidemic vertigo, and acute labyrinthitis represents a semantic difference." They believe that it is a self-limited viral infestation, and that all of the syndromes are one.— R.D. Currier, M.D.

Vagal Stimulation for Control of Complex Partial Seizures in Medically Refractory Epileptic Patients

Wilder BJ, Uthman BM, Hammond EJ (Veterans Affairs Med Ctr, Gainesville, Fla)
PACE 14:108–115, 1991 13–11

Chronic intermittent stimulation of the vagus nerve is currently under investigation for the treatment of medically intractable complex partial seizures (CPS). Nine patients were studied for 4–16 months. They were maintained on constant dosages of antiepileptic drugs; EEGs and ECGs were obtained and clinical laboratory tests and gastric analysis performed over a 6-week baseline period. The neurocybernetic prosthesis (NCP) was then implanted. It was connected to 2 spiral electrodes wound around the left vagus nerve, and vagal stimulation was begun after a 4-week placebo period.

Stimulation parameters were increased stepwise every month until the patients were being stimulated for 3-second periods at 20–50 Hz with 1–2 mA of current at 250–500 μsec pulses. Three months after implantation, a second 4-week placebo period was begun. Thereafter, vagal stimulation was resumed. Self-stimulation with magnetic activation was permitted for 1 minute at onset of an aura.

All patients tolerated the implantation and stimulation well. None complained of pain or discomfort, nor did any patient experience important changes in daily activities, sleep habits, eating, swallowing, or breathing. No remarkable changes were noted in blood pressure or heart rate. Six patients had a significant decrease in the frequency, intensity, or duration of seizures.

Chronic intermittent vagal stimulation appears to be a safe, effective adjunct treatment for medically intractable partial seizures. The patients in this series tolerated NCP implantation and stimulation well without serious changes in physiology or life-style. Adverse effects were limited to a tingling in the throat or hoarseness during stimulation.

▶ Well, this is a new one. If someone had asked me to rate vagal stimulation as an effective means of controlling seizures it would have been far down the list. It's weird, but here it is. Wilder's group found that it helped 6 of 9 patients and did not cause ulcers. We will hear more of it. The same issue of *PACE* contains notes from Utah and Canada on the same subject.—R.D. Currier, M.D.

Toward a Rational Therapeutic Strategy for Arachnoiditis: A Possible Role for D-Penicillamine

Grahame R, Clark B, Watson M, Polkey C (Guy's Hosp, London)
Spine 16:172–175, 1991 13–12

A trial of D-penicillamine was undertaken in 26 patients having radiculographic and/or operative evidence of chronic adhesive spinal arachnoiditis (CASA). During a 6-month crossover trial patients received up to 500 mg of D-penicillamine daily, or a matching placebo.

Nine patients withdrew, 1 because of worsening symptoms and 1 because of a rash. Thirteen of the 17 patients who completed the trial had no clear preference for active drug or placebo. One other patient preferred placebo. There was some objective evidence favoring D-penicillamine, but the small number of patients precluded statistical assessment. Adverse reactions in patients who remained in the study were generally mild and were less frequent with D-penicillamine than with placebo. A minority of patients with CASA may benefit from D-penicillamine therapy, but much more work is needed to determine how to select patients for treatment and to specify the optimal dosage.

▶ The authors point out that D-penicillamine, an inhibitor of fibroblast activity and collagen synthesis, has a history of successful use in scleroderma, morphea, and primary biliary cirrhosis. So, why not try it in arachnoiditis?

Their study was a randomized, double-blind, 6-month, crossover trial of 17 patients. Three of the patients given D-penicillamine preferred it strongly, 1 patient preferred placebo, and 13 of the 17 had no preference.

The world certainly needs a treatment for this disorder and D-penicillamine would seem a fit substance for a larger cooperative trial. But let's think up other substances to try in therapy of this miserable disease.— R.D. Currier, M.D.

NEUROSURGERY

ROBERT M. CROWELL, M.D.

Introduction

In a year filled with remarkable advances in clinical neuroscience, the results reported by the North American Symptomatic Carotid Endarterectomy Trial (NASCET) were arguably the most spectacular. In February 1991, in San Francisco, Dr. Barnett and colleagues triumphantly announced that, with overwhelming statistical significance, carotid endarterectomy yielded better clinical results than medical treatment for symptomatic carotid stenosis of 70%–99%. The investigators are credible, the randomization procedure impeccable, the statistical analysis impressive, and the results irrefutable. Moreover, the tighter the stenosis, the greater the benefit. So far, the study cannot address the subject of lesser stenosis. Further work is required to determine the anticipated threshold of stenosis below which surgery does not confer clinical benefit. Hats off to Barnett and colleagues—carotid endarterectomy is back!

Magnetic resonance imaging continues to make rapid progress. Computer software and clever physical techniques are developing at a breakneck pace. For example, fast echoplanar techniques seem likely to provide extremely rapid studies (measured in a few seconds for each sequence), with even higher quality images. Perhaps even more impressive is the emergence of MR angiography (MRA). Using techniques to eliminate signals from all tissues but arteries, investigators have been able to produce routine programs for MRA sequence. This has reached clinical application in the General Electric "Advantage" program, which has been implemented in a number of centers. Although these angiographic studies do not provide all of the information present on cut film studies, very frequently MRA comes quite close. Aneurysms as small as 3 mm have been visualized, and cervical carotid and intracranial stenosis also can be seen. The precise indications remain to be determined for MRA, but is seems very likely that these studies will supplement and, in some cases, supplant standard angiographic examinations. Magnetic resonance imaging of the spine has now shown the spinal canal, intervertebral disk, and paravertebral structures with great reliability. It appears that nerve roots can be visualized for clinical studies as well. Very often it is possible to omit myelography and proceed with surgery.

Skull base surgery is advancing rapidly but still seeks precise indications. Dolenc has established cavernous sinus surgery to be as safe and often as effective as skull base surgery, but as Al-Mefty notes, cranial nerve palsies (which can occur in up to 30% of patients with tumors in the cavernous sinus) are highly undesirable. New understanding of skull base anatomy and the application of microsurgical techniques have led to the remarkable skull base bypass (saphenous interposition between petrous and supraclinoid internal carotid artery) reported by Fukushima. These surgical procedures are remarkable technical tours de force, but indications have yet to be established.

Radiosurgery is coming into its own. With the increasing use of radiosurgery by heavy ion, gamma knife, and linear accelerator technique, substantial numbers of good results are being reported in a variety of conditions. This YEAR BOOK reviews good results from radiosurgery applied to meningiomas, metastases, and arteriovenous malformations. Here again, indications remain to be established. In a number of cases the interesting problem arises of whether "radical" skull base surgery or "conservative" radiosurgery can offer the best results. Only properly designed scientific clinical trials can give relevant answers.

Endovascular technique continues its astounding ascent. Perhaps most spectacular is development of the Gulielmi detachable coil, a soft, pliable wire coil device that seems very promising for the thrombosis of aneurysms. Theron's new angioplasty system for carotid stenosis has posted encouraging results. Zeumer's group has reported good results for intra-arterial thrombolysis of intracranial emboli. Hieshima's team has reported encouraging results after the endovascular treatment of dural arteriovenous malformations.

Robert M. Crowell, M.D.

14 Diagnostics

MRI

Fast Imaging
Hesselink JR, Martin JF, Edelman RR (Univ of California, San Diego; Harvard Med School)
Neuroradiology 32:348–355, 1990   14–1

Gradient-echo (GRE) pulse sequences represent a useful adjunct to standard spin-echo sequencing in MRI of the brain and spine. Gradient-echo techniques enhance the signals of flowing fluids and make vascular lesions more conspicuous. In addition, they demonstrate chronic hemorrhage and calcification more sensitively. Steady-state methods produce a myelographic effect that helps in assessing spinal degenerative disorders.

Both acute and chronic hemorrhage are paramagnetic and produce marked magnetic susceptibility effects. A small hemosiderin deposit may be the only evidence of an old contusion or a cryptic arteriovenous malformation. If there is calcification, hypointense areas on GRE sequences match the hyperdense areas on CT scans. Rapid MRI helps to image vascular structures by both detecting chronic hemorrhage and sensitively demonstrating blood flow. Also, GRE sequencing is helpful in cases of suspected arterial occlusion.

Gradient-echo scans of the spine are less sensitive to CSF motion than T2-weighted spin-echo images and have a better signal-to-noise ratio for a given imaging time. Further, GRE images are especially helpful in evaluating the cervical spine, where effacement of the hyperintense thecal sac demonstrates any abnormality within the spinal canal.

▶ The fast MR scanning technique of GRE imaging is quite useful to enhance the signal of flowing fluids and to increase the conspicuousness of vascular lesions. This approach is particularly warranted for angiographically occult lesions and sinus thrombosis.— R.M. Crowell, M.D.

The Clinical Applications of Echo Planar Imaging in Neuroradiology
Worthington BS, Mansfield P (Univ of Nottingham, England)
Neuroradiology 32:367–370, 1990   14–2

A complete examination by conventional MRI methods may take as long as 1 hour. The total examination time is drastically reduced with ultra–high-speed echo planar imaging (EPI). Also, EPI allows dynamic phenomena, such as flow in the vascular and CSF compartments of the brain, to be studied in real time.

With EPI, a complete 2-dimensional image may be acquired in a single shot lasting for 64–128 ms. The whole k-space is sampled as a continuous trajectory. A train of gradient echoes, each corresponding to a line in the k-plane, is formed by a rapidly switching G_y frequency-encoding gradient. In 128 ms plus the inversion time, EPI can obtain high-quality 128 × 128 transverse axial inversion recovery images.

The results currently obtained by EPI compare favorably with those of MRI. Benefits of EPI include speed, the ability to study CSF dynamics in real time, better patient tolerance, and elimination of the need to sedate children undergoing the procedure.

▶ Our neuroradiologic colleagues come up with adaptations of MRI practically every month. According to the experts, EPI has the advantages of speed, assessment of CSF dynamics in real time, better patient tolerance, and elimination of the need to sedate children. Practical experience in the field by neuroclinicians is needed to confirm this encouraging report.—R.M. Crowell, M.D.

MR Imaging of Brain Surface Structures: Surface Anatomy Scanning (SAS)
Katada K (Fujita Health Univ Hosp, Toyoake, Japan)
Neuroradiology 32:439–448, 1990   14–3

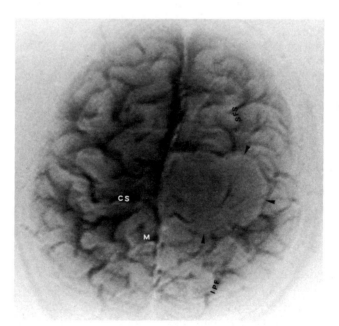

Fig 14–1.—Meningioma in the high parietal region. On parietal SAS image, right precentral and postcentral gyrus cannot be identified because of compression of the large parasagittal meningioma (*arrowheads*). (Courtesy of Katada K: *Neuroradiology* 32:439–448, 1990.)

Surface anatomy scanning (SAS) is an MRI technique that permits direct, noninvasive visualization of brain surface structures. It is based on a long echo time of more than 200 ms, long recovery time spin-echo sequencing, and thick slices.

Sixty-seven patients were examined by SAS, including 16 with intracranial neoplasms and 9 with cerebral infarction. All but 9 of 85 brain images were of good quality. Intracranial lesions were accurately localized by SAS in 37 of 55 cases (Fig 14–1). Abnormal gyral patterns were detected in 5 of 6 patients suspected of having migration anomalies. The examination was helpful in planning surgery in several instances. Among the lesions detected, in addition to stroke tumor, were vascular malformations and focal brain damage.

Cortical sulci and gyri are demonstrated effectively by SAS. Most of the sulci and fissures of the brain surface are clearly visualized by this technique. Surface anatomy scanning is contraindicated when a cardiac pacemaker or surgical clips are present. A severe mass effect can obliterate the sulci and thereby impede visualization of a lesion. Nearly all MR systems can be equipped with SAS without having to modify the hardware.

▶ The special MR technique of SAS seems helpful in the localization of cortical and subcortical lesions, particularly around the motor strip.—R.M. Crowell, M.D.

Magnetic Resonance Imaging of Optic Nerve Meningiomas: Enhancement With Gadolinium-DTPA

Zimmerman CF, Schatz NJ, Glaser JS (Univ of Miami)
Ophthalmology 97:585–591, 1990   14–4

Magnetic resonance imaging is starting to replace contrast-enhanced CT as the procedure of choice for assessing intracranial meningiomas. However, some authors believe that MRI is inferior to contrast-enhanced CT in detecting intracranial meningiomas, because these tumors are isomagnetic to brain. Gadolinium-diethylenetriaminepentaacetic acid (Gd-DTPA) is a paramagnetic contrast agent used to enhance MRI in patients who have optic nerve sheath meningiomas with suspected intracranial extension.

Six patients were studied with Gd-DTPA–enhanced MRI. In all 6 patients the intraorbital and intracranial tumors were isointense to cortical gray matter on T1-weighted studies without contrast. After Gd-DTPA, mild enhancement of the intraorbital tumor was seen in 3 patients, and vivid enhancement of the intracranial tumor was seen in 5 patients. The intracranial extension could not be seen definitively on MRI without Gd-DTPA in 4 cases. Two patients had proton density and T2-weighted studies, and the intraorbital tumor remained nearly isointense in both. In 1 case, the intracranial tumor was suggested on T2-weighted studies but was poorly defined.

Both CT and MRI, when used with contrast enhancement, can delineate intraorbital and intracranial optic nerve meningiomas extremely well. Magnetic resonance imaging may permit better visualization of the intracanalicular optic nerve and the optic chiasm, free from bony artifact and with better soft tissue differentiation.

▶ This study illustrates how MRI is attaining study-of-choice status for virtually all intracranial lesions.—R.M. Crowell, M.D.

Magnetic Resonance Imaging With Aneurysmal Subarachnoid Hemorrhage: Comparison With Computed Tomography Scan
Matsumura K, Matsuda M, Handa J, Todo G (Shiga Univ of Med Science, Ohtsu, Japan; Nagahama Red Cross Hosp, Nagahama)
Surg Neurol 34:71–78, 1990   14–5

The MRI findings were reviewed in 27 consecutive patients with aneurysmal subarachnoid bleeding before they underwent surgery and in 33 patients who had undergone direct aneurysm surgery. Large or giant aneurysms were present in 3 patients who had not undergone surgery. Five patients in the surgical group had unruptured aneurysms.

Magnetic resonance imaging proved to be at least as accurate as CT scanning in detecting acute subarachnoid hemorrhage. It was superior to CT in demonstrating both blood in the ventricles or in the posterior fossa subarachnoid space and transependymal migration of the CSF. Ischemic lesions, especially fresh lesions resulting from delayed vasospasm, were much better shown by MRI than by CT. Nonferromagnetic clips did produce significant artifacts, but the areas of artifacts was consistently smaller with MRI and it was possible to assess structures closer to the clips.

Magnetic resonance imaging holds an important place in the management of patients with aneurysmal subarachnoid hemorrhage. In many cases, MRI demonstrates aneurysms more sensitively than CT does, with or without contrast enhancement. Periventricular hyperintensity in the acute phase of subarachnoid hemorrhage often may indicate transependymal migration of CSF.

▶ Once again, a comparative study indicates that MRI is superior to CT in assessment of aneurysmal subarachnoid hemorrhage. Unfortunately, the availability of MRI for immediate scanning is somewhat limited, and often CT scan remains the most convenient method of study.—R.M. Crowell, M.D.

Angiography

Intraoperative Digital Subtraction Angiography and the Surgical Treatment of Intracranial Aneurysms and Vascular Malformations
Martin NA, Bentson J, Viñuela F, Hieshima G, Reicher M, Black K, Dion J, Becker D (Univ of California, Los Angeles)
J Neurosurg 73:526–533, 1990   14–6

Intraoperative digital subtraction angiography was done after 105 operations in 101 patients treated from March 1985 to July 1989 for an intracranial aneurysm or arteriovenous malformation (AVM). Most patients underwent transfemoral selective arterial catheterization. A radiolucent operating table and head-holder were generally used.

Excellent contrast resolution was achieved. The average time needed for the intraoperative examination was 45–60 minutes. In 5 aneurysms the clips were repositioned after angiography showed an inadequate result. A residual malformation nidus and arteriovenous shunting were seen in 5 patients. In all 5 patients, further exploration demonstrated the residual malformation, which then was resected.

Postoperative angiography showed that the intraoperative study was falsely negative in 3 cases. Three studies in patients with AVMs were falsely positive. One patient had a symptomatic cerebral embolism during intraoperative digital subtraction angiography, and 1 had a femoral artery thrombus. Two patients had intracerebral bleeding after operation.

Intraoperative digital subtraction angiography is recommended for use in surgery to excise an intracranial AVM, to treat a large or giant intracranial aneurysm, and to treat an aneurysm in a site in which all adjacent arterial branches may be difficult to visualize well.

Intraoperative Angiography and Temporary Balloon Occlusion Facilitating Surgical Obliteration of a Traumatic Carotid Cavernous Fistula: A Case Report
LeRoux PD, Elliott JP, Eskridge JM, Mayberg M (Univ of Washington)
Surg Neurol 34:260–265, 1990   14–7

Moderate and severe head injuries can be complicated by posttraumatic carotid cavernous fistula (CCF). Management aims for both occlusion of the fistula and maintenance of patency of the internal carotid artery. Traumatic CCF was managed successfully by a direct surgical approach after endovascular balloon occlusion failed.

Woman, 76, experienced a brief loss of consciousness after falling down the stairs. One month later she was hospitalized with a 2-week history of progressive swelling and reduced vision in 1 eye. Computed tomography showed a left globe markedly proptotic with posterior tenting. There was periorbital edema and swelling of the intraorbital contents and extraocular muscles, with prominent distention of the superior ophthalmic vein. Cerebral angiography showed a slow-flow carotid cavernous fistula. Many attempts at balloon occlusion were made, but all failed because of the small fistula opening and relatively slow flow. A direct surgical approach was then attempted. Intraoperative angiography enabled surgical identification of the fistula and confirmation of its obliteration. Temporary balloon occlusion of the cavernous carotid artery facilitated dissection, bleeding control, and carotid blood flow.

In this case, a traumatic CCF was treated successfully with surgery after failed endovascular balloon occlusion. The combination of surgery, intraoperative angiography, and interventional radiology may improve the outcome of intracavernous vascular lesion treatment.

Selective Cerebral Intraarterial DSA: Complication Rate and Control of Risk Factors

Grzyska U, Freitag J, Zeumer H (Univ Clinic Hamburg–Eppendorf, Germany)
Neuroradiology 32:296–299, 1990   14–8

Approximately 2,800 cerebral vessels were examined by digital subtraction angiography (DSA) in 1,095 consecutive patients. The procedure incorporated intra-arterial contrast injection and on-line digital imaging, which lowers the intravascular evaluation time. The contrast agent was 150 mg of iodine per millimeter of Iopromide. Comparable numbers of patients were assessed for tumor, intracranial hemorrhage, or suspected aneurysm-malformation, and ischemic cerebrovascular disease.

The incidence of persistent neurologic deficit in this series was .09%. Another .45% of patients had transient deficits. The overall complication rate was .9%. No patient required surgical evaluation of hematoma. The only persistent neurologic deficit was hemianopia.

Careful supervision of trainees will limit complications from DSA. The average fluoroscopy time per vessel is a useful measure of a given radiologist's investigational skill. This represents the time the catheter is in possibly dangerous regions.

▶ This remarkable study indicated a single persistent neurologic deficit in 1,095 patients (.09%). The authors ascribe this very low complication rate to technical progress in the area of DSA operator experience and the use of iso-osmotic contrast media. They also suggest the use of fluoroscopy time per vessel as an objective measure of neuroradiologic expertise.—R.M. Crowell, M.D.

Ultrasound

Transcranial Doppler in the Evaluation of Vasospasm After Subarachnoid Hemorrhage

Kaech DL, Despland PA, de Tribolet N (Ctr Hosp Univ Vaudois, Lausanne, Switzerland)
Neurochirurgie 36:279–286, 1990   14–9

Changes in cerebral blood flow velocity (BFV) determined with transcranial Doppler ultrasonography are used in the diagnosis of cerebrovascular disorders. After subarachnoid hemorrhage, an increase in BFV in the middle cerebral artery to more than 100 cm/s is considered diagnostic for vasospasm. A recent study reported that a 25% reduction in the arterial diameter of the middle cerebral artery corresponds with a 56% reduction in vessel lumen, resulting in a 178% compensatory increase in BFV. However, this compensatory increase in BFV can occur only if the peripheral and collateral vessels have normal vasodilatory capacity. Compensatory increases in BFV also may be limited by stenosis or spasm of the internal carotid artery.

To determine how transcranial Doppler ultrasound BFV measurements correlate with clinical and angiographic findings after subarachnoid hemorrhage, 33 men and 32 women aged 20–73 years were monitored 4–7 times per week. The patients were divided into 4 groups: 18 had BFVs of less than 100 cm/s; 19 had BFVs of 100–150 cm/s; 23 had BFVs of 150–200 cm/s; and 5 had BFVs of more than 200 cm/s. Angiographic data were available for 61 patients. Before operation, 7 patients died; 49 patients underwent craniotomy for clipping of an aneurysm, and 9 patients had subarachnoid hemorrhage of unknown origin.

After a follow-up period of 3 months to 2 years, 37 of the 65 patients had good results, 16 had permanent neurologic deficits, and 12 died. There was angiographic evidence of vasospasm in 17 patients. The BFVs correlated closely with angiographic findings, eliminating the need for preoperative angiography. But the BFVs did not correlate with clinical status, except in patients with BFVs of more than 200 cm/s and in patients who had an increase in BFV of at least 100 cm/s within 3 days. Transcranial ultrasonography underestimated the extent of vasospasm of the middle cerebral artery if associated vasospasm of the internal carotid artery was present. In a few patients with loss of autoregulation, a neurologic deficit was present after a hypotensive phase, BFVs remained within the normal range. Doppler ultrasound had limited relevance in patients without vasospasm and in patients with asymptomatic vasospasm. Future transcranial Doppler studies should include monitoring of the pulsatility index.

▶ This is another study demonstrating a close correlation of cerebral BFV as determined by transcranial Doppler ultrasonography and angiographic findings of vasospasm. This supports the concept that transcranial Doppler can be used in evaluation of patients with vasospasm.

In our clinic we have adopted the use of transcranial Doppler ultrasonography to watch for spasm in patients thought, on the basis of early CT scanning after subarachnoid hemorrhage, to have a high likelihood of intracranial vasospasm. We also use this technique to monitor patients under treatment for vasospasm (hypertension, hypervolemia, hemodilution). On the other hand, if a patient is to undergo angioplasty, we use cerebral angiography to monitor the patient both before and after that procedure.—R.M. Crowell, M.D.

Imaging of Cerebral Arterio-Venous Malformations by Transcranial Colour-Coded Real-Time Sonography
Becker GM, Winkler J, Hoffmann E, Bogdahn U (Julius-Maximilians-Univ Würzburg, Germany)
Neuroradiology 32:280–288, 1990   14–10

Transcranial color-coded real-time sonography (TCCS) can provide 2-dimensional sonograms of the parenchyma and vascular cerebrum in most individuals. The results of TCCS examination were reviewed in 2 patients aged 22 and 31 who had intracranial arteriovenous malformations (AVMs). The patients were examined with an ultrasound phased-array system with a 3.5-MHz phased-array transducer and a 2.25-MHz transducer, both with a scanning range of 90 degrees. Perception of the Doppler frequency spectrum and the B-mode image were analyzed simultaneously.

In the 2-dimensional B-mode image, the AVMs were depicted as echodense areas with interspersed zones of lower density. The images correlated well with findings on MRI. Major afferent feeding vessels, venous drainage, and vascular convolution of the lesions were shown clearly by color coding of the intravascular flow phenomena. The blood supply of the angioma from the contralateral internal carotid artery and other hemodynamic information was well demonstrated by color coding of intravascular flow direction, which included analysis of the Doppler frequency spectrum. Transcranial color-coded sonography findings agreed with those of angiography in both cases.

Transcranial color-coded sonography is a noninvasive, mobile, and rapid technique for diagnosis and follow-up of cerebral AVMs. It may also be useful in disclosing the main complications of such lesions. Future applications of TCCS may include screening and follow-up of long-term results of therapy.

Cerebral Blood Flow Velocities in the Anterior Cerebral Arteries and Basilar Artery in Hydrocephalus Before and After Treatment
Nishimaki S, Yoda H, Seki K, Kawakami T, Akamatsu H, Iwasaki Y (Japanese Red Cross Med Ctr, Tokyo)
Surg Neurol 34:373–377, 1990   14–11

Doppler sonographic measurements of cerebral blood flow velocities are useful in evaluating the need or effect of ventriculoperitoneal shunt operations in hydrocephalus. Cerebral blood flow velocity studies with pulsed Doppler sonography were performed on 11 occasions in 7 patients with hydrocephalus to evaluate the need of treatment accurately, even in mild progressive hydrocephalus. Pourcelot's index of resistance (PI), which shows cerebral vascular resistance, was measured in the anterior cerebral arteries (ACA) and basilar artery (BA) before and after shunting or drainage procedures, and the PI ratio (PI-ACA/PI-BA) was calculated.

Mean values of the PI-ACA, PI-BA, and PI ratios before treatment were significantly higher than after treatment and those in normal infants. Before treatment, the mean value of PI-ACA was significantly higher than that of PI-BA. After treatment, the mean value of PI-ACA was significantly less than that of PI-BA, for a 16% decrease in the PI-ACA value in contrast to only an 11% decrease in the PI-BA value. All PI ratios were at least 1 (mean, 1.03) before treatment and decreased to less than 1 (mean, .96) afterward and in normal infants. The mean PI ratio before treatment was significantly higher after treatment and that in normal infants. These data show that the PI ratio is a useful tool for evaluating the need or effect of treatment in hydrocephalus.

▶ These are interesting observations, indicating that the index of resistance in the ACA dropped by 16% after ventriculoperitoneal shunting, whereas the same index in the BA dropped by only 11%. The precise meaning of such changes remains to be clarified. Further studies are needed to establish the role of this sort of study in the clinical evaluation of patients undergoing ventriculoperitoneal shunting.— R.M. Crowell, M.D.

Cerebral Blood Flow

Sequential Changes of Cerebral Blood Flow After Aneurysmal Subarachnoid Haemorrhage

Matsuda M, Shiino A, Handa J (Shiga Univ of Med Science, Ohtsu, Japan)
Acta Neurochir (Wien) 105:98–106, 1990   14–12

The reduction of cerebral blood flow (CBF) after subarachnoid hemorrhage correlates with the severity of neurologic deficits. To examine specific sequential changes in CBF and relate them to outcome, 226 CBF measurements were performed in 96 patients with aneurysmal subarachnoid hemorrhage. Factors analyzed included preoperative neurologic grade, symptomatic vasospasm, and patient age. Factors were related to good, fair, or poor outcome. The remote effect of subarachnoid hemorrhage on CBF in some patients with good outcome also was studied.

Global CBF was significantly reduced during the first week after subarachnoid hemorrhage. Patients with good outcomes had less reduction in CBF than did those with fair or poor outcomes. Patients with good outcomes had progressive improvement in CBF during the subsequent 3 weeks. In a few of these patients the CBF decreased further during the second week but increased steadily thereafter. In contrast, patients with fair or poor outcomes had CBF well below normal values for at least 3 months after subarachnoid hemorrhage. Older age also correlated with persistently reduced CBF for as long as 1 year after subarachnoid hemorrhage.

Older patients require special management, even when they are in apparently good clinical condition, as the CBF threshold to ischemia diminishes with age. Single-photon and positron tomography and stable-xenon CT should provide more detailed information about regional CBF changes that could be helpful in the management of patients with subarachnoid hemorrhage and cerebrovascular disease in general.

▶ This interesting and informative report describes multiple serial CBF studies done with xenon washout technique on patients after subarachnoid hemorrhage. Not surprisingly, the investigators report diminished CBF after subarachnoid hemorrhage in patients in good condition as well as in those with severe neurologic deficit. In the weeks following subarachnoid hemorrhage there was a tendency to return toward normal in patients with mild deficit and even in those who had symptomatic vasospasm. Of rather substantial interest is the fact that older patients had a clearly different CBF pattern as compared with younger patients. Statistically significant differences between blood flow in patients younger than 60 years and older than 60 years were demonstrated at all times following subarachnoid hemorrhage, but particularly in the 2 weeks after the event. In light of the concept that the CBF threshold for ischemia diminishes with age, this is particularly ominous for patients in this older age group.

This is a nice demonstration of how CBF determinations may be helpful in the study of patients with subarachnoid hemorrhage and in their clinical management. Incidentally, Yonas and colleagues at Pittsburgh have established that such studies can be performed reliably in a standard CT scanner, with good reproducibility and regionality.— R.M. Crowell, M.D.

Continuous Postoperative Monitoring of Cortical Blood Flow and Intracranial Pressure
Carter LP, Grahm T, Bailes JE, Bichard W, Spetzler RF (Univ of Arizona, Tucson; Barrow Neurological Inst, Phoenix)
Surg Neurol 35:36–39, 1991   14–13

A technique was developed for continuous postoperative monitoring of cortical blood flow (CoBF) and intracranial pressure. The thermal diffusion CoBF monitoring system consists of a CoBF probe with a pressure port for monitoring intracranial pressure in the subarachnoid space. The flow probe with pressure port is left in contact with the cortex after closing the craniotomy. Previous experimental studies have confirmed the accuracy of this system compared with radioactive xenon clearance and hydrogen clearance methods for measuring CoBF. A total of 32 patients undergoing craniotomies for aneurysm, arteriovenous malformations (AVMs), tumor, or trauma were monitored.

Technique.—The probe is placed on the cortex in a region of interest away from any major vessel, usually in the territory of the ipsilateral middle cerebral artery, and tied in place with a suture through the dura mater or the scalp. The probe is left resting on the cortex at closing of the craniotomy. On completion of monitoring, the probe is removed from the scalp as if removing a subdural drain. Postoperative monitoring is continued for 2–4 days.

Two severely head-injured patients had flows approaching 0 and were eventually declared brain dead. Correlation with stable xenon was not possible because of the variability of cortical flow and the artifact created by the metal probe. This technique may benefit patients with aneurysmal subarachnoid hemorrhage, AVMs, brain tumors, or head trauma, as acute reductions in postoperative blood flow from vasospasm, edema, or reduced perfusion pressure are readily detected and the effects of treatment can be observed easily.

▶ This interesting technique correlated both cerebral blood flow and intracranial pressure in postoperative neurosurgical patients. The advantage of the technique is its ability to sequentially monitor regional cerebral blood flow and intracranial pressure over time. This would be of obvious advantage in assessing the impact of various interventions, e.g., hypertension, hemodilution, alteration of Pco_2, and the like. The disadvantage of the technique is its lack of spatial resolution—that is to say, one is able to monitor only a single point at a time and important changes outside the field of study could be missed. Thus correlation with spatially sensitive techniques, such as stable xenon washout, would be particularly appropriate. Future application will give some further idea of the usefulness of this particular approach.—R.M. Crowell, M.D.

Monitoring of Cortical Blood Flow During Temporary Arterial Occlusion in Aneurysm Surgery by the Thermal Diffusion Method
Ohmoto T, Nagao S, Mino S, Fujiwara T, Honma Y, Ito T, Ohkawa M (Kagawa Med School, Kagawa, Japan)
Neurosurgery 28:49–55, 1991   14–14

When temporary arterial occlusion is necessary during aneurysm surgery, the consequent reduction in cerebral blood flow varies with the collateral circulation. Cortical flow was monitored during operation in 12 patients who had surgery for ruptured aneurysms of the anterior circulation and required temporary arterial clipping. A thermal diffusion flow probe was used. In all cases, surgery was done within 10 days of onset of subarachnoid bleeding.

Cortical flow was most reduced with clipping of the middle cerebral artery. Transient hyperflow followed the release of arterial occlusion. In occluding the common carotid and intracranial carotid, cortical blood flow decreased from 60% to 80% of the baseline value. One patient had an ischemic infarction when the cortical flow was 30 mL/100 g/min and another had infarction when occlusion for 23 minutes produced a cortical flow of 34 mL/100 g/min.

Monitoring the cortical blood flow allows dissection to be expedited when flow values fall to less than 30 mL/100 g/min. Direct measurements of cortical flow can help to determine the time that temporary occlusion of a major artery will be tolerated.

Other

Complications of Lateral C1–2 Puncture Myelography
Katoh Y, Itoh T, Tsuji H, Matsui H, Hirano N, Kitagawa H (Toyama Med and Pharmaceutical Univ, Toyama, Japan)
Spine 15:1085–1087, 1990   14–15

Lateral C1–C2 puncture myelography is a widely used investigative procedure for cervical spinal cord disorders. The technical complications of the procedure were evaluated in 112 patients who underwent lateral C1–C2 puncture myelography in a 5-year period.

Technical complications occurred in 10 patients (9%). Spinal cord puncture and dye injection were the most serious complications and occurred because of inappropriate handling of the needle during dye injection in 3 patients. Puncture between the occiput and C1 occurred in 3 patients, all in the neck hyperextension position. In these patients the puncture level was misconceived between the occiput and C1 because the axis of the x-ray beam was not directed parallel to the coronal axis of the atlas. Injection of dye into the epidural space occurred in 3 patients, and extradural vertebral venous plexus puncture occurred in 1.

Because lateral C1–C2 puncture may cause major vessel injury in cases of anomalous vertebral or posterior inferior cerebellar arteries, a review of 164 vertebral angiograms was undertaken. The vertebral arteries were located anterior to the spinal canal at the C1–C2 level in 96% of radiographs. However, the vertebral artery passed over the middle area of the C1–C2 canal in 2% and was in the posterior one third of the spinal canal in another 2%. The incidence of vertebral artery puncture may depend on its meandering with cervical rotation and mobility. Thus, a lateral C1–C2 puncture to the anterior third of the subarachnoid space carries the most dangerous risk of vascular injury.

Technical complications of lateral C1–C2 puncture myelography include spinal cord puncture and contrast injection, puncture between the occiput and C1, and blood vessel puncture. These complications depend largely on the positioning of the patient's neck (hyperextension) and misdirection of the x-ray beam.

▶ This interesting report documents that serious neurologic complications can occur with C1–C2 puncture for myelography. With the advent of modern contrast materials, the frequency of serious reactions from myelography has become extremely low. However, utilization of this method by personnel who may be less familiar with C1–C2 puncture suggests that the technique be restricted to those with suitable training and experience. Ordinarily, the best technique is puncture ventral to the spinal cord with patients in the supine position. Only meticulous care in the details of this puncture will yield satisfactory results.—R.M. Crowell, M.D.

Cerebrospinal Fluid Endothelin-1 and Endothelin-3 Levels in Normal and Neurosurgical Patients: A Clinical Study and Literature Review
Kraus GE, Bucholz RD, Yoon K-W, Knuepfer MM, Smith KR Jr (St Louis Univ)
Surg Neurol 35:20–29, 1991   14–16

Endothelins are a recently discovered family of structurally related, potent, long-lasting vasoconstrictor peptides. Human plasma endothelin-1 (ET-1) and endothelin-3 (ET-3) levels have been determined in health and disease. Levels of ET-1 and ET-3 in the CSF were measured in 5 different groups of patients: 24 normal patients undergoing myelography for back or neck pain, 4 patients with subarachnoid hemorrhage, 2 with severe head injury, 2 who underwent temporal lobectomy for intractable epilepsy, and 1 who sustained a gunshot wound to the spine with ensuing paraplegia. Of the 2 patients with severe head trauma, 1 died 30 minutes after the CSF sample was obtained. All CSF samples were analyzed by radioimmunoassay.

The mean CSF ET-1 concentration in normal controls was 20.2 pg/cm^3 (range, 11.8−28.2 pg/cm^3). The mean CSF ET-3 concentration in normal controls was 31.6 pg/cm^3 (range, 16−62 pg/cm^3). Patients with subarachnoid hemorrhage had significantly increased ET-3 levels compared with control values. Values of CSF ET-1 in these patients did not differ significantly from control values. None of the other patients had statistically significant differences in ET-1 or ET-3 values compared with controls.

Increased ET-3 levels in the CSF appeared to correlate with neurologic deterioration and, in patients with subarachnoid hemorrhage, with evidence of vasospasm and cerebral ischemia. Although both trauma patients had extremely poor neurologic outcomes and increased ET-3 levels in the CSF, the difference did not reach statistical significance. Further study is needed to determine whether ET-3 is a causative factor promoting neuronal damage, or is an epiphenomenon.

▶ Endothelin is a naturally occurring vasoconstrictor peptide that has been found in relation to vasospasm. This study demonstrates that CSF levels of ET-3 are elevated in patients with symptomatic cerebrovascular vasospasm, but not in controls. Further studies are required to determine whether this agent is causally related to vasospasm as well, and whether such determinations might have clinical usefulness.—R.M. Crowell, M.D.

15 Techniques

Direct Surgery

The Transoral Approach for the Management of Intradural Lesions at the Craniovertebral Junction: Review of 7 Cases
Crockard HA, Sen CN (Natl Hosps for Nervous Diseases, London; Univ of Pittsburgh)
Neurosurgery 28:88–98, 1991   15–1

Intradural lesions ventral to the neuraxis of the craniovertebral junction (CVJ) are relatively inaccessible. Data were reviewed on 7 patients with lesions confined to the intradural space in whom surgery was performed through the transoral route. This approach provides an unencumbered but circumscribed view of the ventral aspect of the CVJ without the necessity for brain retraction. There were schwannomas in 2 patients, meningiomas in 3, an aneurysm of the anterior inferior cerebellar artery in 1, and neurenteric cyst in 1.

Technique.—Patients were placed in a left lateral decubitus position with the head slightly extended. Various methods were used to deal with the soft and hard palates. The posterior pharyngeal mucosa was incised in the midline, with the tubercle of the atlas used as a landmark. Then muscles were elevated from the anterior surface of the clivus, the anterior arch of C1, and the anterior surface of C2.

Both patients with schwannomas were without recurrence at 3 years and 6 years postoperatively, but 2 of 3 patients with meningiomas died, and the th.rd had evidence of tumor growth. In the remaining patients, 1 had abducens palsy that resolved within 4 months postoperatively, and the other had normal neurologic findings at 4-month follow-up. Cerebrospinal fluid leakage in 3 patients was caused by either malfunction of the lumbar drain or the lumboperitoneal shunt, and 3 had difficulties caused by velopharyngeal incompetence. Posterior spinal fusions were necessary in 2 patients after tumor removal; 2 other patients had slight anterior slippage that did not require fusion.

Schwannomas and aneurysms are amenable to cure by the transoral approach. Preoperatively, patients should undergo external carotid and vertebral arteriography. Meningiomas are difficult to remove by this approach, however. Postoperative measures should include the use of fibrin adhesive and prolonged CSF hypotension to avoid CSF leakage. In se

213

lected patients, morbidity from the transoral approach can be kept within acceptable limits.

▶ This interesting review of 7 cases adds intradural lesions to the cranioverte-bral pathology treated by the authors using the transoral approach. Thus a very extensive background with this kind of surgery is available to the authors.

As documented here, the ventral approach to the clivus allows for direct vi-sualization and extirpation of tumors. Problems of wound closure, CSF leakage, and meningitis required vigorous efforts with fibrin glue sealant, multilayer clo-sure, and CSF diversion. Gram-negative meningitis complicated some cases. It is clear that there is merit to this general approach for the most satisfactory exposure of certain midline intradural tumors. It is also abundantly clear that this is very difficult surgery and should be limited to surgeons with special ex-perience in this area.

With regard to the basilar-AICA aneurysm, only 1 angiographic view is pro-vided, but this suggests that a far lateral suboccipital approach or combined supra/infratentorial approach with tentorial section might also have provided good exposure of this lesion for clip obliteration.— R.M. Crowell, M.D.

Surgical Approach to a Large Basilar Artery Bifurcation and Upper Basilar Trunk Aneurysm: Case Report
Lupret V, Vidović D, Negovetić L, Novak M (Clinical Hosp "Dr M Stojanović"; Central Inst for Tumors and Allied Diseases, Zagreb, Yugoslavia)
Surg Neurol 33:404–406, 1990   15–2

Basilar artery aneurysms constitute 5% of all aneurysms. Multiple an-eurysms involving the basilar artery bifurcation, P1 segment of the poste-rior cerebral artery, and the superior cerebellar artery have not been re-ported. A double aneurysm of the basilar artery was observed at the basi-lar artery bifurcation and upper basilar artery trunk between the poste-rior cerebral artery and superior cerebellar artery.

Woman, 49, was admitted because of sudden onset of headache followed by nausea, vomiting, and left oculomotor nerve palsy. Computed tomography showed a hyperdense region in the ambient cistern highly suggestive of a basilar artery aneurysm. Four-vessel angiography revealed 2 aneurysms, 1 at the basilar artery bifurcation oriented superiorly and the other at the P1 segment of the pos-terior cerebral artery and superior cerebellar artery on the left side, posterolater-ally oriented. They measured 1.5 × 1.2 cm and 1.2 × .8 cm, respectively. A left pterional craniotomy was done, and the aneurysms were clipped successfully. The patient was able to resume normal activities.

This is the first reported case of multiple basilar artery aneurysms at the basilar artery bifurcation and the upper basilar artery trunk. A pteri-onal approach from the left side provided enough exposure of the neu-rovascular relationships and enough maneuverability to dissect and oc-clude both aneurysms.

Surgical Approaches to the Cavernous Sinus: A Microsurgical Study

Inoue T, Rhoton AL Jr, Theele D, Barry ME (Univ of Florida)

Neurosurgery 26:903–932, 1990

15–3

Various surgical approaches to the cavernous sinus were investigated in 25 adult cadaver heads, using magnification of 3 times to 40 times. Bony relationships were assessed in dry human skulls.

Methods. The superior intradural approach is directed through a frontotemporal craniotomy and the roof of the cavernous sinus. This procedure may be combined with an extradural approach to remove the anterior clinoid process and unroof the optic canal and orbit. The superomedial approach is directed through a supraorbital craniotomy and subfrontal exposure of the sinus wall adjacent to the pituitary gland. A lateral intradural approach is directed below the temporal lobe to the lateral wall of the cavernous sinus. The lateral extradural approach exposes the internal carotid artery in the floor of the middle fossa proximal to the cavernous sinus. An inferomedial operation exposes the medial sinus wall by the transnasal-transsphenoidal route. There also is a combined lateral and inferolateral approach in which the infratemporal fossa is opened to expose the full course of the petrous carotid artery and the lateral wall of the cavernous sinus.

The site and type of lesion dictates the approach to the cavernous sinus; no single method can provide access to all parts of it. The superior approach is best for the anterior vertical and clinoid segments and the anterior parts of the lateral and posterosuperior venous spaces. A lateral approach best exposes the lateral surface of the posterior vertical and horizontal segments and the lower part of the anterior bend, as well as the cranial nerves in the sinus wall. It also provides good visualization of the origin of the meningohypophyseal trunk and the artery of the inferior cavernous sinus.

▶ Since the pioneering work of Dolenc, neurosurgeons have increased dramatically the frequency and extent of microsurgery in the cavernous sinus, formerly considered an inviolate structure. Excellent results have been obtained, especially in attack on cavernous carotid aneurysms and certain tumors involving the cavernous sinus. The precise indications, however, for such cavernous procedures remain to be well defined, especially in view of the existence of alternative therapies, e.g., balloon catheter occlusion of the internal carotid artery for cavernous aneurysms, with or without bypass grafting.

For the surgeon bold enough to enter this area, mastery of the local anatomy is critical. This comprehensive microsurgical opus from Rhoton's group provides the neuroanatomical basis of knowledge for such approaches to the cavernous sinus. In addition to the narrative provided by this important report, the prospective cavernous microsurgeon also should obtain hands-on, personal, direct experience in the autopsy laboratory before embarking on such an ambitious mode of surgery.— R.M. Crowell, M.D.

Neurovascular Methods

Exposure of the Intracavernous Carotid Artery in Aneurysm Surgery

Ohmoto T, Nagao S, Mino S, Ito T, Honma Y, Fujiwara T (Kagawa Med School, Japan)
Neurosurgery 28:317–324, 1991   15–4

For aneurysms at the site at which the internal carotid artery (ICA) penetrates the roof of the cavernous sinus, the roof is the most difficult obstacle to surgical exposure. There are various approaches to proximal intradural and distal intracavernous aneurysms of the ICA.

Seven consecutive patients seen in a 4-year period had direct surgery of ICAs necessitating exposure of the extradural portion of the ICA by incision of the roof of the cavernous sinus. Four patients had large carotid-ophthalmic aneurysms with the neck attached to the roof of the cavernous sinus, 2 had aneurysms arising from the siphon knee with the dome pointing upward and extending into the carotid cistern, and 1 had a giant carotid-ophthalmic aneurysm extending deeply into the cavernous sinus with an extradural origin of the carotid artery. Four carotid-ophthalmic arteries were ruptured.

The pterional intradural approach to the ICA was used. In the 4 pa-

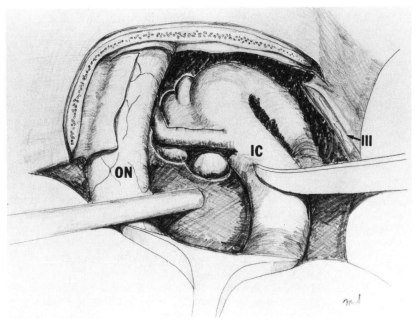

Fig 15–1.—Final exposure of the intracavernous aneurysm. The aneurysm and the horizontal portion of the intracavernous carotid artery were exposed between the optic nerve and the third nerve. The medial wall of the cavernous sinus is covered with oxidized cellulose (*ON*-optic nerve; *IC*-internal carotid artery; *III*-third nerve.) (Courtesy of Ohmoto T, Nagao S, Mino S, et al: *Neurosurgery* 28:317–324, 1991.)

tients with large carotid-ophthalmic aneurysms, the anterior clinoid process and roof of the optic canal were removed, allowing easy access to the pericarotid ring. After dissection of the anteromedial part of this ring to expose the extradural portion of the ICA proximal to the neck and creation of a space between the wall of the cavernous sinus and the extradural portion of the ICA, clipping the neck was easy. In the remaining 2 aneurysms, the optic strut was removed, the lateral wall and roof of the cavernous sinus were opened, and the neck clipped (Fig. 15–1). Wide exposure of the anterior siphon knee was gained by opening the lateral wall anterior to the third nerve. In all 7 cases the operation was successful. One patient was left with a visual field defect, but there were no disturbances of ocular movement.

For proximal intradural and distal intracavernous carotid aneurysms, extended opening of the roof of the cavernous sinus anterior to the posterior clinoid process allows exposure of the horizontal portion of the intracavernous ICA and the entire aspect of the aneurysm. Once exposure is obtained, the operation can proceed easily while the anatomical orientation in the operative field is confirmed.

▶ This very nicely illustrated article demonstrates that intracavernous surgery for aneurysms can be performed very satisfactorily by an intradural approach. The authors demonstrate that for intracavernous carotid and carotid-ophthalmic aneurysms in this area, detailed knowledge of the anatomy of the zone permits removal of the anterior clinoid process and optic strut, with incision of the lateral wall and roof of the cavernous sinus, thus providing wide exposure of the genu and the horizontal portion of the ICA in its intracavernous segment, without injury to the intracavernous structures. The results bespeak success. There is clear advantage to having within the operative field both the aneurysm and proximal control in the event of premature aneurysmal rupture. This is clearly a nice alternative to the extradural Dolenc technique.—R.M. Crowell, M.D.

Petrous Carotid-to-Intradural Carotid Saphenous Vein Graft for Intracavernous Giant Aneurysm, Tumor, and Occlusive Cerebrovascular Disease
Spetzler RF, Fukushima T, Martin N, Zabramski JM (Barrow Neurological Inst, Phoenix; Mitsui Mem Hosp, Tokyo; Univ of California, Los Angeles)
J Neurosurg 73:496–501, 1990   15–5

Internal carotid artery (ICA) occlusion for the management of intracranial aneurysms is associated with both immediate and delayed risks. In 1986, Fukushima performed a petrous carotid (C_5) to intradural ICA (C_3) saphenous vein bypass in a patient to trap a giant cavernous aneurysm. This bypass procedure has since been performed in 15 women and 3 men aged 42–76 years.

Technique.—A saphenous vein graft of sufficient length is harvested from the upper thigh. The proximal portion of the vein provides a good match in diameter for the C_5 and C_3 segments of the ICA. The saphenous vein is anastomosed to the

C_5 portion of the ICA between a temporary proximal clip and a permanent distal clip. In most cases the anastomosis is end to side. The other end of the graft is then anastomosed to the ICA, end to side, between the ophthalmic and posterior communicating arteries. Permanent clips are left distal to the anastomosis and proximal to the ophthalmic artery on the ICA, trapping it in the cavernous sinus. With removal of the temporary clips, the C_5 portion is connected to the C_3 portion by the saphenous vein graft.

The patency rate in this series was 17 of 18 patients. After the bypass, cranial nerve deficits improved significantly in all patients (except in association with radical cavernous sinus resection). The Fukushima bypass technique, with its short, large-caliber venous graft entirely within the skull, has several advantages over other methods and is recommended in patients whose intracavernous ICA must be sacrificed.

▶ The skull-base bypass devised by Fukushima and reported in 18 cases here is a technical tour de force whose place remains to be established. Patency was obtained in 17 of 18 cases, an impressive result. On the other hand, postoperative complications included stroke, temporary left hemiparesis, temporary increase in third nerve palsy, and decreased hearing (2 cases).

This approach should be compared to alternative treatment. Many patients tolerate carotid occlusion with sequelae. Modern testing with tolerance test occlusion by balloon catheter technique can be checked by the clinical response to induced hypotension or by xenon blood-flow determinations, with regard to long-term tolerance. In patients who tolerate test occlusion, the likelihood of late complications is extremely small. In such patients, balloon occlusion of the ICA with a short postocclusion course of heparin constitutes a highly effective and low-risk method of occlusion of the aneurysm. Experience at London (Ontario) and at Massachusetts General Hospital support this point of view. Patients so treated may leave the hospital within 3 or 4 days after the procedure. Interestingly, patients may recover function of cranial nerves in the cavernous sinus after such an approach. In patients who do not tolerate temporary carotid occlusion, obviously, revascularization will be required before occlusion. Whether extracranial-intracranial bypass or C_5–C_3 anastomosis is superior remains to be established by careful follow-up studies.—R.M. Crowell, M.D.

Shunt for Bypass Graft of the Cavernous Carotid Artery: An Anatomical and Technical Study

Al-Mefty O, Khalil N, Elwany MN, Smith RR (Univ of Mississippi)
Neurosurgery 27:721–728, 1990   15–6

The intracavernous carotid artery may be seriously injured in the course of removing a tumor or vascular lesion from the cavernous sinus, or it may have to be totally isolated. A saphenous vein graft bypass of the cavernous carotid artery is a way of reestablishing carotid circulation in this setting. There is, however, a high risk of ischemia if the collateral circulation is poor. In this case the vein bypass may be used for permanent vascularization with carotid cerebral circulation maintained via an operative shunt.

This approach was evaluated in 10 bypass procedures done on 5 cadaver heads. Shunting was from the intrapetrous to the supraclinoid carotid artery with separate arteriotomies (type A); from the intrapetrous to the supraclinoid carotid, using the same arteriotomy for the graft and shunt tube (which passes through the graft), type B; or from the internal carotid in the neck to the supraclinoid carotid (type C).

The type A shunt promptly restores blood flow without the need for additional temporary occlusion, but technical difficulties were sometimes encountered. The type B shunt is more easily introduced, and more space is available; however, it was harder to remove the shunt tube. The type C shunt was the easiest to perform but the added length of the shunt tube is a disadvantage. A balloon shunt may be the best way of securing the shunt and controlling back-bleeding.

A prototype shunt catheter now is available that is similar in concept to the Pruitt-Inahara shunt catheter. In live surgery there will be a risk of cerebral embolization, requiring consideration of heparin treatment.

▶ This imaginative anatomical study demonstrates the possibility of several techniques for revascularization of the internal carotid after occlusion of the cavernous portion of that vessel. A saphenous vein was used as an interposition graft in each case, either from the petrous or the distal cervical carotid artery.

Potential problems with the shunt can be considered an important source of complications with this technique. The use of intraoperative heparin might be considered. Samson has reported such utilization, and we have used it as well, in an effort to maintain normotension during the 2 hours after injection of 5,000 units of heparin USP intravenously. When this is carried out in the early portion of the procedure, we have not found it necessary to reverse the heparin at the end of the operation with external carotid-saphenous-middle cerebral bypass grafts. In 8 cases we have not experienced an intracranial hemorrhage.

The other question that is raised is the need for utilization of a shunt during cross-clamping of the carotid. Preoperative balloon occlusion of the internal carotid can tell one whether the patient actually requires ongoing flow. In only 10% or so of patients will a neurologic deficit be observed during such a maneuver in normotension. This maneuver might be even safer if the patient were monitored with intraoperative EEG to detect any change in electrophysiology during cross-clamping.

Finally, the question of indications for such a procedure remain controversial: In many patients, occlusion of the carotid artery can be carried out with short- or long-term adverse sequelae. In that instance, balloon catheter occlusion might be performed without the need for such a bypass (see Abstract 15–5 on this same general topic). (Then, of course, the patient may not need a bypass.)—R.M. Crowell, M.D.

Effects of Repeated Temporary Clipping of the Middle Cerebral Artery on Pial Artery Diameter, Regional Cerebral Blood Flow, and Brain Structure in Cats

Sakaki T, Tsunoda S, Morimoto T, Ishida T, Sasaoka Y (Nara Med Univ, Kashihara, Nara, Japan)

Neurosurgery 27:914–920, 1990

15–7

Intervals of cerebral ischemia and recirculation may occur occasionally during neurosurgical vascular repair when the major arterial trunk needs to be temporarily clipped to control excessive unexpected bleeding. The effects of single occlusions of varied duration were reported previously in an animal model of cerebral ischemia. The effects of repeated ischemic insults of defined duration and frequency, as would occur with repeated temporary clipping of the major arterial trunk, were assessed.

In the first experiment, a single 20-minute or 1-hour occlusion of the middle cerebral artery was performed in each of 5 cats. In addition to direct observation of cerebral edema and infarction, video imaging was used to determine the pial arterial diameter, and autoradiography was used to measure regional cerebral blood flow. After a 20-minute occlusion, no abnormal changes were seen 5 hours after recirculation. After a 1-hour occlusion, pial arteries were dilated by 45% and regional cerebral blood flow had increased to more than twice the resting cortical values.

In the second experiment, three 20-minute occlusions of the middle cerebral artery within a 1-hour interval were performed in 20 cats, of which 10 were given thiopental to protect the brain; 10 were left untreated. In cats without barbiturate protection, the pial arteries were dilated by 40% and regional cerebral blood flow had decreased to about 70% by the end of the experiment. In contrast, there were only trivial changes in cats that had been pretreated with thiopental. Because repeated temporary clipping of the major arterial trunk during neurosurgical operations may cumulatively cause brain damage, leading to postoperative neurologic deficits, barbiturates should always be administered whenever repeated clipping becomes necessary.

▶ This interesting study points out that, in cats, repeated temporary occlusion of the middle cerebral artery for 20 minutes causes pial artery dilation, decreased cerebral blood flow, and brain damage. These changes are not seen with barbiturate treatment. The authors conclude that temporary trunk artery occlusion, if repeated for more than 20 minutes, may lead to brain damage and should be treated with barbiturates.

The results are certainly intriguing. It is not clear whether the damage is caused by microemboli or inadequate perfusion. Moreover, it is not clear that such damage would actually occur in patients undergoing similar treatment. Nonetheless, there is a strong suggestion that prolonged ischemia, even with interruption of occlusion, may be followed by brain damage. Nor is the best treatment obvious: The present study suggests that barbiturates may be quite helpful, bolstering the claims of other authors that this is the best way to protect during temporary occlusion (1). Another approach is the utilization of mannitol, as advocated by Suzuki, which has proved effective in 60 cases treated in our unit.

Nonetheless, the overall message is important: Intermittent vascular occlusion during surgery may lead to more deleterious cerebral ischemia than single continuous vascular occlusion of the same duration.—R.M. Crowell, M.D.

Reference

1. Dermott MW, et al: *Neurosurgery* 25:54, 1989.

Controlled Hypotension With Adenosine or Sodium Nitroprusside During Cerebral Aneurysm Surgery: Effects on Renal Hemodynamics, Excretory Function, and Renin Release

Zäll S, Edén E, Winsö I, Volkmann R, Sollevi A, Ricksten S-E (Univ of Gothenburg; Univ of Stockholm; Sahlgren's Hosp, Gothenburg, Sweden)
Anesth Analg 71:631–636, 1990   15–8

Adenosine can be used to produce controlled hypotension, particularly during cerebral aneurysm surgery. However, in animal experiments, intrarenal infusion of adenosine decreased renal blood flow (RBF), glomerular filtration rate (GFR), and urine flow, and inhibited renin secretion. Fifteen patients with cerebral aneurysm were studied to evaluate their response to adenosine and compare it to the response to sodium nitroprusside (SNP).

Eight patients were randomly assigned to receive adenosine, 20 mmol/L, 5.3 mg/mL in 5% mannitol, and 7 to receive SNP, 100 μg/mL for induced hypotension. Patients were premedicated with diazepam and atropine before induction of anesthesia with thiopental followed by fentanyl. Fentanyl and droperidol were used as required to maintain anesthesia. Mechanical hyperventilation with 70% nitrous oxide was initiated to maintain the PCO_2 at about 30 mm Hg. Measurements of GFR and RBF were made by standard ^{51}Cr-ethylenediaminetetraacetic acid and paraaminohippuric acid renal clearance methods. Blood and urine samples were obtained before and after a dose of mannitol during normotension, during hypotension, and during normotension after clipping of the aneurysm.

Both groups had a 25% to 30% reduction in mean arterial pressure to approximately 60–70 mm Hg during the hypotensive period. Adenosine resulted in a 91% decrease in GFR and a 92% decrease in RBF, along with a pronounced increase in renal vascular resistance. In comparison, SNP reduced GFR by 24% and RBF by 36%, with no effect on renal vascular resistance. Renin secretion was increased by SNP but not by adenosine. The RBF increased over baseline after discontinuation of adenosine but not SNP; the GFR returned to baseline in both groups after discontinuation of the hypotensive agents. Reversible disturbances in atrioventricular conduction occurred in 4 patients given adenosine.

In patients undergoing surgery for cerebral aneurysm, the use of adenosine to induce hypotension prevents renin release and induces a reversible renal vasoconstriction. This vasoconstriction affects mostly the pre-glomerular resistance vessels and thereby decreases RBF and GFR. Aden-osine should be used only for short periods and should not be given to patients with impaired renal function.

▶ These studies demonstrate that adenosine is highly effective in reducing the mean arterial pressure for intracranial aneurysm surgery. On the other hand, this agent reduces the RBF and GFR quite significantly. Thus adenosine should be used for this purpose only briefly, and probably not at all in patients with disturbed renal function.

The potential dangers of this approach are evident. In most patients we cur-rently avoid systemic hypotension and instead utilize temporary intracranial ar-terial clips as needed to protect against aneurysm rupture in the dissection and obliteration of intracranial aneurysms.—R.M. Crowell, M.D.

Electrothrombosis of Saccular Aneurysms Via Endovascular Approach: Part 1. Electrochemical Basis, Technique, and Experimental Results
Guglielmi G, Viñuela F, Sepetka I, Macellari V (Univ of Rome; Univ of California, Los Angeles; Target Therapeutics, San Jose, Calif)
J Neurosurg 75:1–7, 1991   15–9

Intra-aneurysmal electrothrombosis by an endovascular approach be-came feasible when soft microcatheters were developed, as these may be passed atraumatically into an aneurysm. A soft detachable platinum coil, soldered to a stainless steel delivery wire, may be placed within an aneu-rysm in a controlled manner.

Technique.—Angiography is done via the common carotid to explore the an-eurysm, induced in swine by applying a low positive direct current to the delivery guidewire. The tip of a no. 2.2 F microcatheter having a 70- to 90-degree curve is introduced into the aneurysmal neck. Passage of a current detaches the platinum coil within the aneurysm within 4–12 minutes through electrolysis of the steel wire closest to the thrombus-covered coil. With the coil in position, a current of .5–2 mA is applied using a battery-operated generator.

Angiograms obtained 2–6 months after embolization confirmed permanent oc-clusion of the aneurysms as well as patency of the parent vessel. There were no angiographic signs of untoward distal embolization. The coil did not migrate out-side the aneurysm. These preliminary findings suggest that microcatheter-induced electrothrombosis may be a suitable means of occluding intracranial aneurysms without the need for surgery.

Electrothrombosis of Saccular Aneurysms Via Endovascular Approach: Part 2: Preliminary Clinical Experience
Guglielmi G, Viñuela F, Dion J, Duckwiler G (Univ of Rome; Univ of California, Los Angeles)
J Neurosurg 75:8–14, 1991   15–10

Fifteen patients had thrombosis of a high-risk intracranial saccular aneurysm by an endovascular approach, using a detachable platinum coil and intra-aneurysmal electrothrombosis. Several aneurysms were considered to be inoperable, and other patients were medically unsuited to surgery. Five aneurysms involved the basilar bifurcation and 3 were intra-cavernous in location.

From 70% to complete thrombosis was achieved in all patients. In all but 1 the parent artery was preserved. One patient deteriorated temporarily but no permanent neurologic deficit developed, and there were no deaths. In all cases the parts of the aneurysm filled with coils underwent thrombosis.

This approach may prove to be a viable alternative to the treatment of patients with high-risk intracranial saccular aneurysms. Aneurysms may be occluded in the acute phase of subarachnoid hemorrhage. Long-term follow-up is necessary.

▶ Dr. Guglielmi and colleagues have created an extremely exciting new approach: detachable thrombogenic platinum coils that can be extended via endovascular techniques into intracranial aneurysms. This microcoil system has several specific advantages: The coil is very soft (being doubly coiled) and cannot penetrate the aneurysm wall; the mechanical characteristics of the coil permit it to be laid down in a series of loops filling the fundus back to the neck; and the detachable feature permits one to detach the coil completely at the neck of the aneurysm. Also, if the coil is improperly positioned before detachment, it can be removed. Several coils can be positioned within an aneurysm to achieve the desired effect. Postoperative x-ray studies demonstrate that anatomical packing of the lesion, often without chinks, is possible. Experimental work in swine has demonstrated a high effectiveness and low failure rate. Preliminary experience in 15 cases has been very encouraging (now up to 27 cases reported in Boston in June 1991).

In brief, these coils look extremely promising and merit immediate controlled careful evaluation. It is too early to say what the precise indications and limitations may be. It is not too early to say that it seems highly likely that these coils will indeed find a place in the established armamentarium for the treatment of intracranial aneurysms.—R.M. Crowell, M.D.

Endovascular Therapy

Endovascular Treatment of Intracranial Aneurysms: Present and Future From a Series of 92 Cases
George B, Aymard GA, Godin P, Merland J-J, Mourier KL, Cophignon J (Hôp Lariboisière, Paris)
Neurochirurgie 36:273–278, 1990   15–11

Data on 92 patients who underwent endovascular detachable balloon embolization in the treatment of intracranial aneurysms over a 10-year period were reviewed. Of the 92 patients, 48 had embolization of a parent vessel and 44 were treated by selective occlusion of the aneurysm with salvage of the parent vessel. There were 31 giant aneurysms, 38 vertebrobasilar aneurysms, and 27 cavernous carotid aneurysms. Endovascular embolization was limited to patients with inoperable intracranial aneurysms or patients in whom conventional surgery posed too great a risk. In the early years, beginning in 1978, parent vessels were always occluded. Later, selective occlusion was attempted by primary intention and the parent vessel was occluded only when selective occlusion failed. All patients except the last 5 were treated within 3–8 weeks after subarachnoid hemorrhage; the last 5 patients were treated within the first 3 days after subarachnoid hemorrhage.

Of the 48 patients who underwent parent vessel occlusion, 2 died of ischemic complications, 3 had ischemic complications and survived, and 5 had unsatisfactory results because of incomplete occlusion. Of the 44 patients who had selective embolization, 5 died, 3 of aneurysmal rupture during or after balloon placement; 10 had secondary balloon deflation, 2 with severe meningeal hemorrhage; and the procedure failed in 10 patients. The results were rated as good if the aneurysm was no longer visible on arteriography and if there were no serious treatment-associated complications. By this definition, 19 (43%) patients with selective embolization treatment and 41 (85.4%) with parent vessel embolization had good results.

The results obtained in this series should not be compared with those from surgical series, as neither the locations nor the types of aneurysms treated were comparable with those commonly treated by conventional surgery. The aneurysms encountered in this series generally are the most difficult to treat. Whereas these difficult aneurysms normally account for only 3% to 8% in any surgical series, they accounted for more than 65% in this series. Thus the results obtained in this series seem quite acceptable.

▶ This concise article presents the work of Merland and his group in Paris. As stated by the authors, these patients were essentially deemed inoperable, and therefore the results of balloon treatment cannot be compared directly with surgical results. Note that there were 31 giant aneurysms, 38 vertebral basilar aneurysms, and 27 cavernous carotid aneurysms.

There were some spectacular successes with obliteration of inoperable lesions. On the other hand, there were 10 patients whose lesions were impossible to treat. There were 3 fatal ruptures and 2 late deaths among those with intra-aneurysm occlusion. In 10 cases late balloon deflation occurred, in association with subarachnoid hemorrhage in 2. If one considers angiographic obliteration and no early clinical sequelae as a good result, parent vessel occlusion led to 85% good results and intra-aneurysmal occlusion to 43% good results. (Obviously, these 2 figures cannot be compared directly because occlusion of the aneurysm was the principal aim in recent years, with parent vessel occlusion carried out only as a second and last resort.)

These results may be compared with those of endovascular treatment of intracranial aneurysms reported from other centers. Moret has reported successful balloon treatment in more than 100 cases with approximately a 20%

morbidity/mortality rate. Shcheglov has reported more than 700 cases of aneurysmal obliteration, with impressive results in most cases. Hieshima has reported encouraging results using a silicone system in California.

It is of importance to note that most of the treated cases thus far reported in the literature have been patients with aneurysms after subarachnoid hemorrhage or patients with unruptured aneurysms. The present study, however, includes 5 aneurysms that were treated in the first 3 days after subarachnoid hemorrhage, demonstrating that this technique can be applied successfully at this early stage.

Endovascular treatment of aneurysms presents an encouraging possibility for obliteration of these lesions without direct surgery. However, to establish the appropriate role for this approach, precise data are needed regarding efficacy, including long-term studies to assure lasting obliteration and safety. The technique will have to be compared against surgical treatment for aneurysms in similar locations, for difficulty in performance, and for clinical grade. Only in this fashion can we determine precisely the best utilization of endovascular treatment.

An additional chapter in this saga concerns the recent development of thrombogenic coils for endovascular treatment of aneurysms. Hilal coils have serious problems with failure to obliterate and with migration into parent vessels, but the newer coils (Guglielmi Detachable Coils) introduced by Vinuela's group at UCLA appear to be more effective and safer. More experience is needed here.

It is my opinion that the future holds a place for both surgery and the endovascular treatment of aneurysms. Surgery offers the benefits of direct visualization of the aneurysm and its neck for precise obliteration of the entire lesion. Also, multiple aneurysms can be treated in the same sitting. The small aneurysm is rather straightforward to treat. By contrast, endovascular treatment offers the advantage of awake-monitoring of the patient during treatment, enabling one to perform parent-vessel occlusion if required. The larger aneurysms, especially giant aneurysms, are attractive for treatment by endovascular means. There is an obvious advantage of endovascular treatment—a procedure that doesn't involve opening the skull is more acceptable to patients. We must work with our neuroradiologic interventional colleagues to define the appropriate uses for these promising new techniques.—R.M. Crowell, M.D.

Endovascular Occlusion of Vertebral Arteries in the Treatment of Unclippable Vertebrobasilar Aneurysms
Aymard A, Gobin YP, Hodes JE, Bien S, Rüfenacht D, Reizine D, George B, Merland J-J (Univ of Paris VII; Lariboisière Hosp, Paris)
J Neurosurg 74:393–398, 1991   15–12

Technological advances in the endovascular treatment of aneurysms make it possible to occlude either the parent vessel or, selectively, the aneurysmal sac. A group of 121 patients with intracranial aneurysms were treated by the endovascular technique. Twenty-one patients with vertebrobasilar aneurysms were referred for endovascular treatment because of failed surgery, a poor risk for surgery, or unclippable aneurysms. Six patients had sustained subarachnoid hemorrhage, 10 had compressive symptoms secondary to mass effect, 4 had subarachnoid hemorrhage and mass effect, and 1 patient had evidence of medullary stroke.

Thirteen of the 21 patients had good results and 6 had partial thrombosis of their aneurysms. There was 1 treatment failure and 1 death.

Endovascular occlusion, which does not require general anesthesia and allows continuous neurologic monitoring, is a relatively safe and effective alternative for aneurysms untreatable by other means. Test occlusion before balloon detachment can be used to evaluate the clinical reaction to arterial occlusion and to assess the collateral blood supply.

▶ The group from Lariboisiere Hospital in Paris describes their experience with hunterian balloon arterial occlusion of the vertebral artery in patients with unclippable aneurysms. The balloons were placed at the level of C1 or just beyond takeoff of the posterior inferior cerebellar artery. Overall, the results were quite good, with cure in 13 patients and 70% to 80% thrombosis in most of the others. One patient rebled and died, and another in whom occlusion was not possible worsened and died. The treatment was more effective for more proximally located aneurysms, and distal vertebral occlusion appeared to be more effective than proximal. The precise technique for effective tolerance test occlusion has not been established. This experience indicates that vertebral artery occlusion for an unclippable aneurysm is often effective and should be considered when surgery is deemed unsafe.—R.M. Crowell, M.D.

Endovascular Coil Embolization of Unusual Posterior Inferior Cerebellar Artery Aneurysms

Dowd CF, Halbach VV, Higashida RT, Barnwell SL, Hieshima GB (Univ of California, San Francisco)
Neurosurgery 27:954–961, 1990   15–13

To determine the role of endovascular coil embolization in the treatment of intracranial aneurysms, data were reviewed on 3 women who underwent transarterial platinum coil embolization because of unusual posterior inferior cerebellar artery (PICA) aneurysms. One patient had a partially thrombosed, irregular bilobed fusiform aneurysm arising from the posterior medullary segment off the right PICA. The second patient had an aneurysm of PICA origin with the dome directed medially into the brain stem. The third patient had an aneurysm with a broad-based neck arising from the distal left vertebral artery at the PICA origin. A previous attempt at surgical clipping in this patient had failed. Transarterial detachable balloon embolization was not possible in any of these patients.

Endovascular platinum coil embolization successfully obliterated the aneurysm in all 3 patients. At discharge, 2 patients were neurologically intact. The third patient had persistent cerebellar signs and was discharged with right-sided dysmetria, but able to walk with a walker. These data indicate experience that the use of endovascular coil embolization of unusual intracranial aneurysms is feasible.

▶ This interesting report documents the successful obliteration of 3 PICA aneurysms with endovascular coils of the Hilal type. On short-term follow-up, total obliteration of the aneurysm was possible, as proved by postocclusion angiography.

This type of coil occlusion of aneurysms has been discussed previously by Mullan et al. (1), but recanalization of aneurysms with recurrent subarachnoid hemorrhage led to abandonment of this technique as a direct neurosurgical procedure. More recent utilization of such coils by endovascular technique has been described by Hilal and co-workers (2), but incomplete obliteration of lesions was a continuing problem. In addition, Knuckey recently reported 5 aneurysms treated in this fashion, with 2 incomplete obliterations and 1 instance of migration of coils into the parent vessel with occlusion, massive infarction, and fatal endema (AANS Annual Meeting, 1991).

The method has been further advanced by the development of a new coil developed by Vineula and colleagues at UCLA. This very soft, highly thrombogenic floppy coil can be introduced transvascularly by layers into an aneurysm for complete thrombosis. Initial results are encouraging, but long-term follow-up studies are needed to establish the efficacy and safety of this technique. (Also see Abstract 15–11.)

Overall, these approaches offer encouraging preliminary results, but long-term follow-up is required to establish the indications.— R.M. Crowell, M.D.

References

1. Mullan S, et al: *J Neurosurg* 22:539, 1965.
2. Hilal SK, et al: *Radiology* 173:250, 1989.

Temporary Balloon Occlusion of a Proximal Vessel as an Aid to Clipping Aneurysms of the Basilar and Paraclinoid Internal Carotid Arteries: Technical Note
Shucart WA, Kwan ES, Heilman CB (New England Med Ctr, Boston)
Neurosurgery 27:116–119, 1990   15–14

Temporary intraoperative balloon occlusion was used to treat a basilar artery aneurysm and 3 large paraclinoid aneurysms of the internal carotid artery. Intraoperative angiography confirmed optimal clip placement in these cases. Excellent proximal vascular control was achieved. The carotid artery did not have to be exposed in the neck.

Woman, 39, had recurrent dizziness and a feeling of pressure in the back of the head. Neurologic findings were negative, but contrast CT showed a round dense lesion in the area of the right paraclinoid internal carotid artery. Angiography demonstrated a large bilobate paraclinoid aneurysm of this vessel. The carotid artery was exposed by a right pterional craniotomy. A coaxial catheter system was inserted under fluoroscopic guidance. A nondetachable balloon attached to the catheter tip then was advanced to the C1–C2 level and, after thiopental intravenously, the balloon was inflated with metrizamide to occlude the artery. The aneurysmal neck was clipped and the aneurysm aspirated. Occlusion lasted for 3 minutes. Only a transient mild third nerve palsy was present postoperatively.

Temporary balloon occlusion of the proximal vessel is a useful adjunct in treating aneurysms of the basilar and proximal internal carotid arteries. The maneuver precludes the need for cervical dissection of the internal carotid artery.

► This nice study indicates the utility of intraoperative angiography and interventional balloon techniques during aneurysm surgery. As several groups now have demonstrated, intraoperative angiography can identify incompletely clipped aneurysms or inadvertently occluded parent vessels to allow repositioning of the aneurysm clip in 5% to 10% of cases. The additional utility of temporary balloon occlusion of the parent vessel is a logical further step that provides for proximal control of the aneurysm's circulation without the need for additional neck incisions or the application of intracranial clips, which cause some risk and reduction of working room in the operative field. The group from Dallas has used a related technique, namely, catheter aspiration of the internal carotid artery from a proximally placed catheter for collapse of giant paraclinoid aneurysms during surgical correction.—R.M. Crowell, M.D.

Management of Hemorrhagic Complications From Prospective Embolization of Arteriovenous Malformations
Purdy PD, Batjer HH, Samson D (Univ of Texas, Dallas)
J Neurosurg 74:205–211, 1991   15–15

The role of endovascular embolization in the treatment of cerebral arteriovenous malformations (AVMs) remains controversial. Although endovascular embolization is often used in conjunction with surgery in the treatment of intracranial AVMs, there is commonly little interaction between neurosurgeons and neuroradiologists in the various phases of management. Potentially catastrophic intracranial hemorrhage occurred during or after endovascular embolization in 7 patients.

All 7 patients had at least 1 endovascular embolization procedure using polyvinyl alcohol particles. In addition, occlusion of proximal feeding vessels was carried out with the use of platinum microcoils in 2 patients; detachment of an endovascular balloon was attempted in 1 patient. Hemorrhage occurred in 3 patients when the catheter penetrated the subarachnoid space. In 1 patient a large feeding vessel ruptured during balloon inflation, resulting in a lethal hemorrhage. The other 3 patients experienced delayed intraparenchymal hemorrhage (Fig 15–2). All but 2 patients underwent craniotomy. There were 4 good and 3 poor outcomes.

Hemorrhagic complications of embolization of an intracranial AVM cannot be managed conservatively, particularly when accompanied by intraparenchymal hematoma. The complications encountered in these 7

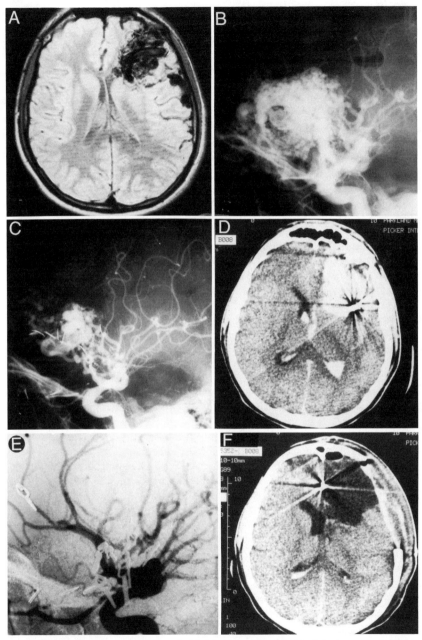

Fig 15–2.—A, pretreatment MRI reveals left frontal AVM involving the lateral ventricle. **B,** left internal carotid angiogram shows major irrigation by left middle cerebral artery branches. **C,** angiogram after the second embolization procedure confirms reduction in filling of the AVM. **D,** emergency CT following sudden headache and obtundation reveals a large frontal hematoma. **E,** left carotid angiogram obtained postoperatively confirms complete AVM excision. **F,** postoperative CT scan illustrates the extent of frontal resection. (Courtesy of Purdy PD, Batjer HH, Samson D: *J Neurosurg* 74:205–211, 1991.)

cases underline the importance of interdisciplinary cooperation that should start at the time of diagnostic studies.

▶ The authors have forthrightly described the complications associated with preoperative embolization of AVMs. The occurrence of 7 life-threatening hemorrhages among 63 cases (11%) represents a substantial rate of complications. Perforation of catheters into the subarachnoid space and rupture of a feeding vessel with a balloon are certainly catastrophic events, and it may be that technical advances can prevent such occurrences. On the other hand, the delayed bleeding in 3 patients after embolization is more difficult to avoid, unless it be by case selection on as yet undetermined criteria. The aggressive management by immediate craniotomy was often life-saving. Certainly, the advantage of a team approach involving interventional radiology and neurosurgery is much commended.—R.M. Crowell, M.D.

Percutaneous Transvenous Catheterization and Embolization of Vein of Galen Anuerysms

Casasco A, Lylyk P, Hodes JE, Kohan G, Aymard A, Merland J-J (Univ of Paris VII; Lariboisière Hosp, Paris; Inst de Investigaciones Neurologicas Doctor Raul Carrea, Buenos Aires)
Neurosurgery 28:260–266, 1991   15–16

Vein of Galen aneurysm (VGA) is a rare intracranial vascular malformation. Percutaneous transvenous catheterization and embolization of a VGA was carried out in 7 patients.

Cerebral arteriograms showed multipedicular VGAs in all patients. All direct fistulas were fed by the posterior choroidal artery from the internal carotid artery or by the posterior artery of the corpus callosum. There was an intervening arterial-arterial network between the posterior thalamoperforating arteries and the wall of the venous aneurysm in 6 patients. Primary treatment in 5 patients was with percutaneous transvenous embolization, and the transvenous approach was used in combination with incomplete transarterial embolization or with the transtorcular approach in 2. Treatment was through the jugular vein in 6 patients and the femoral vein in 1

Angiographic and clinical examinations demonstrated that 5 total and 2 partial occlusions of the VGA were achieved. The venous approach allowed measurement of intra-aneurysmal pressure during treatment, guiding the amount of occlusion to be accomplished during each treatment session, thus preventing the normal perfusion breakthrough phenomenon. There were no complications secondary to catheterization, but 1 guidewire perforation occurred during the transtorcular approach, causing fatal massive hemorrhage.

Percutaneous transvenous catheterization and embolization is superior to transarterial embolization or surgery in the treatment of multipedicular VGAs. The percutaneous approach offers all of the advantages of the transtorcular approach, but avoids both sinus manipulation and potentially bloody surgery. There remains, however, a risk of aneurysm perforation with the guidewire.

▶ This article describes the experience of Merland's group in VGAs. The data support the contention that transvenous catheterization may be superior to the transarterial method.— R.M. Crowell, M.D.

Revascularization of Brain Arteriovenous Malformations After Embolization With Brucrylate
Fournier D, Terbrugge K, Rodesch G, Lasjaunias P (Toronto Western Hosp; Ctr Hosp et Univ, Angers, France; Hôp de Bicêtre, Le Kremlin Bicêtre, France
Neuroradiology 32:497–501, 1990   15–17

Therapeutic embolization of brain arteriovenous malformations (AVMs) with brucrylate has recently gained wider acceptance, but the role of this procedure remains to be properly evaluated, and the risk of revascularization has been questioned. Of 52 brain AVMs embolized with brucrylate, 9 were localized in the occipital lobe. Angiographic follow-up ranged from 1 to 4 years. Two embolized occipital AVMs showed revascularization at 2 years and 6 months, respectively. Embolization completely obliterated the AVM in 1 patient, and the nidus was reduced by 95% in the other.

Because the occipital lobe is richly vascularized, it is more likely than other parts of the brain to produce strong collateralization that will lead indirectly to revascularization of embolized AVMs. Such revascularization of an AVM nidus and development of extensive collaterals after incomplete obliteration of large brain AVMs have been reported previously. The presence of collaterals could also explain the rarity of visual defects related to occipital AVMs.

These 2 patients with revascularization underscore the need for long-term angiographic follow-up within the first 5 years to assess direct or indirect reconstitution of the nidus. Transdural angiogenesis should also be considered as another source of supply. Clinicians should always study the external carotid system during follow-up.

▶ This report again calls attention to the fact that brucrylate injected into an AVM can recanalize. This fact, coupled with the apparent toxicity of this agent, has led many, including our group at Massachusetts General Hospital, to switch to Avicryl (N-butyl-cyanoacrylate). This agent provides for long-lasting embolization, and the toxicity appears to be small. We consider it preferable to polyvinyl alcohol, a more easily administered and probably safer material, but one known to recanalize very readily. The problem of recanalization should especially be noted in cases in which surgical excision is not appropriate; when radiosurgical obliteration is super-added to embolotherapy, one has to keep in mind that recanalization may change the picture dramatically over the course of time.— R.M. Crowell, M.D.

Failure of Transluminal Angioplasty in the Treatment of Myointimal Hyperplasia of the Internal Carotid Artery: Case Report

Culicchia F, Spetzler RF, Flom RA (Barrow Neurological Inst, Phoenix)
Neurosurgery 28:148–151, 1991   15–18

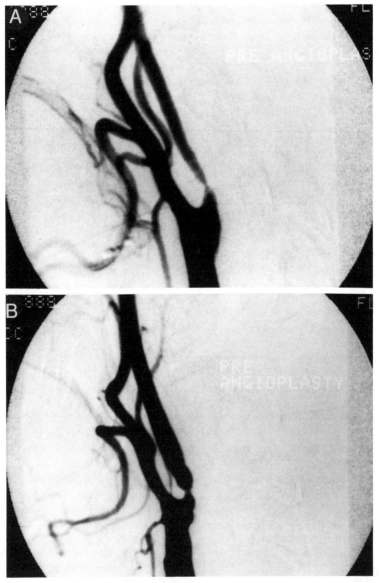

Fig 15–3.—Angiograms of the right (**A**) and left (**B**) carotid artery, 8 months after surgery. (Courtesy of Culicchia F, Spetzler RF, Flom RA: *Neurosurgery* 28:148–151, 1991.)

Percutaneous transluminal angioplasty (PTA) has been suggested as an alternative to surgical correction of recurrent stenosis of the carotid artery after carotid endarterectomy for atherosclerosis. The long-term results were assessed in a patient who underwent PTA for bilateral recurrent stenosis of the carotid artery resulting from intimal hyperplasia.

Man, 59, with a history of hypertension and transient weakness in the left arm, underwent microsurgical carotid endarterectomy with primary closure on the right side. A similar procedure was performed on the left side 1 week later. Postoperative angiography confirmed excellent reconstruction of the vessels. However, noninvasive Doppler studies performed 8 months later revealed high-grade stenosis in both carotid arteries, and angiography showed intimal hyperplasia at the sites of the endarterectomies (Fig 15–3). With PTA, 2–4 dilations were performed on each stenosis, resulting in excellent reconstitution of the vessel lumen. There were no complications, and the patient was discharged the next day. A carotid angiogram obtained 6 months after initial follow-up revealed a recurrent, high-grade stenosis at the same level in both carotid arteries. The patient underwent reconstruction of the vessels with vein patch. The postoperative course was uneventful.

Although initial results of dilatation with PTA were excellent, stenoses later developed at the same sites. Apparently, failure of PTA and treatment of myointimal hyperplasia of the ICA produces additional myointimal hyperplasia.

▶ This interesting report describes the failure of angioplasty in the management of recurrent carotid stenosis. The authors suggest that this was a case of recurrent myointimal hyperplasia, and this may well be the case. On the other hand, Sundt's extensive experience indicates that about half of such restenoses will be some other entity, either atherosclerosis, subacute thrombosis, or a combination of effects. In any event, angioplasty was unsuccessful, with prompt recurrence in a few months' time.

With the advent of new balloon systems (such as the Theron triple-lumen system with distal balloon to prevent internal carotid artery embolization), it is highly likely that substantial further investigation of the problem of angioplasty of carotid stenosis will be carried out in the next few years. Whether this will equal or surpass the clinical effectiveness and safety of carotid endarterectomy as described by the North American Symptomatic Carotid Endarterectomy Trial must await collection of data. Surely, this should go forward very cautiously, because we now know that carotid endarterectomy is safe and effective, as compared with medical treatment, for symptomatic stenosis of 70% or greater.—R.M. Crowell, M.D.

Direct Endovascular Thrombolytic Therapy for Dural Sinus Thrombosis
Barnwell SL, Higashida RT, Halbach VV, Dowd CF, Hieshima GB (Univ of California, San Francisco)
Neurosurgery 28:135–142, 1991   15–19

Clinical findings in dural sinus thrombosis range from asymptomatic incidental findings to courses leading to death. A transjugular local infusion of urokinase delivered through a percutaneously introduced catheter was used to treat symptomatic dural sinus thrombosis in 3 patients aged 51–71 years. All 3 patients had dural arteriovenous fistulas, 2 in the transverse sinus and 1 in the inferior petrosal sinus. Patients underwent complete cerebral angiography and sinus venography. Urokinase was infused locally through a Tracker of EDM infusion catheter. During infusion, serial venograms were obtained once or twice a day to assess the degree of thrombolysis. Patients, who were initially given heparin, were switched to warfarin therapy for 6 weeks.

In 1 patient the initial transfemoral venous approach was discontinued because of infection. Infusion for thrombolysis was maintained for 4–10 days. Clinical signs and symptoms improved, and there was angiographic evidence of clot lysis and dural sinus recanalization. In the third patient, angiography revealed partial resolution of a clot in the torcular herophili and transverse sinus, but the patient had no clinical improvement.

Transjugular local infusion of urokinase can be used effectively for treatment of symptomatic, thrombosed dural sinuses. Because lysis is selective, the danger of systemic hemorrhagic complications is reduced.

▶ The authors report 2 of 3 cases with clinical improvement and the third with angiographic improvement after transvenous thrombolytic therapy with endovascular technique. It is of great interest that thrombosis present for 2 days was reopened in this fashion. Most certainly, this form of treatment should be tried further to gain a more secure notion of efficacy and risk. It should not be forgotten that such thrombosis is often associated with dural arteriovenous malformations, and bleeding might complicate such treatment.—R.M. Crowell, M.D.

Stereotaxic Surgery

Treatment of Intractable Arterial Hemorrhage During Stereotactic Brain Biopsy With Thrombin: Report of Three Patients
Chimowitz MI, Barnett GH, Palmer J (Cleveland Clinic Found)
J Neurosurg 74:301–303, 1991.   15–20

Arterial hemorrhage is an uncommon but serious complication of stereotactic brain biopsy. Between June 1987 and November 1989, 165 consecutive patients underwent CT- or MRI-guided stereotactic brain biopsy at the Cleveland Clinic. Data on 4 (2.4%) patients in whom arterial hemorrhage developed were reviewed.

Arterial hemorrhage was refractory to conventional methods of hemostasis in all 4 patients. Craniotomy was performed in patient to control the hemorrhage. In the other 3, thrombin, .5–2 cc (5,000 units per cc), was injected slowly through the biopsy cannula, resulting in immediate resolution of the hemorrhage. Postoperatively, 2 patients who received thrombin, 1–2 cc, were slow to awaken. In 1 patient CT showed multiple infarcts, and transcranial Doppler ultrasound studies showed increased blood flow velocities in multiple cerebral arteries, suggesting diffuse vasospasm. The other patient had a moderate-sized frontal hematoma with increased intracranial pressure. Mild neurologic deficits persisted in both patients. In contrast, the third patient treated with thrombin, .5 cc, had an uneventful postoperative course.

Thrombin is highly effective in controlling intractable arterial hemorrhage during stereotactic brain biopsy. However, it should be used cautiously as thrombin may induce cerebral vasospasm.

▶ Arterial hemorrhage was controlled with thrombin during stereotactic brain biopsy in 3 cases. All 3 patients survived, 2 with mild deficits. It may be that vasospasm complicated these cases.—R.M. Crowell, M.D.

Direct Stereotactic Intracerebral Injection of Monoclonal Antibodies and Their Fragments: A Potential Approach to Brain Tumor Immunotherapy
Liebert M, Wahl RL, Lawless G, McKeever PE, Taren JA, Beierwaltes WH, Brasswell R (Univ of Michigan)
Am J Physiol Imaging 5:55–59, 1990   15–21

The blood-brain barrier limits the delivery of monoclonal antibodies (Mab) to brain tumors. Direct stereotactic injection of the Mab into the brain was done in an attempt to circumvent this problem. An antimelanoma intact Mab and its antigen-binding fragments (Fab), which do not react with normal rat brain, were radioiodinated and injected into rats intracerebrally or intravenously. The animals were killed 5 days after injection. Intracerebral delivery of intact antibody was 101 times higher than intravenous delivery. There was a 14:1 ratio of radioantibody in injected cerebrum to blood. With Fab fragments delivered intracerebrally, the radioantibody ratio in injected cerebrum to blood was 242:1 at 5 days post injection, with a 680-fold delivery advantage over intravenous injection.

Direct intracranial injection of Mab, and especially of Fab fragment, is a feasible means of delivering radiolabeled Mab or Fab fragments to brain tumors. It may also be of value in the treatment of other accessible solid tumors. Further research is needed to confirm these findings.

▶ This communication shows that direct stereotactic injection of Mabs can be done safely in animals, with a vast increase in radioantibody dosage over intravenous administration. This is a clever idea that may have real benefit for clinical treatment.—R.M. Crowell, M.D.

Brain Damage from ¹²⁵I Brachytherapy Evaluated by MR Imaging, a Blood-Brain Barrier Tracer, and Light and Electron Microscopy in a Rat Model
Bernstein M, Marotta T, Stewart P, Glen J, Resch L, Henkelman M (Toronto Western Hosp; Univ of Toronto)
J Neurosurg 73:585–593, 1990   15–22

To gain a better understanding of the time course and specific pathophysiology of interstitial brachytherapy brain damage, ^{125}I seeds of mid to high activity were placed in a bone trough parallel to the midline on the cerebrum of male rats. The seeds were not implanted because the surgical trauma in such a small volume as the rat cerebrum would produce too great an artifact. An 80-Gy radiation dose was administered to an area having a 5.5-mm radius. The integrity of the blood-brain barrier (BBB) was assessed acutely, and at 3, 6, 9, and 12 months after brachytherapy with the use of MRI before and after gadolinium enhancement, leakage of horseradish peroxidase (HRP), electron microscopy, and light microscopy.

Significant tissue damage was seen at radiation doses of more than 295 Gy. Areas of BBB disruption appeared to increase up to the 6-month time point and to stabilize or decrease thereafter. All visible BBB damage was seen in tissue specimens that had received radiation doses of more than 165 Gy. The BBB disruption indicated by gadolinium-enhanced MRI was greater than that indicated by leakage of HRP. Why gadolinium enhances a larger area than HRP after the same circulation times is unclear.

The time course of ^{125}I brain damage in this rat model was similar to that reported by other studies. The area of BBB disruption appeared to progress from time 0 to 6 months and to stabilize or decrease thereafter, suggesting that the pathophysiologic substrate of BBB disruption must be capable of some degree of repair. The time course of brain damage closely approximated the situation in human brain tumor brachytherapy.

▶ This imaginative experimental study provides quantitative data on the BBB and its damage after ^{125}I brachytherapy in rats. The study confirms the extent of BBB disruption occurring with significant radiation doses over a 6-month time course. Some questions arise: What is the basis for the differences between gadolinium-enhanced MRI and leakage of HRP? This question concerns the reliability of gadolinium positivity in clinical MRIs to detect BBB damage. Moreover, the rat model may reflect the clinical situation. This approach in a primate model may be productive of clinically important data.—R.M. Crowell, M.D.

Radiation

In Vivo Biological Effects of Stereotactic Radiosurgery: A Primate Model
Lunsford LD, Altschuler EM, Flickinger JC, Wu A, Martinez AJ (Univ of Pittsburgh)
Neurosurgery 27:373–382, 1990   15–23

The safe delivery of single-fraction, small-volume irradiation through a closed skull requires accurate knowledge of radiation tolerance. A baboon model was developed in which to evaluate the destructive effects of stereotactic radiosurgery.

Three adult baboons received 150 Gy in a single fraction to the caudate nucleus, thalamus, or pons, using the 8-mm collimator of the gamma unit. Xenon-enhanced CT, MRI, and somatosensory and brain stem evoked potential studies were carried out, and myelin basic protein was determined in the CSF.

A lesion detectable by MRI developed at the target site within 45–60 days after irradiation. When a lesion encroached on auditory pathways, brain stem evoked potentials deteriorated before imaging changes were evident. Levels of myelin basic protein in the CSF increased after imaging changes developed. Autopsies confirmed the presence of well-demarcated radionecrosis at the site of radiation exposure.

This model is useful for investigating the in vivo biologic effects of radiosurgery. More knowledge of radiation tolerance of the brain stem, cranial nerves, and basal cerebral vasculature may make safer and more effective radiosurgical treatment possible for patients with tumors and vascular malformations.

▶ This important article is the first in a series relative to the study of gamma knife radiosurgery in a primate model. The authors have thoughtfully chosen an extensive battery of neurologic, physiologic, radiologic, and neuropathologic investigations of standardized gamma knife lesions to the brain. They intend to carry this further in a wide-ranging future study.

This study confirms the findings of Steiner et al. (1) that a dosage of more than 140 Gy causes lesions of the brain when delivered as single-fraction focused radiation. A number of interesting effects were uncovered during the various tests. Most striking, however, is the larger volume of the lesion in the thalamus (13 mm) compared to those in both the caudate and the pons (8 mm). This may represent an important difference in the susceptibility of various structures to the effects of gamma ionizing radiation. On the other hand, it is also possible that there is significant variability between animals, and even between species. Thus one must be extremely cautious in interpreting data, particularly small numbers of observations and most especially in nonhuman subjects, without the various influences of targeted pathology, intercurrent illness, and variable age. Nonetheless, this is an important start, and one hopes that a better understanding of the dose-response curve of focused radiosurgery will emerge.—R.M. Crowell, M.D.

Reference

1. Steiner L, et al: *Acta Neurochir (Wien)* 52:173, 1980.

Stereotactic Radiosurgery of Meningiomas

Kondziolka D, Lunsford LD, Coffey RJ, Flickinger JC (Univ of Pittsburgh)
J Neurosurg 74:552–559, 1991   15–24

Surgical resection of a meningioma from its dural attachment can produce long-term disease-free survival, but it may be associated with neurologic deficits. Also, although incomplete resection can preserve neurologic function, meningiomas may recur. Single-fraction precisely guided multi-

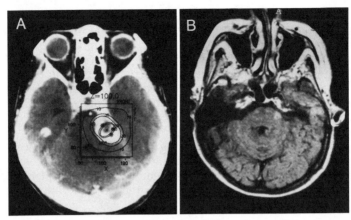

Fig 15–4.—A, CT scan with contrast enhancement showing a left tentorial meningioma treated at the 50% isodose line (2 isocenters) of irradiation; marginal dose 18 Gy). **B,** MR (T1-weighted spin-echo) image with gadolinium-diethylenetriamine pentaacetic acid enhancement showing a marked decrease in tumor size at 10 months after radiosurgery. (Courtesy of Kondziolka D, Lunsford LD, Coffey RJ, et al: *J Neurosurg* 74:552–559, 1991.)

ple photon-beam irradiation (stereotactic radiosurgery) is an effective adjuvant treatment for patients with tumors in high-risk locations or residual meningiomas, or for patients who are poor medical risks. Stereotactic surgery was used in 50 patients with meningiomas and management strategies and initial results were evaluated.

The radiosurgical dose with the 201-source cobalt-60 gamma knife was dependent on tumor size and location. Three patients had neurologic complications compatible with delayed radiation injury. At 6–12 months after treatment, a decrease in tumor size was noted in 4 patients, whereas 22 had no change (Fig 15–4). Between 12 months and 36 months after treatment, a reduction in tumor volume was seen in 13 of 24 patients; 9 had no change. The actuarial 2-year tumor growth control rate was 96%. Follow-up over years is necessary to evaluate treatment fully, but radiosurgery appears to be an effective primary treatment alternative in selected patients with symptomatic meningiomas.

▶ This careful presentation from the Pittsburgh group documents that radiosurgery for meningiomas can lead to reduction in tumor size as well as loss of CT enhancement. Decreasing tumor size was seen in two thirds of the tumors followed for 24–36 months. Two instances of neurologic worsening and a single permanent third nerve complicated the treatment. Overall, this is an encouraging report, but certainly much longer follow-up is needed to know for certain what the role of radiosurgical treatment will be in this group of patients. Moreover, the precise indications remain uncertain, particularly in that most interesting group of patients with tumors in the area of the cavernous sinus. It's worth noting that this general approach contrasts sharply with the aggressive approach of tumor resection from the cavernous area, which can now technically be carried out.—R.M. Crowell, M.D.

Stereotactic Single High Dose Radiation Therapy of Benign Intracranial Meningiomas

Engenhart R, Kimmig BN, Höver K-H, Wowra B, Sturm V, Van Kaick G, Wannenmacher M (Univ Clinic of Radiology, Heidelberg, Germany; German Cancer Research Ctr, Heidelberg; Univ Clinic of Neurosurgery, Heidelberg; Univ Clinic of Neurosurgery, Cologne, Germany)
Int J Radiation Oncology Biol Phys 19:1021–1026, 1990   15–25

About 15% of all intracranial and 25% of all intraspinal neoplasms are meningiomas. The standard therapy for meningiomas is surgical resection. Postoperative radiotherapy improves long-term local control of subtotal resected or recurrent meningiomas. Treatment with a single high dose of radiation delivered stereotactically to the tumor volume was evaluated in 17 patients with intracranial meningiomas.

Radiosurgery was indicated by unresected tumors, gross disease remaining despite surgery, and recurrences. Multiple noncoplanar arc irradiations from a 15-MeV linear accelerator were used. Coupled with secondary tungsten collimators, this technique permitted a high concentration of the dose in the target volume, with a very steep dose gradient at the field borders. A single irradiation dose of 10–50 Gy was delivered.

Four patients died. One death was tumor related and not attributable to treatment, 1 death was treatment related, and the other 2 resulted from intercurrent diseases. The 13 survivors had no evidence of tumor relapse at a median follow-up of 40 months. Late severe effects did occur: 5 patients had a large area of brain edema, concurrent in 3 with tumor necrosis.

Intracranial meningiomas can be treated with a high single dose of radiation therapy with good expectations for prolonged, disease-free survival. Definitive conclusions on the optimal dose and target volume cannot yet be drawn. However, single doses of 20–30 Gy appear to be sufficient to arrest further tumor growth. To minimize neurologic effects, doses of more than 30 Gy and target volumes of more than 40 cm^3 are avoided.

▶ In this study of 17 patients with meningioma, radiosurgery was carried out with doses of 10–50 Gy. The follow-up data show 1 treatment-related death and substantial brain edema in 5 cases. The investigators suggest that a dosage of 20–30 Gy appears to be sufficient to arrest further tumor growth, but to minimize neurologic effects target volumes should be 40 cm^3 or less.

These results should be compared with the slow rate of growth for asymptomatic lesions and the results of radiosurgery (as reported by the Pittsburgh group elsewhere in this volume).—R.M. Crowell, M.D.

Combined Radiosurgery and External Radiotherapy of Intracranial Germinomas

Casentini L, Colombo F, Pozza F, Benedetti A (Ospedale Civile, Vicenza, Italy)
Surg Neurol 34:79–86, 1990   15–26

Although irradiation is an effective treatment for intracranial germinomas, modalities and dose planning reported by different authors have varied. Another therapeutic approach was developed consisting of single-dose stereotactic irradiation to the tumor mass, followed by standard extended fields in refracted doses.

Five males and 1 female aged 12–29 years were treated with combined radiosurgery and external radiotherapy. Radiosurgery doses at the target point ranged from 10 to 12.5 Gy. Whole brain irradiation, done in 5 cases, was given in doses of 24–36 Gy in 12–20 sessions. Spinal irradiation was done in 2 cases, with 27 Gy and 24 Gy delivered in 17 sessions and 12 sessions, respectively. The patients were followed for 1–58 months after treatment.

One patient died 5 weeks after radiosurgery. However, 4 patients were clinically normal at their last follow-up examination. The sixth had slight improvement in his initial visual disturbances.

In most of the cases described, a single dose of stereotactic irradiation reduced the tumor volume within a few days. External whole brain irradiation in 5 patients and spinal irradiation in 2 were done to prevent tumor cell seeding.

Stereotactic Radiosurgery of Angiographically Occult Vascular Malformations: Indications and Preliminary Experience

Kondziolka D, Lunsford LD, Coffey RJ, Bissonette DJ, Flickinger JC (Univ of Pittsburgh)
Neurosurgery 27:892–900, 1990   15–27

Stereotactic radiosurgery has been used effectively in the treatment of angiographically demonstrated lesions, but its role in the treatment of angiographically occult lesions is not well defined. Data on initial experience with stereotactic radiosurgery in the treatment of occult vascular malformations (AOVMs) were reviewed.

During a 32-month period, 24 adults underwent gamma knife stereotactic radiosurgery in the treatment of AOVMs identified on MRI as being located in a region of the brain where microsurgical removal was considered too risky. Only patients who had sustained 2 or more hemorrhages were included in the study. The mean time from diagnosis to treatment was 3 years. All patients underwent high-resolution subtraction angiography to exclude venous angiomas. There were 11 AOVMs in the pons/midbrain, 4 in the medulla/pons, 3 in the thalamus, 2 in the basal ganglia, 3 deep in the temporal lobe, and 1 within the precentral gyrus.

There were no immediate postoperative complications and no nausea or vomiting. Each patient received a single intravenous dose of methylprednisolone, 40 mg, immediately after delivery of the radiosurgical dose. All patients left the hospital within 24 hours after radiosurgery. Follow-up MRI was at 3, 6, and 12 months after radiosurgery and at 6-month intervals thereafter.

During a follow-up interval of 4–24 months, 19 patients either improved or remained clinically stable without recurrence of hemorrhage; 5 patients with large AOVMs had temporary worsening of preexisting neurologic deficits suggestive of delayed radiation injury. One patient had another hemorrhage 7 months after radiosurgery, which caused left hemiparesis. She improved progressively with high-dose corticosteroid therapy but mild left hemiparesis persisted. Another patient required microsurgical excision and a ventriculoperitoneal shunt. This patient remains totally disabled and requires long-term medical care. These initial data indicate that stereotactic radiosurgery can be performed safely in patients with AOVMs located in deep, critical, or relatively inaccessible cerebral locations.

▶ The authors treated 24 adult patients with deep angiographically AOVMs in which 2 or more hemorrhages had occurred. Patients with surgically amenable lesions were excluded. Nineteen patients either improved or remained stable without recurrence of hemorrhage; 5 patients had worsening, suggesting delayed radiation injury. In 1 of these cases all symptoms resolved, but in the other 4 symptoms persisted and in 1 were markedly disabling.

The authors conclude that the data demonstrate the safety of this approach, but certainly a 21% complication rate must be regarded as substantial. Whether this is better than the natural history of the condition or the results of microsurgical excision has not been demonstrated. It should be noted that, on the basis of unacceptable complications, Steiner has decided against treating such lesions with radiosurgery.—R.M. Crowell, M.D.

The Long-Term Side Effects of Radiation Therapy for Benign Brain Tumors in Adults

Al-Mefty O, Kersh JE, Routh A, Smith RR (Univ of Mississippi)
J Neurosurg 73:502–512, 1990   15–28

The risks of intracranial radiotherapy may be warranted for patients with malignant tumors but not necessarily for those with benign tumors. The complications of radiotherapy were reviewed in 58 adults treated between 1958 and 1987 for benign intracranial tumors. Forty-six patients had pituitary adenomas. The other lesions included 5 meningiomas, 4 glomus tumors, 2 pineal-area lesions, and 1 craniopharyngioma. The mean age at the time of radiotherapy was 48 years. An average of 4,984 cGy was delivered in an average of 27 fractions in 46 days. The mean follow-up was about 8 years.

Twenty-two patients had what were thought to be long-term or delayed side effects of irradiation. Two patients had visual disturbances and, in 6 cases, hypopituitarism was diagnosed. Seventeen patients had changes of delayed brain necrosis, severe in 4; 3 patients had diffuse atrophy. In 1 patient a clival tumor developed 30 years after irradiation for acromegaly in addition to changes of radiation necrosis (Fig 15–5). Con-

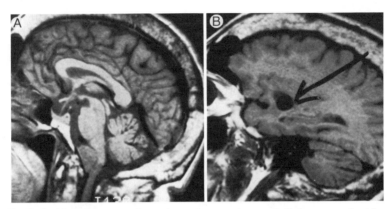

Fig 15–5.—Magnetic resonance images in a patient treated nonsurgically for acromegaly with an estimated 4,000 cGy of irradiation in 20 fractions at the age of 32 years. **A,** sagittal image demonstrating a clival tumor in the irradiated field. **B,** image showing a large cystic area in the irradiated field *(arrow).* (Courtesy of Al-Mefty O, Kersh JE, Routh A, et al: *J Neurosurg* 73:502–512, 1990.)

siderable delayed sequelae of cranial irradiation occur in adults given "safe" treatment for benign brain tumors.

▶ This important study provides information on 58 patients with benign tumors who received radiation therapy. The radiation dosage averaged about 5,000 cGy. Pituitary deficiency occurred in 6 patients, with evidence of parenchymal changes in 21. Although the report does not clearly indicate the extent of symptoms associated with the radiographic or autopsy parenchymal changes, it appears that in at least half of these cases there was significant neurologic impairment. This occurred in patients with radiation dosage of as low as 3,500 cGy. In addition, 2 secondary neoplasms were reported within the field of the radiation. The contribution overall points out that radiation for benign neoplasms is not an entirely benign treatment, and delayed consequences (as long as 15 years after treatment) must be anticipated.—R.M. Crowell, M.D.

Reduction in Radiation-Induced Brain Injury by Use of Pentobarbital or Lidocaine Protection
Oldfield EH, Friedman R, Kinsella T, Moquin R, Olson JJ, Orr K, DeLuca AM (Natl Inst of Neurological Disorders and Stroke; Natl Cancer Inst, Bethesda, Md)
J Neurosurg 72:737–744, 1990   15–29

If neural activity during radiation exposure influences tissue damage in the brain, as it does in ischemic neural injury, agents that suppress brain cell activity might protect against adverse radiation effects. Rats were exposed to whole-brain irradiation during pentobarbital- or lidocaine-induced anesthesia; the results were compared with those in unmedicated animals and others anesthetized with ketamine. Shielding prevented damage to respiratory and digestive tissues.

At 7,500 rad of whole-brain irradiation, survival rates differed significantly in pentobarbital-treated and control animals. Anesthetic doses of pentobarbital and lidocaine provided comparable protection against early radiation toxicity. Ketamine anesthesia was ineffective. No significant differences in body temperature were noted. There were no histologic differences in the brain between awake and pentobarbital-treated animals.

Pentobarbital protects the rat brain against acute irradiation toxicity, presumably through a general suppressive effect on brain synaptic activity or metabolism. Nevertheless, it is late, delayed toxicity that limits the radiation dose and thereby compromises tumor control. Whether barbiturates can control late toxicity remains to be determined.

▶ This clever study compares the survival of rats after brain radiation with 7,500 rad and anesthetization with either phenobarbital, 30 mg/kg, and ketamine, or no medication whatever. After 45 days, 45% of the phenobarbital-treated group survived; none of the untreated animals survived beyond 13 days. This remarkable difference strongly suggests that barbiturate produces a protective effect against radiation-induced brain injury. Although further studies will be needed to expand and confirm these observations, the findings suggest that barbiturate anesthesia might be used to enhance the radiation effects against intracranial lesions such as tumors and arteriovenous malformations.— R.M. Crowell, M.D.

A Histological and Flow Cytometric Study of Dog Brain Endothelial Cell Injuries in Delayed Radiation Necrosis
Yamaguchi N, Yamashima T, Yamashita J (Kanazawa Univ, Japan)
J Neurosurg 74:625–632, 1991   15–30

Delayed radiation necrosis of the CNS may occur months to years after therapeutic irradiation. The changes in the cell cycle and DNA injury of the cerebral endothelial cells after irradiation have never been studied in detail. A histologic and biochemical study was done in dogs, with special attention to vascular endothelial cell injuries.

Nineteen dogs received a single 15-Gy dose of irradiation to the head; 6 dogs served as controls. The animals were killed 3, 6, 9, 12, 15, or 30 months after irradiation, and the brains were resected immediately. Specimens of the brains were then prepared for light and electron microscopy. Acridine orange was used to stain capillary endothelial cells, and flow cytometry was done to investigate the cell ratios in the reproductive phase. To demonstrate changes in the DNA of endothelial cells, Feulgen hydrolysis and computer analysis of the hydrolysis curves were done.

Light microscopy 6 months after irradiation showed spongy degeneration of brain tissue with small cell infiltration, particularly in the frontal white matter. Foci of necrosis appeared at 9 months and developed until 15 months. In the necrotic area, blood vessels were narrowed with endothelial hyperplasia and proliferation. No new areas of necrosis were seen at 30 months. Electron microscopy showed increased pinocytosis in the capillary endothelial cells in the necrotic area. Increased infoldings and euchromatin were seen in the nuclei. Cell ratios in the reproductive phase ranged from 14.5% to 23.3% in the irradiated dogs compared with 6.4% in the control animals. Production of apurinic acid, which correlates with transcriptional activity of DNA, was lowest at 3 months and highest at 9 months after irradiation.

The pathogenesis of delayed radiation necrosis appears to be affected greatly by impairment in the microcirculation. The timing of necrosis is closely correlated with the cell cycle of the vascular endothelial cells.

16 Tumors

Gliomas

Biological Significance of Tissue Plasminogen Activator Content in Brain Tumors

Sawaya R, Rämö OJ, Shi ML, Mandybur G (MD Anderson Cancer Ctr, Houston)
J Neurosurg 74:480–486, 1991   16–1

Plasminogen activators (PAs), serine proteolytic enzymes that convert plasminogen to the active proteinase plasmin, have a role in normal and neoplastic physiologic events. The 2 major types, tissue PA (t-PA) and urokinase PA (u-PA), differ in tissue distribution and catalytic, molecular, and immunologic properties. Earlier studies have indicated that there may be a difference in the immunologic identity of the PA present in benign and malignant tumors.

The t-PA content of normal and brain tumor tissue was analyzed using activity and immunologic assays, and the results were correlated with specific biological parameters. The 6 tissue categories represented in 130 brain tumor tissue samples and 7 normal samples were glioblastomas, metastatic brain tumors, meningiomas, low-grade gliomas, neurinomas, and normal tissue. The t-PA content in benign tumors was 3 times higher than that in malignant tumors, and there was an inverse relationship between the tissue content of t-PA and the presence and degree of tumor necrosis and peritumoral brain edema (Fig 16–1). There was no signifi-

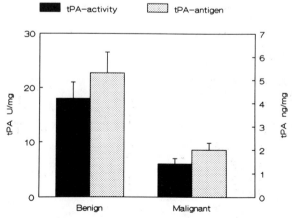

Fig 16–1.—Tissue plasminogen activator (t-PA) activity *(dark block)* and antigen content *(shaded block)* of benign and malignant brain tumors. Both parameters were significantly higher in benign brain tumors (*P* < .0006 and *P* < .001, respectively). (Courtesy of Sawaya R, Rämö OJ, Shi ML, et al: *J Neurosurg* 74:480–486, 1991.)

cant correlation between tissue t-PA content and patient age and sex, steroid use, or plasma t-PA level, or duration of symptoms.

Benign brain tumors are associated with a high t-PA content, whereas malignant neoplasms have less t-PA than normal brain tissue. Tumor necrosis and peritumoral edema correlate inversely with the t-PA content of the tumor. Pharmacologic manipulation of t-PA may affect the growth of certain types of brain tumor as well as their treatment.

▶ This careful study establishes the reduction of t-PA in malignant brain tumors and relative preservation in benign lesions. An interesting inverse relationship of tumor necrosis and peritumoral edema was noted with t-PA contact. Tissue plasminogen activator is important to microvascular perfusion and tissue oxygenation, and it may well be that pharmacologic manipulation of t-PA plays a role in tumor treatment.— R.M. Crowell, M.D.

Malignant Astrocytoma in South Australia: Treatment and Case Survival
North B, Reilly P, Blumbergs P, Roder D, Esterman A (Royal Adelaide Hosp; Inst of Med and Veterinary Science; South Australian Health Commission, Adelaide, Australia)
Med J Aust 153:250–254, 1990   16–2

Kernohan grades III and IV astrocytomas are always fatal, but the short-term survival has been improved by postoperative radiotherapy, and adjunctive chemotherapy is under investigation. To assess the outcomes of past management and establish a baseline, results in a series of 285 patients seen in a 9-year period with these tumors were reviewed. The series included 176 men and 109 women (median age, 57 years); 44% were 55–69 years of age.

The tumor was located in the parietal lobe in 27% of patients, the frontal lobe in 24%, and the temporal lobe in 19%. Patients were treated by biopsy only, biopsy with radiotherapy, decompression, or decompression with radiotherapy. Supplementary information on the tumor was collected on 18 patients who survived for 2 years and on 18 age- and sex-matched controls. Univariate analysis, relative case survival, and proportional hazards regression analysis were performed.

Treatment was biopsy only in 38% of patients; 34% were treated by decompression with radiotherapy, 16% by biopsy with radiotherapy, and 12% by decompression. Patients younger than 40 years of age were treated mostly by decompression with radiotherapy. The median survival was 24 weeks, with a 1-year survival of 25% and a 2-year survival of 15%. Two-year survival was 53% for patients less than 40 years old, compared with 5% for patients 70 or more years of age; this was thought to result in part from the more aggressive treatment of younger patients. Factors related to longer survival, in addition to age and treatment mode, were longer duration of symptoms before diagnosis and frontal lobe tumor. After adjustment for tumor location, no other variable was a significant predictor of survival.

Long-term outcomes for grades III and IV malignant astrocytomas are still very poor despite recent advances in treatment. The effects of these treatments on quality of life, as well as survival, need to be considered.

▶ This report gives further data supporting the concept that older patients with astrocytoma do worse than younger patients. The interesting new point here is that, as the Australian investigators indicate, this apparent difference in biology may be related to the fact that older patients in general were often treated conservatively, whereas younger patients were treated more aggressively.—R.M. Crowell, M.D.

Human Glioblastoma Cells Release Interleukin-6 In Vivo and In Vitro
Van Meir E, Sawamura Y, Diserens A-C, Hamou M-F, de Tribolet N (Univ Hosp, Lausanne, Switzerland)
Cancer Res 50:6683–6688, 1990   16–3

How the brain modulates the host immune system is not well understood. Interleukin-6 (IL-6) has been widely studied in the acute-phase response to infections, inflammation, and tissue injuries. The role of its production by human cancers, however, is still obscure. The release of IL-6 by glioblastomas was investigated.

An IL-6-dependent cell line was used to test for IL-6 bioactivity in 20 glioblastoma cell lines. All but 1 line released IL-6. When cells from the line that did not release IL-6—the LN-229 line—were treated with interleukin 1β or tumor necrosis factor α, there was a significant induction of IL-6 production and secretion. Five of the 6 lines tested showed various amounts of IL-6 mRNA. Interleukin-6 mRNA was found in the LN-229 line only when the cells were treated with IL-1β or tumor necrosis factor α. Glioblastoma cells produced IL-6 in vivo also. Interleukin-6 activity was noted in 11 of 13 CSF specimens and in 5 of 5 tumor cyst fluids; IL-6 mRNA was found in 4 of 4 tumors. Immunohistochemical analysis demonstrated IL-6 in the tumor cells of 15 of 20 glioblastoma sections.

This study demonstrates the in vivo production of IL-6 by human glioma cells for the first time. Biologically active IL-6 is released by almost all glioblastomas in vivo as well as in vitro. The increased levels of serum acute-phase proteins and immune complexes in patients with glioblastoma may result from this secretion.

▶ In this nicely done study from the Lausanne group, the production of IL-6 by human glioma cells is demonstrated for the first time. The physiologic and clinical significance of this production remains to be elucidated by further immunologic studies.—R.M. Crowell, M.D.

Increasing Annual Incidence of Primary Malignant Brain Tumors in the Elderly

Greig NH, Ries LG, Yancik R, Rapoport SI (Natl Inst on Aging, Bethesda, Md; Natl Cancer Inst, Bethesda)
J Natl Cancer Inst 82:1621–1624, 1990   16–4

Cancer has been recognized to occur relatively frequently in the elderly, as has been highlighted in recent epidemiologic studies. Data from the National Cancer Institute (NCI) Surveillance, Epidemiology, and End Results (SEER) Program were reviewed for the years 1973 through 1985.

The total age-adjusted cancer incidence rose by 10.7% during the review period, for an average rate of .9% per year. Primary malignant brain tumors were nearly twice as frequent in 1985 and in 1973 in persons aged 75–79 years, nearly 4 times as frequent in those aged 80–84, and 5 times as frequent in those aged 85 and more. Both men and women exhibited an age-related increase in malignant brain tumors. The incidence rates changed little in younger persons during the same period. The most frequent tumor types in the elderly were glioblastoma multiforme and astrocytoma. Medulloblastomas are rare in the elderly. The apparent increase in malignant brain tumors seen in the elderly in the past 2 decades may be a real effect, or may be related to the wide use of CT.

▶ This important presentation documents, on the basis of national incidence statistics, a dramatic increase of 200% to 500% for primary brain tumors in patients older than age of 75 between 1973 and 1985. The authors suggest that these changes may be attributable to an increase in detection since the introduction of CT scanning, or reflect a true increase in incidence independent of diagnostic advances. In all events, these data are quite important for neurologists and neurosurgeons, who are the primary physicians for most of these patients.— R.M. Crowell, M.D.

Tumors of the Cerebral Aqueduct: Presentation of 5 Cases and Review of the Literature

Rilliet B, Reverdin A, Haenggeli CA, Pizzolato GP, Berney J (Hôp Cantonal Univ, Geneva, Switzerland; Ctr Méd Univ, Geneva)
Neurochirurgie 36:336–346, 1991   16–5

Tumors of the aqueduct of Sylvius are a rare cause of cerebral stenosis. No more than 48 cases have been reported in the literature, all of them diagnosed at autopsy. The introduction of MRI has radically changed the diagnosis of aqueductal tumors because cases are now diagnosed during the patient's lifetime. Five additional patient's were seen.

One patient, a woman aged 77 years, died of fibrinous pericarditis 2 days after admission. Autopsy of the brain revealed moderate triventricular dilatation and a small subependymoma that completely obstructed the aqueduct. The other 4 patients ranged in age from 14 to 26 years

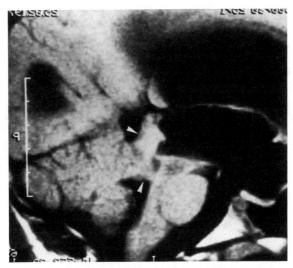

Fig 16—2. Magnetic resonance imaging, sagittal view, T1-weighted image: huge hydrocephalic, space-occupying lesion in mesencephalic tectum and tela choroida superior, isotense with brain tissue. *Arrows* show amputation of superior part of fourth ventricle by this mass. (Courtesy of Rilliet B, Reverdin A, Haenggeli CA, et al: *Neurochirurgie* 36:336–346, 1991.)

when their tumor was first diagnosed. All 4 patients had signs of chronically elevated intracranial pressure caused by triventricular hydrocephalus. In all 4 patients, MRI clearly demonstrated the aqueductal lesions.

In 1 of the 4 patients, a boy aged 14 years with a lifelong history of severe headaches, MRI showed a lesion that occupied the mesencephalic tectum and Vieussen's valve and amputation of the superior part of the fourth ventricle (Fig 16—2). To relieve the pressure, the hydrocephalus was drained surgically. Cytologic examination did not reveal any tumor cells. At follow-up for 18 months MRI showed no change in tumor size.

The other 3 patients were also treated conservatively to relieve the symptoms of hydrocephalus. Radiation therapy of aqueductal tumors was not attempted in any of them because all remained clinically stable and MRI showed no sign of tumor growth after a mean follow-up of 3.7 years. Because tumors of the aqueduct of Sylvius appear to be very slow-growing lesions, providing symptomatic relief by draining the hydrocephalus and monitoring by MRI appear to be appropriate measures. Further information on long-term follow-up is needed.

▶ The authors point out that aqueductal tumors can now be diagnosed nicely with MRI. Their results in 5 cases suggest that many of these lesions will be very gradually progressive and thus are probably of glial origin without malignant characteristics. In such a setting, shunting appears reasonable for hydrocephalus. On the other hand, it is now possible to explore this area, with low morbidity, for definitive biopsy diagnosis and gross total resection. We recently encountered a 21-year-old patient in whom gross total resection led to normal neurologic results after 1 year of follow-up. Treatment should be individualized for these patients.—R.M. Crowell, M.D.

Interstitial Chemotherapy With Drug Polymer Implants for the Treatment of Recurrent Gliomas
Brem H, Mahaley MS Jr, Vick NA, Black KL, Schold SC Jr, Burger PC, Friedman AH, Ciric IS, Eller TW, Cozzens JW, Kenealy JN (Johns Hopkins Hosp; Univ of Alabama, Birmingham; Northwestern Univ; Univ of California, Los Angeles; Duke Univ; et al)
J Neurosurg 74:441–446, 1991   16–6

Malignant gliomas account for about half of the 9,000 new cases of primary brain tumors reported in the United States annually. The standard treatment of resection followed by external beam irradiation provides a median survival time of less than 1 year, but the tumor is refractory. The chemotherapeutic agent nitrosourea BCNU (carmustine) has been effective; however, its use is limited by its systemic toxicity and its serum half-life of 15 minutes. Because tumor recurrence is usually within 2 cm of the initial tumor margin, a biodegradable polymer wafer to deliver BCNU directly to the tumor site was tested.

Three groups totaling 21 patients with recurrent malignant glioma were treated with increasing amounts of BCNU in drug-impregnated polymer wafers. The mean survival time was 48 weeks from reoperation and 94 weeks from the original operation. Eighteen of 21 patients lived for more than a year from the time of initial diagnosis and 8 lived for more than 1 year after intracranial implantation of the polymer. Monitoring revealed no systemic effects of BCNU.

Interstitial chemotherapy with BCNU was well tolerated and safe. Implantation prolonged local exposure with minimal systemic exposure. A placebo-controlled clinical trial will measure the effect of the second treatment dose on survival of patients with recurrent malignant glioma.

▶ This interesting study indicates that wafers impregnated with BCNU can be placed in the bed of a resected glioma for local intensive postoperative chemotherapy. The technique is safe, and trials are now underway to assess efficacy.—R.M. Crowell, M.D.

Interstitial Thermoradiotherapy of Brain Tumors: Preliminary Results of a Phase I Clinical Trial
Stea B, Cetas TC, Cassady JR, Guthkelch AN, Iacono R, Lulu B, Lutz W, Obbens E, Rossman K, Seeger J, Shetter A, Shimm DS (Univ of Arizona, Tucson; Barrow Neurol Inst, Phoenix)
Int J Radiat Oncol Biol Phys 19:1463–1471, 1990   16–7

The prognosis of patients with intracranial gliomas is extremely poor. Even with treatment, the median survival of patients with glioblastoma multiforme (GBM) is only 8–12 months. A phase I clinical trial was initiated to assess the feasibility, tolerance, and morbidity associated with interstitial thermoradiotherapy in the treatment of high-grade supratentorial brain gliomas.

The study population included 4 men and 10 women aged 21–69 years, 11 of whom had a biopsy-proven GBM; 3 had an anaplastic astrocytoma. Five patients had recurrent GBM. Only patients with a life expectancy of at least 3 months and a Karnofsky performance status of at least 50 were included. Hyperthermia was delivered via thermally regulating ferromagnetic implants afterloaded into stereotactically placed plastic catheters. Heat treatments with a desired target temperature ranging from 42° to 45° C were administered immediately before interstitial irradiation. At completion of hyperthermia, the catheters were afterloaded with iridium 192, which delivered a variable radiation dose of 14–50 Gy. Patients with previously untreated tumors were given supplemental external beam radiotherapy at 40–41.4 Gy. The median number of treatment catheters implanted per patient was 19. In addition, each patient had 2–5 thermometry probes inserted for temperature measurements.

All 14 patients underwent at least 1 attempt at hyperthermia, but 2 patients could not complete heat treatment because of poor tolerance. Both completed the iridium 192 brachytherapy portion of the protocol. Five of the remaining 12 patients received a second heat treatment at completion of brachytherapy. A total of 175 intratumoral points were monitored, of which 83 (47%) had time-averaged mean temperatures >42° C (Fig 16–

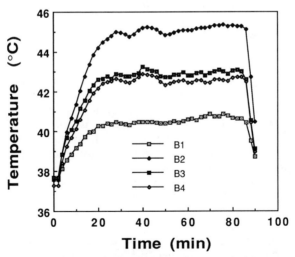

Fig 16–3.—Temperature profiles during a hyperthermia treatment of a left temporoparietal GBM. Sensors are spaced at 1-cm intervals; B1 is the innermost (deepest) sensor, whereas B4 is the most superficial one (closest to the skull). Note that the middle 2 sensors (B2 and B3) register the highest temperatures, whereas the sensors (B1 and B4) located at the periphery of the tumor register the lowest temperatures. (Courtesy of Stea B, Cetas TC, Cassady JR, et al: *Int J Radiat Oncol Biol Phys* 19:1463–1471, 1990.)

3). Only 12 sensors (7%) exceeded a temperature of 45° C. There were 4 minor complications, which resolved with conservative treatment. One of the 2 patients who had major acute complications died of treatment-associated toxicity.

Five of the 7 patients with primary tumors who completed at least 1 hyperthermia treatment were still alive 7–19 months after diagnosis, 1 patient died of progressive disease at 9 months, and 1 died of treatment-associated complications 2 months after diagnosis. Four of the 5 patients with recurrent disease died 1–5.5 months after treatment. These preliminary results confirm the feasibility of interstitial thermoradiotherapy of brain tumors with the use of ferromagnetic implants.

▶ These results of interstitial thermoradiotherapy of gliomas were encouraging, with minor toxicity and a single demise among 14 patients. Further inquiries are needed, however, before this approach can be used on a routine basis.—R.M. Crowell, M.D.

Radioresponse of Human Astrocytic Tumors Across Grade as a Function of Acute and Chronic Irradiation
Schultz CJ, Geard CR (Columbia Univ)
Int J Radiat Oncol Biol Phys 19:1397–1403, 1990   16–8

The treatment of patients with high-grade astrocytomas remains difficult because long-term survival is rare. In contrast, the 5-year survival among patients with low-grade astrocytomas treated with subtotal resection and postoperative radiotherapy approaches 50%. Because variable sensitivity across tumor grade may contribute to the difference in the behavior of astrocytomas, the radioresponse of human glial tumors across grade as a function of the dose rate of irradiation was studied.

Cell lines derived from 1 low-grade and from 2 high-grade astrocytomas were established in culture. Clonal survival was determined after irradiating the 3 cell lines with cesium 137 gamma rays at a high dose rate of 78 Gy/hr and at a low dose rate ranging from 14 to 79 cGY/hr.

The survival curves of the 3 astrocytic human tumor lines after acute high-dose rate irradiation showed that the low-grade astrocytoma was more radiosensitive than either of the high-grade tumor lines. This finding may in part explain the superior clinical radioresponses obtained when treating low-grade tumors compared with high-grade tumors.

▶ This interesting radiobiological study of astrocytic tumors comes up with some interesting findings: Low-grade tumors were more sensitive than high-grade tumors, and a number of specific dose correlations could be achieved. This kind of study seems likely to help in development of more effective strategies for irradiation of intracranial gliomas.—R.M. Crowell, M.D.

Interstitial Brachytherapy for Malignant Brain Tumors: Preliminary Results

Bernstein M, Laperriere N, Leung P, McKenzie S (Univ of Toronto)
Neurosurgery 26:371–380, 1990   16–9

The outcome of interstitial brachytherapy was reviewed in 46 patients with a histologically proven supratentorial malignant astrocytoma. Only patients aged 18–70 years with a Karnofsky performance score of 70 or better and a maximal CT tumor dimension of 6 cm or less were accepted into the study. Patients stratified by age and Karnofsky score were randomized to receive external radiation with or without an ^{125}I implant (Fig 16–4).

Twenty-three patients have received interstitial implants to date. Eighteen others have been treated for recurrent astrocytoma, and 3 for recurrent solitary metastatic adenocarcinoma. Two other patients were treated as part of initial management for radiation-induced malignant astrocy-

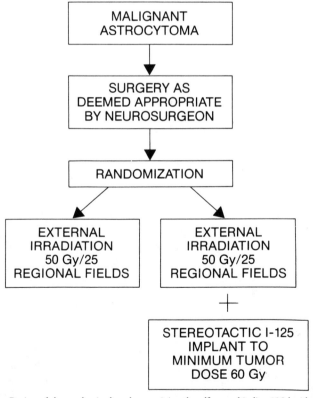

Fig 16–4.—Design of the randomized study examining the efficacy of iodine-125 brachytherapy as part of the initial management for patients with malignant astrocytoma. (Courtesy of Bernstein M, Laperriere N, Leung P, et al: *Neurosurgery* 26:371–380, 1990.)

toma or fibrous histiocytoma. After a maximum follow-up of 31 months, the median survival was 60 weeks for patients given implants and 44 weeks for patients given implants for recurrent astrocytoma. Two of the 3 patients given implants for recurrent solitary metastasis are alive. Significant complications occurred in 22% of the patients; 12 had a second operation after deteriorating.

Interstitial brachytherapy benefits selected patients with recurrent malignant astrocytoma or solitary recurrent metastasis. Its role as part of initial management in patients with malignant astrocytoma remains uncertain. The measure remains palliative for those with tumor cells outside the main treated lesion. In addition, interstitial brachytherapy has significant toxic effects on the brain.

▶ Interstitial radiation of brain tumors has been carried out for at least a decade. The theoretical advantage of placing a very high dose of radiation directly into the tumor remains tantalizing. However, the results to date have not firmly established the indications for this treatment method, if any. This presentation from Toronto offers a thoughtful and careful review of 46 patients with malignant brain tumors treated with interstitial brachytherapy. The data demonstrate a benefit for selected patients with recurrent malignancy in terms of longevity but did not permit identification of a benefit for patients initially treated with this method. It also should be noted that the treatment technique had a 21.7% incidence of complications occurring that were attributable to brachytherapy.

Although it is technically possible for many groups to perform this type of treatment, the indications, benefits, and cost-benefit ratio have not yet been determined. The number of cases required to obtain compelling data on the method is large and the number of cases to be seen in any single center is small, thus it appears highly appropriate to proceed with the development of a single multicenter trial to establish the place (if any) of this type of treatment for malignant brain tumors.—R.M. Crowell, M.D.

Metastases

The Value of Computed Tomographic (CT) Scan Surveillance in the Detection and Management of Brain Metastases in Patients With Small Cell Lung Cancer
Hardy J, Smith I, Cherryman G, Vincent M, Judson I, Perren T, Williams M (Royal Marsden Hosp, Sutton, England)
Br J Cancer 62:684–686, 1990   16–10

Brain metastases are common in patients with small-cell lung cancer (SCLC). Prophylactic cranial irradiation (PCI) can reduce the risk of cranial relapse, but it has not been associated with improved survival and carries the risk of short- and long-term morbidity. A study was done to evaluate the efficacy of serial CT scanning at 3-month intervals, as an alternative to PCI, in the early detection of CNS disease in 127 asymptomatic patients.

Serial CT scanning was done every 3 months for 2 years. Central nervous system metastases were found in 56 patients, or 44%. Metastases were found in 16 patients at diagnosis and in 40 at a median of 4 months after chemotherapy was completed. None of the patients had CNS disease while receiving chemotherapy.

Thirty-six patients were asymptomatic at diagnosis, but clinical CNS relapse developed in 20 between CT scans. Despite prompt radiotherapy, 56% of the patients asymptomatic at diagnosis and 60% of those with CNS relapse died with active CNS disease. There was no significant difference in survival between these 2 groups or between either group and those in whom CNS disease never developed.

In this series, regular CT scanning failed to detect presymptomatic disease in one third of the patients in whom CNS metastases developed. Therefore, regular CT brain scan surveillance, even when done as often as every 3 months and followed by prompt CNS radiotherapy, is not an effective substitute for PCI.

▶ The debate regarding PCI for SCLC goes on. In this study, regular CT scanning failed to detect presymptomatic disease in many patients, and the authors reason that PCI is therefore warranted. Many, however, do not accept the contention that such irradiation leads to an improved outcome.—R.M. Crowell, M.D.

Surgical Treatment of Brain Metastases in Malignant Melanoma
Brega K, Robinson WA, Winston K, Wittenberg W (Univ of Colorado)
Cancer 66:2105–2110, 1990   16–11

The management of patients with metastatic malignant melanoma to the brain presents a significant dilemma because no successful therapy has been reported for preventing or treating malignant melanoma that involves the brain. In a retrospective study the records of 13 patients who underwent 19 craniotomies for resection of metastatic malignant melanoma during a 6-year period were reviewed. Eleven patients had preoperative evidence of extracranial metastases and 8 had more than 1 intracranial metastasis at operation. Intraoperative ultrasound was used in 18 of the 19 craniotomies to minimize surgical trauma to the brain.

The 30-day mortality was zero and the 30-day morbidity was minimal. No patient acquired a new neurologic deficit as a result of surgery, and all patients with preoperative neurologic deficits experienced significant palliative benefit after surgery. The median survival of the 13 patients was 10 months (range, 4–25 months). Seven who were dead at the time of review had a median survival of 10 months (4–18 months).

The surgical treatment of brain metastasis in malignant melanoma may improve survival and the quality of life. The median survival in this series was longer than that reported previously after conventional chemotherapy or cranial radiation. Surgery should be considered in patients who have a life expectancy of 2 or more months, those with life-threatening intracranial metastases even when there is more than 1 metastatic lesion, and in those who have no metastatic disease elsewhere.

▶ Surgical excision of brain metastases in malignant melanoma offers extended longevity and favorable quality of life. This retrospective study offers support to surgical excision of these lesions, which are known to be radioresistant. A prospective study is needed to confirm this impression.— R.M. Crowell, M.D.

Final Report of the French Multicenter Phase II Study of the Nitrosourea Fotemustine in 153 Evaluable Patients With Disseminated Malignant Melanoma Including Patients With Cerebral Metastases
Jacquillat C, Khayat D, Banzet P, Weil M, Fumoleau P, Avril M-F, Namer M, Bonneterre J, Kerbrat P, Bonerandi JJ, Bugat R, Montcuquet P, Cupissol D, Lauvin R, Vilmer C, Prache C, Bizzari JP (Hôp Pitié-Salpétrière, Paris; Hôp St Louis, Paris; Centre R Gauducheau, Nantes; Inst G. Roussy, Villejuif; Centre A Lacassagne, Nice et al)
Cancer 66:1873–1878, 1990   16–12

The incidence of malignant melanoma is increasing worldwide. This virulent form of cancer has a poor prognosis and is resistant to conventional chemotherapy. Data from the French multicenter phase II study of the nitrosourea fotemustine in 169 patients with disseminated malignant melanoma were reviewed.

All 169 patients had histologic evidence of disseminated disease, and some had cerebral metastases. Treatment consisted of a 100 mg/m^2 1-hour intravenous infusion every week for 3 consecutive weeks followed by a 4- to 5-week rest period. Maintenance therapy for those responding or stabilizing included 100 mg/m^2 every 3 weeks until disease progression.

Among 153 evaluable patients, 3 had complete responses and 34 had partial responses, for an objective response rate of 24.2%. Responses occurred in 25% of cerebral metastatic sites, 19.2% of visceral metastatic sites, and 31.8% of nonvisceral metastatic sites. The median response duration was 22 weeks. Previously untreated patients had an objective response rate of 30.7%. Hematologic effects comprised the main toxicity consisting of delayed and reversible leukopenia and/or thrombocytopenia.

Fotemustine appears to be an effective drug in the treatment of disseminated malignant melanoma. It is associated with a promising response rate and activity against cerebral metastases, and causes a minimal amount of extrahematologic toxicity.

▶ This multicenter French trial suggests that fotemustine is effective against disseminated malignant melanoma. The possible combination of this type of chemotherapy with surgical treatment should be considered in selected patients. Further data are required to establish the role of this promising new treatment.— R.M. Crowell, M.D.

Disposition of Cerebral Metastases From Malignant Melanoma: Implications for Radiosurgery
Davey P, O'Brien P (Toronto-Bayview Regional Cancer Ctr)
Neurosurgery 28:8–15, 1991   16–13

Most patients in whom cerebral metastases develop from malignant melanoma die of intracranial tumors rather than from metastatic disease. Whole-brain irradiation has been the treatment of choice for palliation of patients with metastatic disease, but recently there has been increasing use of higher-dose irradiation to small targets within the brain. Data on 41 patients with cerebral metastases from malignant melanoma were reviewed retrospectively to document the disposition of intracranial tumors and to determine whether these patients represent a group in which radiosurgical techniques might be appropriate.

Computed tomographic scans were available for all patients. The location, size, and shape of cerebral metastases were determined. Before starting radiotherapy, 5 patients had undergone surgical decompression and evacuation of the tumor. During the time that cerebral metastases developed, 7 patients were undergoing chemotherapy; 2 others received chemotherapy after whole-brain irradiation, and 2 patients died before irradiation treatment was begun.

Of a total of 206 metastases, there were 6 solitary metastases; 26 patients had 3 or fewer metastases. Only 12 patients had metastases that were not spherical. The median survival of the group was 12 weeks. In 26 of 34 patients, the principal cause of death was progression of the intracranial tumor. Radiation dose-volume histograms demonstrated that a third of the patients had cerebral metastases amenable to a radiosurgical approach.

Eradication of cerebral metastases will not cure most patients with malignant melanoma, but improved control of intracerebral tumors should provide additional palliation. Radiosurgery may be appropriate in patients with limited numbers of small-volume cerebral metastases.

▶ This interesting paper presents a case for radiosurgical treatment of intracranial metastatic melanoma. The basic rationale is that these lesions are relatively radioresistant, thus they require a higher dosage of radiation, and radiosurgery offers the best means to deliver this dose.

Several reservations about this approach: The dose calculations indicate that a minumum tumor dose of 22.5 Gy to 3 targets in the brain with 25-mm collimators may be safe, but current data from Pittsburgh and Boston strongly disagree (a total dose of 18 Gy is suggested as a maximum by the Pittsburgh group). Moreover, a rationale is not proof of efficacy or safety: Only the careful accretion of data from treated patients will help to establish this approach as effective and safe. It is important to keep in mind, as well, that surgical excision of these lesions can produce long-term benefit when the lesion is accessible and careful microsurgical resection is carried out.— R.M. Crowell, M.D.

Meningiomas

Growth Rate of Incidental Meningiomas
Firsching RP, Fischer A, Peters R, Thun F, Klug N (Univ of Köln, Germany)
J Neurosurg 73:545–547, 1990   16–14

Incidental meningiomas, frequently found at autopsy, are now being identified in asymptomatic persons undergoing CT. The growth rate of meningiomas that do not require operative removal is now known, but some observations suggest that it may be quite slow. Data were reviewed on 17 cases of incidentally discovered meningiomas to characterize the growth rate of these tumors.

The diagnosis was verified histologically in only 1 patient. Radiologic findings, together with the age range of the group and the preponderance of women, provided the basis for diagnosis in the remaining patients. Most of the patients had undergone CT to determine the cause of such symptoms as headache and dizziness. Tumor volume was determined by repeat CT scans or MRI.

The median follow-up period was 21 months, and the median annual rate of tumor growth was 3.6%. Two tumors, however, grew at markedly higher rates (18% and 21%), but 1 of these was extremely small (.09 cc^3) at the time of diagnosis. Neither patient age nor initial tumor size appeared to have an influence on the growth rate. Although growth was very slight in some cases, none of the tumors appeared to be shrinking.

No operations were performed in this group of patients, either because the tumor was thought to have no clinical relevance or because the operative risk was considered to be too high. These findings suggest that not all meningiomas need be removed in asymptomatic cases. The tumors should be monitored, however, by repeat CT.

▶ This useful report indicates that on careful serial CT scans, the volume of meningiomas increases annually at a rate of about 3.6% over a mean follow-up of 21 months. On the other hand, 2 tumors grew at markedly higher rates (18% and 21%). No tumor got smaller.

The report suggests that serial scanning is important in the management of these lesions. Not all lesions need to be removed, especially when they are not asymptomatic. Certain lesions grow faster than others and can be identified in this way.— R.M. Crowell, M.D.

Meningiomas Involving the Clivus: A Six-Year Experience With 41 Patients
Sekhar LN, Jannetta PJ, Burkhart LE, Janosky JE (Univ of Pittsburgh)
Neurosurgery 27:764–781, 1990   16–15

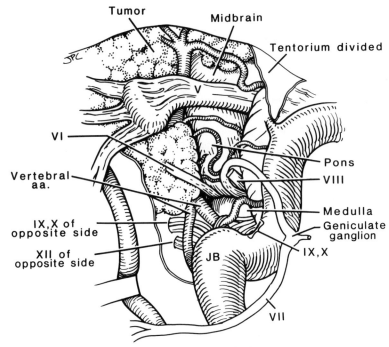

Fig 16–5.—Exposure of a large clival meningioma by a total petrosectomy approach. The encased basilar artery is seen. The petrous ICA has been displaced forward to improve the exposure. Facial nerve reconstruction, as illustrated here, was not possible in another patient because of the absence of a central nerve stump. (Courtesy of Sekhar LN, Jannetta PJ, Burkhart LE, et al: *Neurosurgery* 27:764–781, 1990.)

Meningiomas involving the clivus are a challenging neurosurgical problem. Data were reviewed concerning 41 patients operated on for such tumors between 1983 and 1990. Five patients had giant tumors, 27 had large tumors, and 9 had medium-sized lesions. The patients were evaluated by thin-section, high-resolution CT using soft tissue and bone algorithms.

Many operative approaches were used, including the frontotemporal-transcavernous approach for tumors involving the cavernous sinus and the upper and some of the middle clival region. A frontotemporal or anterior subtemporal approach with zygomatic osteotomy is feasible when the cavernous sinus is not involved. The middle and lower clival region may be exposed by a frontotemporal and preauricular infratemporal approach without having to retract the brain. Other operations include the posterior subtemporal/presigmoid transpetrous approach, total petrosectomy (Fig 16–5), a retrosigmoid operation, and an extreme lateral transcondylar-C1 laminectomy approach.

Total tumor excision was possible in 32 of 41 patients. One patient died operatively and 3 had major neurologic complications ascribed to vascular occlusion in the posterior circulation. Two patients thought to have had total removal had recurrences on follow-up and underwent secondary surgery. Two patients undergoing subtotal excision had evidence of tumor regrowth. Two others had persistent tumor growth despite gamma knife radiosurgery or external radiotherapy.

▶ In 32 of the 41 cases, total removal was achieved. In those cases without total removal, usually those with cavernous sinus involvement, radiosurgery was superadded. The reader is advised that classification of the various meningiomas in this area is a complex subject with several different approaches being described in the literature. In addition, the difficulty of the surgery should be obvious, with these kinds of results being obtainable only in the most experienced hands using extensive monitoring capability. Also, it is worth noting that MR enhancement may certainly occur in the absence of recurrent tumor, thus it may be warranted to follow these patients without early efforts at reoperation.—R.M. Crowell, M.D.

Clonal Analysis of Human Meningiomas and Schwannomas
Jacoby LB, Pulaski K, Rouleau GA, Martuza RL (Massachusetts Gen Hosp, Boston; Harvard Med School)
Cancer Res 50:6783–6786, 1990   16–16

Meningiomas and schwannomas—among the most common tumors of the human nervous system—most often are sporadic and nonheritable. However, occasionally they are seen in association with neurofibromatosis type 2 (NF2), an autosomal dominant genetic disorder. Molecu-

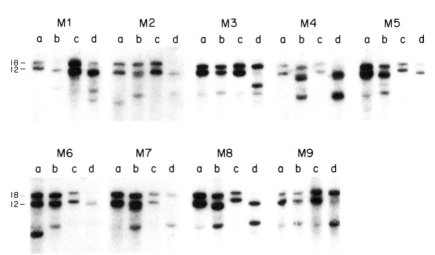

Fig 16–6.—Clonal analysis of meningiomas from patients 1 through 9 using HPRT700 as a probe. DNAs from blood leukocytes *(lanes a and b)* or tumors *(lanes c and d)* were digested with *Bam*HI and *Pvu*II. One aliquot was not digested further *(lanes a and c)*, whereas the other was digested with *Hpa*II (lanes b and d). Left ordinate, restriction fragment size in kilobases. (Courtesy of Jacoby LB, Pulaski K, Rouleau GA, et al: *Cancer Res* 50:6783–6786, 1990.)

lar genetic studies have documented a loss of alteration of chromosome 22 in most of the benign tumors associated with NF2.

Nine meningiomas and 8 schwannomas obtained from females were examined. One tumor occurred in a patient who had NF2; the others were sporadic tumors appearing in the general population. Molecular genetic techniques were used to study X chromosome inactivation to determine whether the tumors arise from a single cell or from multiple cells. The tumors also were screened with polymorphic DNA markers for loss of heterozygosity at several sites on chromosome 22.

In at least 3 of the 9 meningiomas a loss of alleles was noted on chromosome 22 (Fig 16–6). Five tumors retained heterozygosity for the chromosome 22 alleles examined. All of these tumors were monoclonal. At least 7 of the 8 schwannomas examined retained heterozygosity for chromosome 22 loci. Seven of these tumors were monoclonal.

Most, if not all, human meningiomas and schwannomas arise from a single cell. It is not clear whether the locus on chromosome 22 that promotes meningioma formation is the same as that promoting the formation of schwannomas. The molecular mechanisms of these tumors remain to be established.

▶ Dr. Martuza's group continues to provide molecular genetic data for human intracranial tumors. This nice study documents clearly and simply that both meningiomas and schwannomas are monoclonal and thus arise from a single cell abnormality. This type of report shows the power of this basic approach to neuro-oncology.—R.M. Crowell, M.D.

Molecular Genetic Analysis of Chromosome 22 in 81 Cases of Meningioma
Dumanski JP, Rouleau GA, Nordenskjöld M, Collins VP (Ludwig Inst for Cancer Research, Stockholm; Karolinska Hosp, Stockholm; Montreal Gen Hosp; McGill Univ)
Cancer Res 50:5863–5867, 1990 16–17

Meningiomas are primary tumors of the meninges that may originate from any of their constituents. Loss of genetic material from chromosome 22 may be a fundamental event in the tumorigenesis of meningioma. An extensive analysis was made of deletions of genetic material in meningiomas obtained from unrelated patients.

Constitutional and tumor tissue genotypes from 81 patients were compared at 25 polymorphic loci on chromosome 22. Thirty tumors (37%) retained the constitutional genotype along chromosome 22, consistent with no detectable aberrations on chromosome 22 as studied. Forty-two tumors (52%) demonstrated loss of 1 allele at all informative loci consistent with monosomy 22 in the tumor DNA. The remaining 9 tumors (11%) had retained constitutional heterozygosity in tumor DNA at 1 or more centromeric loci and heterozygosity loss at other telomeric loci, a findings consistent with variable terminal deletions of 1 chromosome 22q in tumor DNA.

The localization of breakpoints in these 9 cases with deletions may mean that a meningioma locus is localized distal to myoglobin locus within 22q12.3-qter. Men had a higher percentage of tumors with no detectable aberrations on chromosome 22, which suggests that these tumors in males have preferentially smaller rearrangements on chromosome 22q than those in females, or that there is another mechanism of oncogenesis in male and female cases with no detectable aberrations.

This study confirms the earlier localization of the tentative meningioma gene to the region distal to the myoglobin locus, corresponding to 22q12.3-qter, in extensive material. These findings also suggest that the meningioma and the neurofibromatosis-2 loci are separate entities.

▶ This study confirms localization of the tentative meningioma gene to the distal region of the myoglobin locus, separate from the neurofibromatosis-2 locus.—R.M. Crowell, M.D.

17 Aneurysms

Basic Studies

Angiographic Study of Induced Cerebral Aneurysms in Primates
Kim C, Kikuchi H, Hashimoto N, Hazama F (Fukui Red Cross Hosp, Fukui, Japan; Kyoto Univ Hosp; Shiga Univ of Med Science, Otsu, Japan)
Neurosurgery 27:715–720, 1990   17–1

An animal model of induced saccular cerebral aneurysms was developed in monkeys treated with unilateral carotid ligation, renal hypertension, and β-aminoproprionitrile feeding. By using this model the growth pattern of saccular cerebral aneurysms was studied by repeated angiographic studies in 5 cynomolgus monkeys.

Saccular cerebral aneurysms developed in 3 monkeys; 2 were visualized at 15 months and 1 at 12 months after the operation. One was found at the left internal carotid artery (ICA), 1 was found at the anterior cerebral artery-anterior communicating artery complex, and the third was seen at the right ICA-posterior communicating artery. Autopsy showed that the saccular aneurysm was unilocular in 2 monkeys and bilocular in 1. Fusiform aneurysms were present in 4 monkeys.

Histologically, the walls of the saccular aneurysms were very thin and consisted of fibrous tissue. The conversion of early aneurysmal changes into saccular aneurysms occurred abruptly, and no consistent growth rate was noted. There was no evidence of previous subarachnoid hemorrhage, and the largest aneurysm was bilocular and almost completely thrombosed.

Saccular cerebral aneurysms may grow abruptly from early aneurysmal changes, and multiloculation is closely related to the size of the aneurysm. The development and growth of saccular cerebral aneurysms vary, depending on systemic and focal conditions.

▶ Hashimoto's group continues to provide interesting information on experimental aneurysms produced in the laboratory. This particular communication documents information gleaned from serial angiographic studies in 5 primate aneurysms. Probably the most interesting feature here is the lack of consistent growth from the saccular aneurysm with abrupt conversion of early alterations into full-fledged saccular aneurysms. Also, the development of multilobular and fusiform aneurysms could be demonstrated by this type of study. Further investigations of this type are extremely valuable for learning about the alterations in aneurysms developed in this way. It should be noted that these changes are specifically relevant to the degenerative process of aneurysm formation and may not apply fully to aneurysms that develop on the basis of congenital defects in the arterial wall.—R.M. Crowell, M.D.

Cerebral Blood Flow Patterns at Major Vessel Bifurcations and Aneurysms in Rats

Nakatani H, Hashimoto N, Kang Y, Yamazoe N, Kikuchi H, Yamaguchi S, Niimi H (Kyoto Univ; Nat'l Cardiovasc Ctr Research Inst, Osaka, Japan)
J Neurosurg 74:258–262, 1991 17–2

Saccular cerebral aneurysms have a predilection for arterial bifurcations or the top of an arterial curvature where the bloodstream is likely to impinge. A method was developed of inducing cerebral aneurysms at the bifurcation of major cerebral arteries in male Sprague-Dawley rats.

The left common carotid artery and the posterior branches of both renal arteries were ligated to induce experimental hypertension and produce cerebral aneurysms. Two weeks later the rats were fed β-aminopropionitrile fumarate. Flow patterns of latex particles introduced under a constant flow rate were analyzed with a 16-mm cine-camera and a videocassette recorder. After perfusion and fixation, the anterior cerebral artery (ACA) and the olfactory artery (OA) at the base of the brain were removed under a dissecting microscope and samples of bifurcations containing shallow invaginations and small aneurysms were obtained and analyzed. Similar arterial junctions of untreated rats were also analyzed.

Aneurysms developed most commonly on the ACA at the origin of the OA on the side opposite the carotid ligation. Flow studies in the bifurcations of control rats showed that the apical intimal pad, rather than the apex itself, acted as the flow divider. Small particles tended to accumulate at the region just distal to the apical intimal pad where initial aneurysmal changes are known to occur. The particle accumulation indicated that there was flow stagnation at that site. There was a marked pressure gradient at the proximal end of the aneurysm orifice. Because wall shear

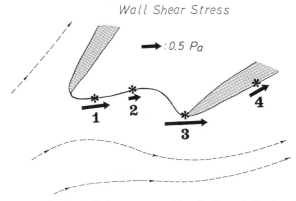

Fig 17–1.—Drawing showing wall shear stress at and just distal to a shallow invagination. The *arrows* indicate the vectors of wall shear stresses. The length of the scale *(uppermost arrow)* represents a wall shear stress of .5 Pa. Wall shear stress was: 1 = .74 Pa; 2 = .34 Pa; 3 = .88 Pa; and 4 = .61 Pa. Note that the wall shear stress was highest at the distal end of the invagination. (Courtesy of Nakatani H, Hashimoto N, Kang Y, et al: *J Neurosurg* 74:258–262, 1991.)

stress was greatest at the distal end of the aneurysmal orifice (Fig 17–1), it may be responsible for the development of aneurysmal lesions.

▶ This study is part of an ongoing effort to develop experimental aneurysms in the laboratory. The work is carefully done, and the results support the degeneration theory of aneurysm causation. The data do not, however, negate a genetic factor in some cases, especially familial cases.—R.M. Crowell, M.D.

Elastic Skeleton of Intracranial Cerebral Aneurysms in Rats
Yamazoe N, Hashimoto N, Kikuchi H, Hazama F (Kyoto Univ; Shiga Univ of Med Science, Ohtsu, Japan)
Stroke 21:1722–1726, 1990   17–3

Electron microscopic studies have suggested that the internal elastic lamina is not the sole causative element of aneurysms; rather, it is a part of the complex architecture of the elastic skeleton. To clarify the changes that take place in the elastic skeleton at various stages of aneurysm for-

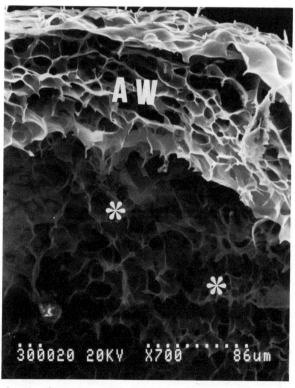

Fig 17–2.—Scanning electron micrograph showing large aneurysm in rat. Thickened aneurysmal wall (AW) was composed of multiple concentric elastic lamellae. On luminal surface fine elastic lamellae were newly formed *(stars)*; ×700. (Courtesy of Yamazoe N, Hashimoto N, Kikuchi H, et al: *Stroke* 21:1722–1726, 1990.)

mation, cerebral aneurysms were produced in 19 male Sprague-Dawley rats by unilateral ligation of the common carotid artery, which induced renal hypertension, and feeding with β-aminoproprionitrile fumarate. After 4–16 weeks the arterial specimens were removed for hot formic acid extraction, freeze drying, and scanning electron microscopy. A control group of 12 age-matched rats was also studied.

The earliest change noted in the experimental animals was loss of folds, both in height and number, protruding from the internal elastic lamina. Loss or disintegration of the elastic skeleton of the intima and then the media occurred. There were then morphological changes of the internal elastic lamina, which were thought to be mainly responsible for aneurysmal formation. It was thought that the risk of rupture was reduced by proliferation of elastic lamellae in aneurysms with thick domes (Fig 17–2).

Aneurysms appear to develop because of disintegration of the complex elastic skeleton of the arterial wall rather than by simple rupture of the internal elastic lamina. This disintegration appears to be related to the functional state of the elastin-producing cells. In rats no enlarged fenestrations are seen in either early or well-developed experimental aneurysms.

▶ A host of studies from Hashimoto's group help to clarify features of aneurysm development in experimental animals. In this particular communication, scanning electron microscopic studies, done at various times during development of aneurysms, show that disintegration of the complex elastic skeleton appears to be the first change leading to aneurysm formation. Further studies of this type will be helpful in elucidating the pathogenesis of experimental aneurysms to throw light on the development of aneurysms in patients.—R.M. Crowell, M.D.

Experimental Isobaric Subarachnoid Hemorrhage: Regional Mitochondrial Function During the Acute and Late Phase

Marzatico F, Gaetani P, Silvani V, Lombardi D, Sinforiani E, Rodriguez y Baena R (IRCCS Policlinico S Matteo, Pavia; Univ of Pavia, Italy)
Surg Neurol 34:294–300, 1990   17–4

Long-term follow-up studies show that patients treated for aneurysmal subarachnoid hemorrhage (SAH) have an increased rate of cognitive disturbances and psychological maladjustments that may be related to the neurotoxic effects of blood deposition in the subarachnoidal space resulting in diffuse encephalopathy. To define the biochemical correlates of this fact, nonsynaptic mitochondrial function was studied in the frontal cortex, occipital cortex, hippocampus, and brain stem after experimental isobaric SAH in rats. The biochemical parameters were measured at 1 hour and 72 hours after the subarachnoidal injection of .07 mL of arterial autologous blood into the cisterna magna.

The intracranial pressure did not significantly increase. Experimental SAH did not significantly affect the nonsynaptic mitochondrial enzymatic activities related to aerobic metabolism at 1 hour and 72 hours. However, SAH caused significant changes in nonsynaptic mitochondrial respiratory parameters. A reversible inhibition of the NADH-oxidative branch of the electron transfer chain was evident only at the frontal cortex at 1 hour after isobaric SAH induction. At 72 hours there was a significant decrease in the respiratory control ratio in all brain areas, which was related primarily to a widespread increase in state 4.

These experimental data suggest that, after SAH, the decrease in cerebral oxidative machinery can be related to severe impairment of mitochondria and is site and time dependent. The increased mitochondrial vulnerability in the delayed phases can be related to neuronal impairment after the initial bleeding and can be one of the biochemical correlates of posthemorrhage encephalopathy.

▶ These studies in rats indicate that, in the absence of increased intracranial pressure, experimental SAH leads to disturbances in mitochonrial enzymatic activities and diminished cerebral oxidative metabolism. Thus SAH causes a direct disturbance of brain metabolism without the need to postulate a change in intracranial pressure. Such factors must be considered in the overall pathophysiology of SAH in a clinical setting.—R.M. Crowell, M.D.

Multiple Arterial Fenestrations, Multiple Aneurysms, and an Arteriovenous Malformation in a Patient With Subarachnoid Hemorrhage
Kalia KK, Ross DA, Gutin PH (Univ of California, San Francisco)
Surg Neurol 35:45–48, 1991   17–5

A patient was treated for an aneurysm of the anterior communicating artery (ACOMA), multiple aneurysms of the middle cerebral artery (MCA), and an arteriovenous malformation (AVM) in association with a fenestrated ACOMA and MCA.

Man, 49, right-handed, experienced the sudden onset of severe headache. Cerebral angiography, CT, and MRI revealed a large, right frontotemporal AVM with feeding arteries from the right MCA and the anterior cerebral artery (ACA), venous drainage of the AVM to the right sylvian veins and the cavernous sinus through the sphenoparietal sinus, 3 aneurysms of the right MCA, an aneurysm of the ACOMA, and a normal vertebrobasilar system. Dissection was performed in 3 stages. At the third operation, dissection into the sylvian fissure revealed a puzzling aneurysm complex that proved to be a fenestrated MCA with the aneurysm contained in the fenestration. Because the aneurysm could not be clipped without risk of rupture, this aneurysm and the distal infundibular were wrapped on all sides with muslin. The patient was discharged neurologically intact.

Congenital and hemodynamic factors may have combined to manifest in the anomalies found in this patient. This combination of vascular pathology has not been reported previously.

▶ This interesting report documents the coincidence of an AVM, aneurysms, and arterial fenestrations in the same patient. The occurrence of aneurysm in association with an AVM is not rare, and most often the aneurysms arise on the major arteries feeding the AVM. Thus an increase in flow through the feeding arteries may be related to the development of aneurysms, suggesting a hemodynamic degenerative mechanism. This mechanism certainly could have been a part of the MCA aneurysms on the right in this case.

The existence of an ACOMA aneurysm in this case, however, would not appear to be related to increased flow to the AVM. Thus a congenital, possibly genetic mechanism, could be at work. The existence of multiple fenestrations in this patient also suggest the possible dysplasticity of vessels, and an underlying genetic mechanism would be likely. It is hoped that gene probe studies in the future will enable us to identify the specific genetic abnormalities in such cases.

The MCA aneurysm in this case was judged too hazardous to be clipped directly by the operating surgeon, and certainly intraoperative judgment is of the greatest importance in such a decision. On the other hand, it is also true that clip obliteration of an aneurysm is the best known treatment to avert future hemorrhage. In some cases, aneurysms related to a fenestration can be clipped appropriately, as in the case of the ACA in this case. Temporary clipping of the MCA can sometimes be helpful in the dissection and safe obliteration of such aneurysms. In this particular case, such a program of temporary clipping might create a special hazard in relation to the AVM. The question of barbiturate treatment during such temporary occlusion and thereafter to prevent reperfusion bleeding comes into the discussion. Clearly, a case of this sort is extremely complex, and the hazards of management are substantial.—R.M. Crowell, M.D.

Autopsy Study of Unruptured Incidental Intracranial Aneurysms
Inagawa T, Hirano A (Shimane Prefectural Central Hosp, Izumo, Japan; Montefiore Med Ctr, Bronx)
Surg Neurol 34:361–365, 1990   17–6

In a series of more than 10,000 autopsies done at Montefiore Medical Center between 1951 and 1987, 84 patients had 102 unruptured aneurysms, for a prevalence of .8%. Sixteen patients had multiple aneurysms. The mean age at death was 67 years. Nearly two thirds were women. Middle cerebral artery and internal carotid artery aneurysms were most frequent.

In this series, unruptured aneurysms were most common in patients aged 60 and older. Fifty-four percent of the aneurysms were 4 mm or less in diameter, whereas 35% measured 5 mm to 9 mm in diameter. Aneurysm size could not be related to age, aneurysm site, or wall thickness.

Small aneurysms may be at a low risk of rupturing, but this low risk probably cannot be explained adequately by morphological features alone. Hemodynamic studies might cast light on why unruptured aneurysms rarely rupture.

▶ This interesting study showed a prevalence of .8% unruptured aneurysms in an autopsy study of 10,259 cases. The incidence of unruptured aneurysms is higher in patients older than 60 years, most common on the middle cerebral artery, somewhat more common in females, and most common in the setting of lesions 9 mm or less (89%). The study suggests that larger lesions may be more likely to rupture, but morphological features alone cannot predict whether rupture will occur.—R.M. Crowell, M.D.

Negative Angiography

Ruptured Cerebral Aneurysms Missed by Initial Angiographic Study
Iwanaga H, Wakai S, Ochiai C, Narita J, Inoh S, Nagai M (Dokkyo Univ, Mibu, Tochigi, Japan)
Neurosurgery 27:45–51, 1990   17–7

The cause of bleeding is not determined in a significant number of patients with subarachnoid hemorrhage (SAH), even when advanced neuroradiologic methods are used. Some of these patients will have further bleeding, and a poor outcome is possible. The CT scans and angiograms of 45 patients with SAH whose initial angiograms were negative for aneurysm were reviewed. They were among 469 patients with SAH who were assessed during a 15-year period. The mean time from onset of SAH to initial angiography was 8 days. Thirty-eight patients underwent angiography a second time within a mean of 16 days after SAH.

Aneurysms were found in 8 patients, 7 on the anterior communicating artery and 1 involving the junction of the internal carotid and posterior communicating arteries. The second angiogram was most often positive in patients in whom a thick layer of subarachnoid blood was observed on CT examination done within 4 days of SAH. Most patients with substantial blood in the basal frontal interhemispheric fissure had an aneurysm of the anterior communicating artery.

Angiography need not be pursued if an early CT study shows no blood, or blood primarily in the perimesencephalic cisterns. However, if subarachnoid blood is present, angiography should be repeated at an early stage. Patients with a negative repeat angiogram can expect a normal life but should know that there is a minor risk of rebleeding.

▶ The authors usefully correlate the amount and distribution of blood on early CT with the presence of aneurysm detected after an initial negative angiogram. They found that thick layering of blood in the basal interhemispheric area was predictive of an aneurysm in the anterior communicating complex. In addition, blood in the perimesencephalic cisterns was unlikely to be associated with a missed aneurysm. The source of hemorrhage in the few patients with new bleeding in spite of complete study was presumed to be from refilling of aneurysmal sacs that were thrombosed at the time of angiography.

A useful recommendation from the study is that, after negative angiography, further evaluation be guided by the initial CT. If the early CT shows no blood, or blood primarily in the perimesencephalic cisterns, no further angiography need be done. If the CT shows subarachnoid blood, particularly in the interhemispheric fissure, repeat angiography is warranted. When the repeat angiogram is negative, patients may be informed that a minor risk of rebleeding exists.

In addition to these points, we have found that exploration of an area with remarkable deposition of blood can sometimes lead to detection at surgery of an aneurysm that was not appreciated on repeated angiography. In addition, we occasionally have repeated angiographic study months after 2 initially negative studies when recurrent symptomatology suggested a possible problem, and on occasion we have found an aneurysm.—R.M. Crowell, M.D.

Subarachnoid Hemorrhage of Unknown Etiology: Early Prognostic Factors for Long-Term Functional Capacity
Oder W, Kollegger H, Zeiler K, Dal-Bianco P, Wessely P, Deecke L (Univ of Vienna)
J Neurosurg 74:601–605, 1991   17–8

Subarachnoid hemorrhage (SAH) of unknown cause has a better early prognosis than aneurysmal or angiomatous SAH, but its long-term outcome is worse than expected. Prognostic factors deserve more attention because specific treatment is impossible. A series of patients with SAH was reviewed to evaluate early prognostic factors for long-term functional capacity.

Seventy-two patients were admitted with a diagnosis of spontaneous SAH during a 9-year period. Of these, 41 had SAH without a demonstrable bleeding source. There were 24 men and 17 women; the mean age at admission was 47.3 years. Thirty-nine patients had a detailed neurologic and psychiatric examination an average of 90.9 months after onset of SAH; the other 2 patients died.

Nineteen patients were able to return to their previous work level, 5 had part-time work, and 4 were unable to work. Moderate disability in activities of daily living was present in 5 patients, and 1 was severly disabled. One patient had rebleeding. Three clinical variables at admission were correlated with an unfavorable outcome: history of hypertension, Hunt and Hess grade greater than II, and focal neurologic deficits. Reduced functional capacity was also predicted by the presence of an organic mental syndrome at discharge. Limitations in functional level were not related to the other variables considered, including sex, age, history of headache, time between SAH and admission, impairments in consciousness, and cognitive deficits. Restrictions in global function, as measured by the Karnofsky Performance Scale, were not predicted by residual neurologic deficits and Glasgow Outcome Scale score at discharge.

Among patients with SAH of unknown cause, those who have no history of hypertension, no focal neurologic deficits, and a Hunt and Hess grade of I or II on admission are at extremely low risk of residual deficit. They can be told that their disease is benign if they have no organic mental syndrome at discharge, and they should be encouraged to resume their normal activities after repeated panangiography.

▶ This report indicates that a large majority of patients with SAH of unknown etiology return to work status (86%). Early prognosis of an unfavorable functional capacity was possible on the basis of 3 factors: history of hypertension, Hunt and Hess grade of greater than 2, and presence of focal neurologic deficits. This prognostic scale does not correlate with the later occurrence of subarachnoid hemorrhage, which is known to be rare.—R.M. Crowell, M.D.

Microsurgery

Direct Surgery for Carotid Bifurcation Artery Aneurysms
Laranjeira M, Sadasivan B, Ausman JI (Henry Ford Neurosurgical Inst, Detroit)
Surg Neurol 34:250–254, 1990   17–9

Surgical treatment of bifurcation of internal carotid artery aneurysms is particularly difficult because of perforating arteries surrounding and adherent to the aneurysm. Although some aneurysms are treated with proximal ligation of the carotid artery, good results can be achieved with appropriate dissection strategy and direct surgery of the aneurysms.

In 18 patients whose aneurysms were treated with direct surgery, 16 outcomes were judged excellent, 1 good, and 1 fair with no mortality. Dissection strategy was determined by aneurysm size and length of the intracranial internal carotid artery. The pterional approach was used in all of the cases. In a small aneurysm, bifurcation of the internal carotid artery can be exposed by dissecting along the artery in a proximal to distal direction. The aneurysm and perforating vessels are identified before the aneurysm is clipped (Fig 17–3). In a large aneurysm or when the intracranial segment of the internal carotid artery is long, the sylvian fissure is opened before dissection of the aneurysm and perforators.

In this series, 94% of the patients who underwent direct surgery in treatment of carotid bifurcation artery aneurysms had a good or excellent result, and there was no mortality. With an appropriate dissection strategy and an understanding of the microanatomy of the perforators, all carotid bifurcation aneurysms can be treated by direct surgery with good results.

▶ Experience with 18 patients indicates that these lesions can be clipped successfully by direct attack. Preservation of perforator vessels is important. For

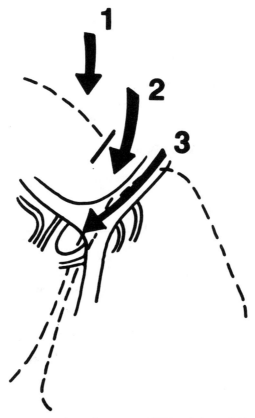

Fig 17–3.—Dissection strategy for small aneurysm: *(1)* The optical nerve is identified. *(2)* The proximal intracranial carotid artery is identified. This is dissected toward the bifurcation. *(3)* The aneurysm and perforators are identified. The aneurysm is clipped. (Courtesy of Laranjeira M, Sadasivan B, Ausman JI: *Surg Neurol* 34:250–254, 1990.)

small aneurysms this can be achieved by following the carotid artery. For large or giant lesions, a wide sylvian split is recommended.—R.M. Crowell, M.D.

Saccular Aneurysms of the Distal Anterior Cerebral Artery
Ohno K, Monma S, Suzuki R, Masaoka H, Matsushima Y, Hirakawa K (Tokyo Med and Dental Univ)
Neurosurgery 27:907–913, 1990   17–10

Forty-two consecutive patients with distal anterior cerebral artery (ACA) aneurysms were studied. Five and 2 aneurysms each, and 1 had 3 lesions (Fig 17–4). Thirty patients had a ruptured distal ACA aneurysm; in 20 of these cases the aneurysm measured less than 5 mm in diameter. Eighteen patients in all had multiple aneurysms. The distal ACA aneurysm caused subarachnoid hemorrhage in 10 patients.

Of the 34 patients who had direct surgery, 30 had excellent outcomes

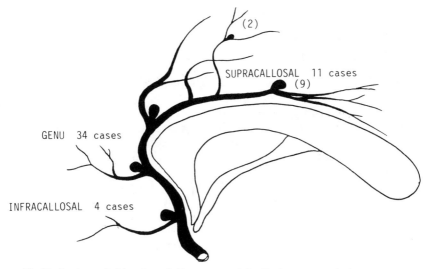

(2)

SUPRACALLOSAL   11 cases
(9)

GENU   34 cases

INFRACALLOSAL   4 cases

Fig 17–4.—Anatomical locations of 49 aneurysms of the distal anterior cerebral artery in 42 patients. (Courtesy of Ohno K, Monma S, Suzuki R, et al: *Neurosurgery* 27:907–913, 1990.)

3 months postoperatively. Overall, 36 of the 42 patients had good outcomes and 2 had poor outcomes. There were 4 deaths. Twenty-six distal ACA aneurysms were managed by clipping the neck. Considerable technical difficulty was encountered in some patients with other aneurysms and in some who had a distal ACA aneurysm with a broad neck.

Distal aneurysms of the ACA are prone to bleeding even if they are not large. Excellent results can be achieved by direct surgery on these aneurysms if this is done at an early stage when the patient is in good neurologic condition.

▶ This nice presentation emphasizes 3 key points about distal anterior cerebral artery aneurysms: (1) they are often present in the setting of multiple aneurysms; (2) they bleed at small sizes in many cases (less than 6 mm in many); (3) with microsurgical techniques, excellent results may be obtained.—R.M. Crowell, M.D.

Long-Term Results of Wrapping of Intracranial Ruptured Aneurysms
Fujiwara S, Fujii K, Nishio S, Fukui M (Kyushu Univ, Japan)
Acta Neurochir (Wien) 103:27–29, 1990   17–11

When clipping ruptured aneurysms is not feasible, reinforcement of the aneurysmal wall is the next best option. Results of long-term follow-up were assessed in a series of patients whose aneurysms were wrapped.

Of 495 intracranial ruptured aneurysms treated during a 23-year period, 29 were treated by wrapping with muscle or gauze and/or coating with bioadhesives. The patients were 15 women and 14 men aged 30–74 years, 10 of whom were treated in the premicrosurgical era. The mean follow-up was 11 years. The most common locations of the aneurysm were the middle cerebral, anterior communicating, and internal carotid arteries, and the most common indication for wrapping was a wide-based neck.

The outcome was good in 19 patients; there was severe disability in 2 and death in 8. Five deaths resulted from rerupture of the aneurysm; in all cases, episodes of rebleeding were fatal. Severe disabilities usually resulted from intraoperative complications in the premicrosurgical era. Most aneurysms that had good outcomes were small; wide-based, large, or giant-type lesions of the middle cerebral artery tended to have a poor outcome.

Wrapping ruptured aneurysms is not a safe alternative to direct operative occlusion. The rate of rebleeding, 17% in this series, is higher than after clipping but lower than after conservative treatment. The indications for wrapping in this series are no longer valid. Given the array of clips for different situations, even large or giant aneurysms can be clipped successfully.

▶ This report adds to the experience with wrapping of intracranial ruptured aneurysms. The suggestion is that this approach led to some protection, albeit incomplete, from rupture. Unfortunately, the wrapping techniques were varied, including muscle, gauze, alpha Aron, and Biobond. Because the effects of the various wrapping agents are known to be different, it is difficult to draw conclusions from a lumping of these results.

Today when clipping is not safely possible, I advise (1) local wrapping with muslin, taking care to avoid muslin touching cranial nerves, and (2) consideration of transvascular obliteration. Note that the surgical exploration can assist endovascular treatment by drawing attention to thin areas (which must be treated) and thick walls (which need not be treated).—R.M. Crowell, M.D.

Giant Carotid-Ophthalmic Artery Aneurysms: Direct Clipping Utilizing the "Trapping-Evacuation" Technique

Tamaki N, Kim S, Ehara K, Asada M, Fujita K, Taomoto K, Matsumoto S (Kobe Univ; Hyogo Med Ctr for Adults, Akashi, Japan)
J Neurosurg 74:567–572, 1991   17–12

The difficulty of clipping giant carotid-ophthalmic artery aneurysms directly has led to the development of various alternative surgical methods. A technique of "trapping-evacuation" was developed to facilitate direct clipping of giant aneurysms of the paraophthalmic region of the internal carotid artery (ICA).

Technique.—After isolation of the common carotid and external and internal carotid arteries in the neck and exposure of the ICA proximally in the cavernous portion outside the dura propria, the aneurysm is prepared for trapping and evacuation. The cervical common carotid and external carotid arteries are temporarily occluded, and the intracranial ICA distal to the aneurysm is clipped temporarily to collapse the aneurysm. Through a catheter in the cervical ICA, blood is simultaneously aspirated from the aneurysm. The proximal end of the aneurysm neck, which must be exposed if clipping is to be successful, is reached by extensive unroofing of the optic canal, removal of the anterior clinoid process, opening of the anterior cavernous sinus, and exposure of the most proximal intradural and genu portions of the ICA.

The procedure was used in 4 patients with giant aneurysms of the paraophthalmic ICA during a 9-year period. All 4 lesions were unruptured and on the right side. All patients had a good postoperative outcome. Important factors in successful operation included preoperative MRI, the ICA balloon occlusion test, and intraoperative measurement of cortical blood flow. The success of clipping was confirmed by intraoperative digital subtraction angiography through the cervical ICA catheter.

The trapping-evacuation technique is safe and effective for use in clipping giant paraophthalmic aneurysms previously considered inoperable. The time needed to accomplish trapping is difficult to determine exactly.

▶ This small series illustrates that intraoperative trapping and aspiration of giant carotid-ophthalmic aneurysms may help with dissection and obliteration. The work of Sampson and Batjer in Dallas supports this approach. Results have been good from the small number of patients reported. On the other hand, modern transvascular treatment can also be effective in this group of patients; Carotid occlusion with balloon technique may completely obliterate the lesion, with or without bypass. To determine the best mode of treatment, further controlled studies are required.—R.M. Crowell, M.D.

Aneurysms of the Posterior Inferior Cerebellar Artery-Vertebral Artery Complex: Variations on a Theme

Salcman M, Rigamonti D, Numaguchi Y, Sadato N (Univ of Maryland)
Neurosurgery 27:12–21, 1990   17–13

Data were reviewed on 17 patients seen between 1982 and 1989 with aneurysms of the posterior inferior cerebellar artery (PICA)-vertebral artery (VA) complex. These aneurysms included those on the distal artery and those at the junction of the vertebral and basilar arteries. Nine additional patients had radiologic records available.

Three of 17 patients in the clinical series were not operated on. All but 1 of the 14 who did have surgery had typical signs of subarachnoid hemorrhage, and 6 patients had focal neurologic deficits. Four patients had evidence of intraventricular hemorrhage alone and 2 had intracerebral hemorrhage. Twelve patients had primary clipping of the aneurysmal neck. One each had trapping of the vertebral artery and proximal ligation of this vessel. Surgery was done acutely in 5 instances. Morbidity resulted chiefly from cranial nerve dysfunction; there were no perioperative deaths. After a mean follow-up of 2 years, 11 of the 13 surviving patients were independent.

A PICA-VA aneurysm should be considered when subarachnoid hemorrhage is suspected but the CT study shows no obvious abnormality. Most of these aneurysms are within 7 mm of the midline; a tortuous, elongated vertebral artery can push the aneurysm across the midline, necessitating a contralateral approach. Preoperative test occlusion of the vertebral artery with a balloon may be very helpful. The surgical results are generally quite good.

▶ This is a good review of aneurysms of the PICA, distal vertebral artery, and vertebral basilar junction. I agree fully with the difficulty of diagnosis and other radiographic points that have been made. The CT scan may not suggest a typical subarachnoid hemorrhage. Both vertebral arteries must be injected to detect distal PICA aneurysms. Repeat angiography may well be warranted if the initial studies are negative.

With regard to operative treatment, the authors are to be congratulated on their excellent results. An alternative approach to the vertebral-PICA lesions is obtained with the method described by Heros (1), involving removal of the condyle and approach from below along the axis of the vertebral artery. I find this a very useful method in this group of lesions. In addition, for the higher lesions, a presigmoid, retrolabyrinthine approach is quite useful. This permits preservation of hearing and the lateral sinus with good working space around the vertebral basilar junction. I prefer this method for aneurysms in this location.

With regard to the timing of surgery, the authors were able to obtain good results with acute surgery in 5 cases. I would caution the possibility of marked posterior fossa swelling in this setting, even in the absence of neurologic signs. I encountered 1 such patient in whom severe cerebellar swelling led to an adverse outcome. In the future, I would retreat from such an approach to return after the swelling is resolved.—R.M. Crowell, M.D.

Reference

1. Heros RC: *J Neurosurg* 64:559, 1986.

Isolated Trigeminal Sensory Loss Secondary to a Distal Anterior Inferior Cerebellar Artery Aneurysm: Case Report
Zager EL (Massachusetts Gen Hosp, Boston)
Neurosurgery 28:288–291, 1991   17–14

Isolated trigeminal sensory loss is an exceedingly rare feature of vascular anomalies of the posterior fossa. In a recent patient, isolated trigeminal sensory loss was caused by a distal inferior cerebellar artery aneurysm.

Woman, 25, had acute onset of right-sided facial numbness and headache, with accompanying nausea, photophobia, and transient diplopia. Except for the meningismus and right-sided facial sensory loss, the rest of the neurologic examination was unremarkable. Magnetic resonance imaging and CT showed an acute hematoma in the right cerebellopontine angle. A 4-vessel cerebral arteriogram failed to demonstrate the abnormality, and MRI also failed to show flow through the aneurysm. On posterior fossa exploration, a large, partially thrombosed fusiform aneurysm of the distal anterior inferior cerebellar artery (AICA) was identified, indenting the pons dorsal to the trigeminal root entry zone. The aneurysm was excised. The patient recovered, but was left with a persistent trigeminal sensory deficit.

Aneurysms of the AICA are rare. Generally, these aneurysms are associated with a cerebellopontine angle syndrome and occasionally with facial sensory loss.

▶ This case has several interesting points. In addition to the fact that trigeminal loss may accompany a distal AICA aneurysm, one notes that the AICA can be sacrificed, at least in some cases, without neurologic sequelae. One could take another tack in such a case: When the angiogram is fully negative, follow-up with repeat angiography at a later time might be appropriate. The chance of recanalization and hemorrhage would appear to be small in these cases. It is also important to remember that negative angiography does not exclude an aneurysm that may be partially or totally thrombosed.—R.M. Crowell, M.D.

Rupture of a Giant Carotid Aneurysm After Extracranial-to-Intracranial Bypass Surgery
Anson JA, Stone JL, Crowell RM (Univ of Illinois, Chicago; Cook County Hosp, Chicago; Massachusetts Gen Hosp, Boston)
Neurosurgery 28:142–147, 1991   17–15

In 4 previously reported patients with ruptured giant aneurysms after extracranial-intracranial (EC-IC) bypass and carotid ligation, rupture may have been caused by changes in pressure/flow dynamics resulting from the bypass. Data were reviewed on an additional patient with a fatal rupture of a previously unruptured giant aneurysm of the bifurcation of the internal carotid artery (ICA) after EC-IC and partial occlusion of the ICA.

Woman, 54, had a 2-year history of severe headache, dizziness, and occasional right-handed clumsiness. A CT scan revealed a hyperdense homogeneous mass in the left frontotemporal region suggestive of a giant aneurysm. A carotid angiogram confirmed a giant aneurysm at the bifurcation of the left ICA and very poor filling of the left middle cerebral artery. The patient underwent a left EC-IC bypass with a saphenous vein graft from the left external carotid artery to the left middle cerebral artery. Surgeons were unable to mobilize the occipital artery for direct anastomosis to the middle cerebral artery or to interpose a vein graft to the middle cerebral artery. After 10 days the graft was patent and there was some improvement in visualization of the M1 segment of the left middle cerebral artery, but the aneurysm was unchanged. Because balloon occlusion was unsuccessful, the ICA was clamped to produce approximately 75% carotid occlusion. After 30 hours the clamp was opened because of suspected hemispheric ischemia. A massive subarachnoid hemorrhage was demonstrated by CT, and the clamp was closed completely. The patient became unresponsive, and the CT scan was suggestive of thrombosis. Increased intracranial pressure unresponsive to treatment and diabetes insipidus developed, and the patient died 1 week later.

Internal carotid artery occlusion supplemented by EC-IC bypass may be an effective treatment for thrombosis of giant ICA aneurysms, but the bypass may cause catastrophic aneurysmal hemorrhage. To minimize hemodynamic stress on the aneurysm, the bypass caliber should be as small as possible consistent with adequate cerebral blood flow after ICA occlusion. Also, complete ICA occlusion should be performed as soon as possible after bypass.

▶ This case again demonstrates that cerebral revascularization may lead to rupture of a giant intracranial aneurysm. The experience with this case and others suggests that (1) A high-flow graft such as the saphenous vein is more likely to cause such rupture; (2) prompt occlusion of the feeding artery will probably reduce the chance of rupture; (3) temporary balloon occlusion of the feeding artery with the patient awake offers a good indicator as to the safety of feeder occlusion; (4) acute occlusion of the feeder artery is probably just as safe as gradual occlusion; and (5) giant aneurysms are perilous in their threat of subarachnoid hemorrhage, even when they are unrupted. In that respect, this patient probably would have done better had the ICA been promptly occluded abruptly, either by balloon or direct clamping, soon after surgical revascularization.—R.M. Crowell, M.D.

Do Control Angiography and CT Scan Lead to a Better Understanding of Postoperative Outcome in Aneurysm Surgery? A Series of 100 Consecutive Cases
Creissard P, Rabehenoina Ch, Sevrain L, Freger P, Hattab N, Tadie M, Clavier E, Thiebot J, Laissy J-P (Hôp Charles-Nicolle, Rouen, France)
Neurochirurgie 36:209–217, 1990   17–16

Until 1982, only CT was routinely used for postoperative follow-up of patients who had been operated on for a cerebral aneurysm. Postoperative arteriography was limited to patients who either did not improve or whose condition deteriorated for unknown reasons. Because arteriography in these patients often revealed clinically unsuspected findings (e.g., vasospasm and thrombosis), the postoperative follow-up protocol was changed in 1983 to include arteriography in all patients who underwent aneurysmal repair.

The usefulness of postoperative CT scanning and arteriography in assessment of the postoperative outcome was evaluated in 52 women and 48 men (mean age, 46 years) who underwent repair of a cerebral aneurysm during a 2-year period. Ninety-three patients had symptoms of subarachnoid hemorrhage (SAH) and 7 were asymptomatic. All patients underwent preoperative and postoperative CT scanning and arteriography. Intravenous infusion of nimodipine in a dose of 2 mg/kg/hr was started before operation and continued until follow-up CT and arteriography were performed 10–12 days after operation. If there was no evidence of vasospasm, the infusion was removed and nimodipine was orally administered for 8 days. If vasospasm was present, nimodipine infusion was continued for another 15 days.

Follow-up arteriography revealed that 2 patients had an incompletely clipped aneurysm of the anterior cerebral artery, which led to reoperation in both patients. Postoperative arteriography also revealed vasospasm in 18 of 93 patients with SAH. Twelve patients had arterial thrombosis; 1 of those patients was completely asymptomatic. Forty-three follow-up CT scans showed abnormalities, including 32 hypodensities and 11 cases of hydrocephalus. Of the 32 hypodensities, 16 were attributable to the initial hemorrhage, 6 to thrombosis, 3 of vasospasm, 4 to hemorrhage plus thrombosis, and 1 to vasospasm plus thrombosis. Twenty-four of the 32 hypodensities were associated with clinical signs of neurologic deficits. The Glasgow Outcome Scores correlated well with initial grading of preoperative CT scans.

Nimodipine reduces the incidence of postoperative vasospasm after repair of a cerebral aneurysm. The use of routine follow-up arteriography is warranted as it identifies postoperative thrombosis and its contribution to outcome.

▶ This very interesting paper presents the results of follow-up angiography after 100 aneurysm surgeries. Not surprisingly, 2 cases had residual aneurysm, and this was remedied by repeat operation. Of substantial surprise, however, was the appearance of 12 arterial occlusions, half of which caused neurologic deterioration. Cerebral vasospasm was a common finding.

The contribution underlines the utility of postoperative angiography in disclosing unexpected aneurysmal remnants, vascular occlusions, or vasospasm. These diagnoses could clearly be beneficial to the patient in terms of guiding therapy. Of note was the absence of morbidity in this series of angiography. This paper thus argues strongly in favor of postoperative angiography for patients undergoing intracranial aneurysm surgery.

It should not be forgotten that aneurysms may recur late. Recanalization of aneurysms can also occur after endovascular balloon occlusion. Therefore, in the presence of symptoms late after aneurysm obliteration, repeat angiography may be warranted.

Another feature of postoperative angiographic study is the present-day possibility of intraoperative angiography. This approach offers the nice advantage of immediate correction of the problem, whether it be residual aneurysm or arterial occlusion. It is important to recognize, however, that this technique does not provide the same clarity of images as standard subtracted magnified views in the angiographic suite. Therefore, in questionable cases studied in the operating room, standard postoperative angiographic studies may also be used for supplementation. It is also worth noting that resolution of even the finest angiographic studies may not pinpoint dysplastic arterial abnormalities: The surgeon can see red dysplastic vessels that may bulge minimally if at all and yet pose a threat of later aneurysmal outpouching. Thus the intraoperative data should be kept in mind in following these patients.

Because of the possibility of late development of difficulties, I believe that patients with intracranial aneurysm should be followed carefully for life.— R.M. Crowell, M.D.

Poor-Grade Aneurysms

Poor Grade Aneurysms (Hunt and Hess Grades IV and V): A Series of 66 Cases

Sevrain L, Rabehenoina Ch, Hattab N, Freger P, Creissard P (Hôp Charles Nicolle, Rouen, France)
Neurochirurgie 36:287–296, 1990   17–17

The prognosis is poor for patients with subarachnoid hemorrhage (SAH) caused by intracerebral aneurysms who are initially classified as clinical grade IV or V on the Hunt and Hess scale. Data were reviewed on all patients who were admitted during a 5-year period with initial poor-grade ruptured intracerebral aneurysms.

During the study period, SAH from ruptured intracerebral aneurysms was diagnosed in 250 patients, of whom 66 (26.4%) were considered in poor clinical grade initially. There were 36 men (mean age, 44.4 years) and 30 women (mean age, 50.5 years), of whom 37 were in grade IV and 29 in grade V. Glasgow Coma Scores ranged from 4 to 7. Assignment of initial clinical grade was based on preoperative arteriography, CT, and clinical examination. Fisher's criteria were used to evaluate the severity of SAH on CT. Contraindications to operation were ruptured aneurysms of the anterior artery or the basilar trunk with important hemorrhage, grade V with bilateral mydriasis, and poor physiologic state.

Surgery was performed on 50 patients within 12 hours after admission. It was not attempted in the other 16 because of bilateral fixed dilated pupils or the presence of major intracerebral hematoma at admission; all 16 patients subsequently died. Poor initial grade was associated with size of the initial hemorrhage in 84.9% of the patients, early seizures in 7.6%, acute hydrocephalus in 1.5%, multiple emboli in 3%, and early diffuse vasospasm in 1.5%. Within a minimum follow-up period of 2 months, 12 patients (18.2%) recovered, 1 had moderate neurologic disability, 4 (6%) had severe disability, 4 were in a vegetative state, and 45 (68.2%) died. The overall mortality rate was 74.2%. The severity of the initial intracebral hemorrhage was the most important determining factor in poor initial clinical grade. However, because some patients recovered unexpectedly, the final outcome could not be predicted preoperatively.

▶ In this series of patients, good recovery was noted in 12 of the 66 despite grade IV or V on admission. The authors found that no specific clinical features preoperatively were predictive of this outcome, and thus advise aggressive treatment for all.—R.M. Crowell, M.D.

Management Morbidity and Mortality in Grade IV and V Patients With Aneurysmal Subarachnoid Haemorrhage

Seifert V, Trost HA, Stolke D (Medical School Hannover, Germany)
Acta Neurochir (Wien) 103:5–10, 1990   17–18

Although early surgery in low-risk patients with aneurysms reduces perioperative management morbidity and mortality, the treatment of patients who are severely injured by initial hemorrhage remains a challenge. To determine whether certain variables of treatment, including early surgery, could be defined that might help to improve the grim outlook for stuporous or comatose patients with a ruptured aneurysm, data were reviewed on 74 patients with aneurysmal subarachnoid hemorrhage (SAH).

All were admitted in Hunt and Hess grade IV or V. Thirty-nine patients were hospitalized within 24 hours of the SAH, 29 between 24 and 72 hours, and 6 later than 72 hours. Ruptured aneurysms were found at the anterior communicating artery complex in 46%, on the middle cerebral artery in 26%, on the internal carotid artery in 16%, and at the vertebrobasilar artery complex in 12%. No surgery was performed in 51% of the cases. Half of those patients were in grade IV on admission and the other half in grade V. The aneurysm was clipped in the remaining cases. Overall, 81% of the patients were in grade IV and 19% in grade V.

Thirty-seven of the 38 patients who had no aneurysm surgery died, for a mortality rate of 97%. The 1 survivor had a grade III Glasgow Outcome Scale (GOS) score. Of the 19 patients in grade IV who had early aneurysm clipping, 53% had a good recovery, 16% were severely disabled, and 31% remained in a vegetative state or died. Of the 10 in grade IV who had delayed surgery, 40% were in grade I or II after surgery, 20% were in grade III, and 40% were in grade IV or V GOS. Early surgery did not produce a good outcome in any of the 4 grade V patients. Two survived in grade III GOS, and 2 died. Of the 3 patients in grade V who survived long enough to have delayed surgery, 1 survived without a deficit, 1 was severely disabled, and 1 died.

Without surgery, patients with poor-grade aneurysms have an almost nonexistent chance of survival. The prognosis of those admitted in grade V is poor whether or not surgery is done and whether it is done early or late. Patients in grade IV have a better prognosis. In these patients, an aggressive surgical approach is justified. Early surgery produces better results than delayed surgery.

▶ In this interesting study of grades IV and V patients with aneurysmal SAH, good results were obtained in 53% of the grade IV cases, whereas there was only a single survivor in grade V after early surgery. The authors conclude that full treatment, including neurosurgery, is warranted for grade IV but not for grade V cases. This jibes with data from Edmonton, but the Phoenix series suggests that some grade V patients can improve with ventriculostomy and go on to a satisfactory outcome. Further experience is needed to establish a program of care, but grade IV patients appear to be reasonable candidates for full treatment.—R.M. Crowell, M.D.

Flunarizine Treatment in Poor-Grade Aneurysm Patients

Fujita S, Kawaguchi T, Shose Y, Urui S (Hyogo Brain and Heart Ctr at Himehi, Hyogo, Japan)
Acta Neurochir (Wien) 103:11–17, 1990   17–19

The calcium antagonist, nimodipine, has given promising results in prophylaxis of delayed ischemic neurologic deficit (DIND) in patients with severe subarachnoid hemorrhage (SAH). The lipophilic calcium antagonist, flunarizine hydrochloride, which has a stronger affinity for the brain and exerts a stronger cerebral protective effect, was tested in 37 patients with DIND, a sequela of SAH. All 37 patients were in Fischer's group III. Results were compared retrospectively with those in an untreated a control group of 37 patients, also in Fischer's group III. The Dosage of flunarizine was 10 mg orally 4 times a day for 4 days, then 3 times a day for 3 days, and twice a day for 14 more days.

In the overall series of patients treated with flunarizine, DIND developed in only 1. Of the untreated controls, 8 died and 10 contracted infections as a result of DIND. Only 1 patient given flunarizine had a permanent DIND, and this was attributable to inadequate administration of the drug. Diffuse severe vasospasm was seen in 57% of the controls who had angiography, compared with 18% of the flunarizine group. No side effects of flunarizine were noted.

Flunarizine appears to be effective in inhibiting the development of severe neurologic deficit resulting from delayed vasospasm in patients with poor-grade aneurysms. Its intense inhibition of intracellular Ca^{2+} overloads may be responsible for its favorable effect on severe delayed vasospasm, especially in very ill patients. Given the absence of adverse reactions, the use of higher flunarizine doses should be investigated.

▶ This retrospective study suggests that patients at high risk from cerebral vasospasm do better when treated with flunarizine, a calcium-channel blocker. Further controlled studies, preferably of a prospective nature, are needed to confirm this observation.—R.M. Crowell, M.D.

Emergent Aneurysm Surgery Without Cerebral Angiography for the Comatose Patient

Batjer HH, Samson DS (Univ of Texas, Dallas)
Neurosurgery 28:283–287, 1991   17–20

The presence of intraparenchymal hematomas sharply increases mortality in patients with aneurysmal hemorrhage. When evidence of the brain stem compression syndrome is seen on CT, most modern hospitals proceed with definitive angiography, which results in further delay before craniotomy. During the past 3 years, 4 comatose patients with CT-documented brain stem compression syndromes underwent emergent operations without definitive angiographic verification.

Because of the degree of brain stem compromise, it was thought unwise to delay craniotomy for diagnostic angiography in all 4 patients. While they were in the emergency room, 2 patients deteriorated rapidly, presumably from new bleeding. The average delay from onset of coma to scalp incision was 3 hours (range, 1.7–6.5 hours). The average delay between arrival in the emergency room and scalp incision was 1.8 hours (range, .75–2.5 hours). All 4 patients underwent hematoma evacuation, aneurysm clipping, lobectomy for decompression, and external decompression. Temporary clipping was required in 1 patient; intraoperative rupture occurred in 2 patients. All 3 patients who survived had significant disability.

Most life-threatening hematomas caused by aneurysmal rupture involve either the temporal lobe, frontal operculum, or mesial frontal lobe, for which the CT scan will suggest a particular anatomical source of hemorrhage. The middle cerebral bifurcation is strongly implicated in parasylvian hematomas either inferior or superior to the sylvian fissure. It is this relatively straightforward anatomical circumstance that focuses and limits the scope of empiric exploration at the time of emergent evacuation. Although definitive angiographic verification should remain the standard practice in all patients with subarachnoid hemorrhage, the delay imposed for diagnostic angiography may be avoided in very critically ill patients to save vital minutes of severe brain stem decompression. Emergent craniotomy with empiric exploration of appropriate subarachnoid cisterns after hematoma decompression may be life-saving in some patients.

▶ This interesting communication raises several questions: (1) Was it worth it? All 3 patients survived with significant disability. Clearly, this is a major concern in the older patient, and thus one should focus mainly on younger patients for this form of treatment. (2) Could intraoperative angiography be helpful? Once the hematoma is partially removed and decompression has been achieved, intraoperative angiography could give some information on the site of the aneurysm and help with the operative attack. It is even possible that endovascular technique might obtain proximal control in certain aneurysms to help the surgeon.—R.M. Crowell, M.D.

The Effect of Continuous Drainage of Cerebrospinal Fluid in Patients With Subarachnoid Hemorrhage: A Retrospective Analysis of 108 Patients
Kasuya H, Shimizu T, Kagawa M (Tokyo Women's Med College)
Neurosurgery 28:56–59, 1991   17–21

Although most patients who undergo continuous CSF drainage (CCFD) after subarachnoid hemorrhage (SAH) have an immediate clinical response, a statistically significant rate of improvement in treated patients has not been demonstrated. The effects of CCFD on vasospasm and hydrocephalus in 108 patients with SAH who underwent surgery for ruptured aneurysms within 48 hours of onset were reviewed. Of the patients, 92 underwent CCFD with cisternal drainage, lumbar drainage, ventricular drainage, or a combination of these procedures. The relationship between the average daily volume of CSF removed before the period of vasospasm and the development of cerebral infarction associated with delayed ischemic symptoms were determined. Drainage was maintained for at least 4 days. The relationship between the total volume of drained CSF and shunt-dependent hydrocephalus also was determined.

Drainage was maintained for a mean of 10.4 days. The total volume of CSF drainage was 2,034 mL, and the average daily volume was 190 mL. The volume and height of CCFD during early stages after SAH were both significantly related to the incidence of cerebral infarction in association with delayed ischemic symptoms from vasospasm. Patients who had a larger volume of drainage from a lower height in the early period after SAH had more later cerebral infarctions. There also was a significant relationship between total volume of drained CSF and shunt-dependent hydrocephalus. Cerebral infarction from vasospasm had a significant association with hydrocephalus.

The removal of large amounts of CSF may induce both cerebral vasospasm and hydrocephalus. A degree of intracranial hypertension sufficient to restore normal CSF circulation, rather than CCFD, may be a preferable method of removing spasmogenic substances from the subarachnoid space in patients with SAH.

▶ The data presented here strongly suggest that continous CSF drainage in patients with SAH leads to an increase in cerebral infarction. The mechanism by which this occurs is not clear. These problems are in addition to the occasional rupture of an intracranial aneurysm that can be induced by lowering the intracranial pressure by CSF drainage. Drainage of the CSF should probably be limited to circumstances in which clinical deterioration with ventricular enlargement provides a clear mandate following SAH.—R.M. Crowell, M.D.

Vasospasm

Sustained Increased Cerebral Blood Flow With Prophylactic Hypertensive Hypervolemic Hemodilution ("Triple-H" Therapy) After Subarachnoid Hemorrhage
Origitano TC, Wascher TM, Reichman OH, Anderson DE (Loyola Univ, Maywood, Ill)
Neurosurgery 27:729–740, 1990   17–22

In patients who initially survive an aneurysmal subarachnoid hemorrhage (SAH), the prevention or treatment of delayed cerebral ischemia remains a challenge. Forty-three patients with nontraumatic, nonhypertensive SAH were treated according to a uniform protocol of prophylactic hypertensive hypervolemic hemodilution ("Triple-H" therapy).

The goals of therapy were to reduce the hematocrit to 30% and increase central venous pressure to 8–12 mm Hg. Albumin 5% was infused to maintain these levels. Labetalol or dopamine infusions were used to maintain systolic blood pressure at 130–150 mm Hg in patients with unclipped aneurysms. Serial cerebral blood flow (CBF) measurements were performed using the ^{133}Xe inhalation technique. Both f_1, representing cortical or gray matter flow, and CBF_{15}, representing the true mean blood flow of gray and white matter, were determined. Craniotomy was performed within 24 hours of instituting the protocol when possible.

Therapeutic goals were attained within the first 24 hours of triple-H therapy, and 93% of the patients had a sustained neurologic grade or improved by at least 1 neurologic grade within 48 hours of therapy. During the first 24 hours of the protocol, the mean increase in CBF was 34.2% for f_1 and 21.2% for CBF_{15}. The maximum mean increase in CBF was 47.2% for f_1 and 30.1% for CBF_{15}. Increases in CBF occurred in all of the patients and were maintained for 21 days after SAH, regardless of neurologic grade on admission, age, sex, or angiographic arterial narrowing.

None of the patients in full compliance with the protocol experienced permanent neurologic deficit, but in 2 patients delayed ischemia and infarction developed because of inability to sustain protocol requirements. Eighty-four percent of all patients, and 87% of all patients who underwent surgery, were discharged capable of following an independent lifestyle.

Prophylactic hypertensive hypervolemic hemodilution is the first treatment protocol that consistently achieves an immediate and sustained increase in CBF after SAH. Triple-H therapy, in combination with early aneurysm surgery, diminishes morbidity and mortality caused by diminished CBF and delayed ischemia after SAH.

Normovolaemic Induced Hypertension Therapy for Cerebral Vasospasm After Subarachnoid Haemorrhage
Otsubo H, Takemae T, Inoue T, Kobayashi Sh, Sugita K (Shinsu Univ, Matsumoto, Japan)
Acta Neurochir (Wien) 103:18–26, 1990   17–23

In the postoperative treatment of subarachnoid hemorrhage (SAH), one should monitor the patient's hemodynamic status as well as the neurologic status. Hypovolemia, which decreases cerebral perfusion, is not uncommon.

Forty-one patients were treated with induced hypertension in management of postoperative vasospasm during a 4-year period. Vasospasm was evaluated angiographically from the first postoperative day to 3 weeks after SAH. Hypertension was induced with dopamine and dobutamine, up to 20 μg/kg/min, to maintain systolic blood pressure at the level of symptom improvement, as neurologic deficits occurred and according to angiographic findings. A Swan-Ganz catheter was inserted for cardiac measurements in 6 patients.

Neurologic deficits improved in 17 of 24 patients in whom hypertension of 25% to 50% over normal systolic pressure was induced. Three of 9 patients who had an increase of more than 50% improved; in the other 6 no effect was observed. There were 4 hemorrhagic infarctions in which blood pressure increased to more than 50% of systolic arterial pressure; CT showed an area of low density before vasospasm occurred. Induced hypertension was not considered in these cases. All 25 patients who had positive results had a clinical grade below III.

Normovolemic-induced hypertension appears to be an effective method of raising the perfusion pressure of cerebral blood flow in patients with cerebral vasospasm after SAH. Hemodynamic monitoring with a triple-lumen thermodilution Swan-Ganz catheter is recommended as a preventive measure. Complications of overhydration, hemorrhagic infarct, and aneurysm rupture may occur.

▶ This study may be added to the many that suggest that normovolemic-induced hypertension may improve neurologic performance in the face of cerebral vasospasm after SAH. Although there is a great deal of suggestive data, it should be pointed out that no adequate controlled study of this problem has ever been performed. This would be difficult to do in today's milieu, in that the approach has been established in many locations as the standard of care.—R.M. Crowell, M.D.

A Study of the Effectiveness of the Iron-Chelating Agent Deferoxamine as Vasospasm Prophylaxis in a Rabbit Model of Subarachnoid Hemorrhage
Vollmer DG, Hongo K, Ogawa H, Tsukahara T, Kassell NF (Washington Univ; Univ of Virginia)
Neurosurgery 28:27–32, 1991   17–24

Delayed ischemia secondary to cerebral vasospasm is a leading cause of morbidity and death after aneurysmal hemorrhage. If heme-bound or free iron is important in the development of cerebral vasospasm in this setting, chelation may counter the arterial narrowing that occurs.

The use of deferoxamine, an iron-chelating agent that readily crosses the blood-brain barrier, was assessed in a rabbit model of cerebral vasospasm, which was induced by instilling autologous blood suboccipitally. Treatment was begun 16 hours before inducing subarachnoid hemorrhage (SAH). The diameter of the basilar artery was monitored.

Treatment with deferoxamine did not alter the caliber of the basilar artery before subarachnoid bleeding. However, after induction of spasm treatment attenuated the vasospasm significantly. These findings support the concept that SAH-induced vasospasm is mediated by iron, possibly through the generation of free radicals. Other recent studies have indicated that a decrease in free radical formation may counter cerebral vasospasm in the rabbit and in the primate.

Impairment of Cerebral Autoregulation During the Development of Chronic Cerebral Vasospasm After Subarachnoid Hemorrhage in Primates
Takeuchi H, Handa Y, Kobayashi H, Kawano H, Hayashi M (Fukui Med School, Fukui, Japan)
Neurosurgery 28:41–48, 1991   17–25

Autoregulation of cerebral blood flow (CBF) was examined during development of chronic cerebral vasospasm in monkeys subjected to simulated subarachnoid bleeding by placement of an autologous blood clot around exposed cerebral arteries. Regional CBF was measured by the hydrogen clearance technique, and somatosensory evoked potentials were recorded. The arterial pressure was lowered incrementally by infusing metaraminol bitartrate.

Vessels near the blood clot were reduced in diameter, compared with those on the other side of the circle of Willis. Parietal CBF on the side of the clot was less than on the other side at mean arterial pressure levels of 40–100 mm Hg and increased at a pressure of 180 mm Hg. Central conduction time was prolonged on the side of the clot when the mean arterial pressure was 40 mm Hg. Autoregulation of CBF appears to be importantly affected by the development of cerebral vasospasm. Decreased cerebral perfusion pressure readily depresses electric brain function in this primate model.

Unusual Aneurysms

Dissecting and Fusiform Aneurysms of Vertebro-Basilar Systems: MR Imaging
Iwama T, Andoh T, Sakai N, Iwata T, Hirata T, Yamada H (Gifu Univ, Japan; Matsunami Gen Hosp, Gifu)
Neuroradiology 32:272–279, 1990   17–26

The MRI findings were reviewed in 3 patients with vertebrobasilar dissecting aneurysms and 2 who had fusiform aneurysms in the same region. Only dilatation of a signal-void area was seen in the latter cases. All patients with dissecting aneurysms, however, had a variety of abnormalities on MR images.

Man, 74, with left-sided motor weakness, was found to have a hyperdense mass in the prepontine cistern on CT scanning. There were multiple lacunar infarcts in both cerebral hemispheres. Vertebral angiography 3 months after the onset showed a fusiform dilatation of the basilar artery (Fig 17–5), with retention of contrast in the dorsal region of the dilatation in the venous phase. A T1-weighted sagittal MR image demonstrated the basilar artery as a linear signal-void mass, with an irregular, hyperintense mass ventral to the vessel, and T2-

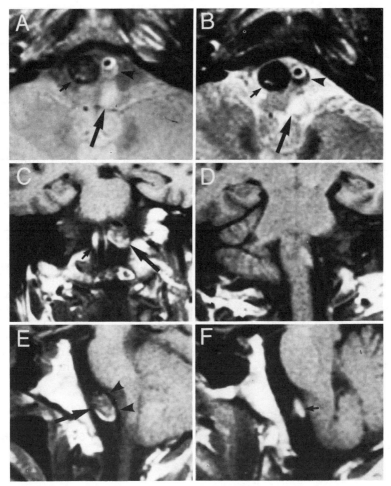

Fig 17–5.—Proton-density (PD)-weighted (**A**) and T2-weighted (**B**) axial images demonstrating 2 lesions in the premedullary cistern. The left lesion is seen to consist of a circle and a crescent-shaped part *(arrowheads)*. The circle is relatively thick and demonstrated as an increased intensity on both PD-weighted and T2-weighted images. The crescent-shaped part is demonstrated as being isointense on the PD-weighted image and as being hypointense on the T2-weighted image. The right lesion is larger than the left and is depicted as being hypointense with an inside vague isointensity on the PD-weighted image and an inner hyperintense spot on the T2-weighted image *(small arrows)*. Pontine infarction is seen as a hyperintense area *(large arrows)*. The T1-weighted coronal (**C**) and sagittal (**F**) images at the plane, including the left vertebral artery, show thickening of the arterial wall as being hyperintense *(small arrows)*. The T1-weighted coronal (**C, D**) and sagittal (**E**) images at the plane including the right vertebral artery depicting an oval mixed-intense mass *(large arrows)* located ventral to the arterial lumen *(arrowheads)*. (Courtesy of Iwama T, Andoh T, Sakai N, et al: *Neuroradiology* 32:272–279, 1990.)

weighted axial images showed a circular hyperintensity surrounded by a hypointense rim (Fig 17–6). The dissecting lumen seen on angiography was not apparent on MR images.

Hematoma was seen in all cases of dissecting aneurysm. In 1 case an intimal flap and a double lumen were demonstrated. Magnetic resonance

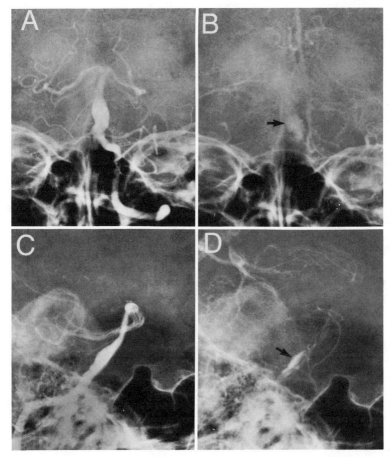

Fig 17–6.—In man aged 74 years, anteroposterior (**A**) and lateral (**C**) views of left vertebral angiogram demonstrate irregular dilatation of basilar artery. Retention of contrast medium is seen in venous phase of angiogram (**B** and **D**) *arrows.* (Courtesy of Iwama T, Andoh T, Sakai N, et al: *Neuroradiology* 32:272–279, 1990.)

imaging is a useful way of demonstrating large dissections and of distinguishing dissecting and fusiform aneurysms.

▶ This lovely study demonstrates the utility of MR in the detailed analysis of complex intracranial aneurysms. The presence of an intimal flap intramural hematoma and a parent artery hematoma can be detected by MR to assist the diagnosis of dissecting intracranial aneurysm.—R.M. Crowell, M.D.

Hemifacial Spasm Caused by a Spontaneous Dissecting Aneurysm of the Vertebral Artery: Case Report
Matsumoto K, Saijo T, Kuyama H, Asari S, Nishimoto A (Okayama Univ, Japan)
J Neurosurg 74:650–652, 1991   17–27

Most dissecting aneurysms of the intracranial arteries are associated with subarachnoid hemorrhage or ischemia, and there are few reports of hemifacial spasm resulting from aneurysm. In what is apparently the first reported case, a spontaneous dissecting aneurysm of the vertebral artery resulted in hemifacial spasm.

Woman, 58, had left hemifacial spasm of 2 years' duration. This sign began around the orbicularis oculi and spread to involve all muscles innervated by the left facial nerve. There were no additional abnormalities on neurologic or physical examination. After inconclusive CT and MRI examinations, a fusiform enlargement of the left vertebral artery, with contrast medium remaining in the venous phase, was found on vertebral angiography. Paramedian suboccipital craniectomy was done to expose a fusiform aneurysm compressing the brain stem and impinging on the root exit zone of the affected nerve. The whitish gray surface and neovascular pattern of the outer wall suggested the diagnosis of dissecting aneurysm. Hemifacial spasm was completely relieved by microvascular decompression of the facial nerve and wrapping of the aneurysm.

Spontaneous dissecting aneurysms are usually associated with subarachnoid hemorrhage and diverse angiographic findings.

▶ This case demonstrates that vertebral artery dissection can cause hemifacial spasm, which is not surprising if the dissection occurs in relation to the nerve entry zone.—R.M. Crowell, M.D.

Infectious Intracranial Aneurysms: Comparison of Groups With and Without Endocarditis
Barrow DL, Prats AR (Emory Univ)
Neurosurgery 27:562–573, 1990   17–28

Twelve patients with infectious intracranial aneurysms were reviewed. Six of them (group A) had associated infective endocarditis and 6 (group B) had other predisposing factors. Three of the latter patients had bacterial meningitis and 3 had fungal aneurysms (Fig 17–7). All group A patients had bacterial aneurysms caused by organisms typically associated with endocarditis, and all 6 had intracranial hemorrhage before the aneurysm was discovered. Three of the 12 patients had 2 aneurysms each. Many group B patients had aneurysms in unusual sites, such as the posterior cerebral artery and vertebral confluence.

All of the patients received antibiotics, and 6 were operated on as well. Four group A patients had surgery. All 6 group A patients survived, 3 with significant neurologic deficits. Only 2 of the 6 group B patients lived, but both had a good neurologic outcome. All patients who were operated on survived, and 4 of the 6 had a good outcome.

An infectious aneurysm does not necessarily have to be operated on. A trial of antibiotic therapy is especially indicated if the aneurysm is unruptured or is in a surgically problematic site, or if multiple aneurysms are

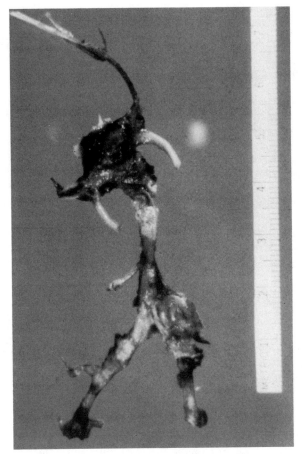

Fig 17–7.—Gross pathologic specimen reveals aneurysms of the vertebral *(lower right)* and basilar *(upper left)* arteries. (Courtesy of Barrow DL, Prats AR: *Neurosurgery* 27:562–573, 1990.)

present. Surgery should be strongly considered if the aneurysm does not resolve, or if it enlarges during antibiotic therapy. Intracerebral hemorrhage with a significant mass effect is a clear indication for surgery.

▶ This is an excellent review of 12 patients with infectious intracranial aneurysms. The authors stress that patients with bacterial endocarditis generally present with intracranial hemorrhage, an unusual location of the aneurysm, and bacterial etiology (often *Streptococcus* or *Staphylococcus*). In another group without endocarditis, the aneurysms tend to occur more proximally and sometimes, because of fever, may be diagnosed before hemorrhage. This latter group has more unusual organisms, including fungal agents, and their prognosis is much worse. It seems likely that we will see more of these patients because of immunosuppression in the era of transplantation and AIDS.

With regard to guidelines for treatment, it may not be necessary to perform angiography every 2 weeks as recommended, because MRI and CT may give enough information about the size of the lesion. Furthermore, one may argue that the aneurysm should not be attacked in every case of hematoma removal, particularly the more proximal aneurysms that do not have a well-defined neck. Delayed treatment of these proximal lesions might lead to thrombosis or fibrosis of the neck, permitting later safer obliteration.—R.M. Crowell, M.D.

Traumatic Intracranial Aneurysms Caused by Missiles: Their Presentation and Management

Haddad FS, Haddad GF, Taha J (American Univ of Beirut Med Ctr, Lebanon; Montreal Neurological Inst)

Neurosurgery 28:1–7, 1991   17–29

Traumatic intracranial aneurysms (TICAs) appear to be more common than a review of the literature would suggest. At the American University of Beirut Medical Center, 15 patients with 19 TICAs as a result of head injuries caused by missiles were seen between 1969 and 1984. Except for the injuries in the patient seen in 1969, all others were incurred during the war in Lebanon, which started in 1975.

Nine patients were civilians and 6 were militia fighters. One patient was injured by a spent bullet; the remaining injuries all resulted from shrapnel. The TICAs were diagnosed by cerebral angiography. All formed on the anterior circulation, 13 on a secondary branch of the middle cerebral artery. The aneurysms were as large as 20 × 10 mm at surgery. There was an average interval of 19.5 days between the injury and diagnostic angiography.

The TICAs usually appear at angiography with a well-defined border, although some may be irregular and lobulated in the early phase. A number of characteristics differentiate TICAs from berry aneurysms. The latter are located most often on large blood vessels at the base of the brain, are found at the bifurcation of arteries, and differ histopathologically from TICAs. The peak incidence for berry aneurysms is in the sixth decade; TICAs occur most often in the second decade, reflecting a population more exposed to missile injuries.

Although some investigators believe that TICAs may disappear in time, that has not been the experience at this center. Not all TICAs appear simultaneously in a given patient, and some may enlarge with time, rupture, and lead to death. Irrespective of the size and location of TICAs, surgical treatment is strongly recommended. In most cases (80%), TICAs are associated with an intracerebral hematoma. The outcome depends on the original injury and the patient's preoperative state.

▶ As noted by the authors, angiography cannot be offered in every instance of head injury. On the other hand, the restriction of angiography to selected patients seems chary, in that the risk of angiographic study in these patients is probably small and the pick-up rate substantial. The authors' recommendation of angiography for those patients with shrapnel injury or low-velocity bullet injury, no exit wound and an associated intracerebral hematoma would appear to be a minimum. Other investigators have suggested angiography for all patients with penetrating intracranial wounds. Certainly, the recommendation that all of these aneurysms be considered dangerous and meritorious of surgical exploration and repair is to be applauded. One should remember that these are not like berry aneurysms; that is to say, because they disrupt the wall of the vessel, the best treatment is trapping and excision rather than clipping.—R.M. Crowell, M.D.

18 Other Hemorrhagic Conditions/AVMs

Brain AVMs

Pregnancy and the Risk of Hemorrhage from Cerebral Arteriovenous Malformations
Horton JC, Chambers WA, Lyons SL, Adams RD, Kjellberg RN (Massachusetts Gen Hosp, Boston; George Washington Univ)
Neurosurgery 27:867–872, 1990   18–1

To determine whether pregnancy increases the risk of hemorrhage from an arteriovenous malformation (AVM), data were reviewed on 451 women with confirmed AVM who underwent proton beam therapy during a 9.5-year period. The 540 pregnancies resulted in 438 live births and 102 abortions. All patients gave a detailed medical history and received a comprehensive neurologic examination; information on subsequent hemorrhage and the obstetric history were obtained by questionnaire, record review, or other means. Hemorrhages and pregnancies occurring after proton beam therapy were not included in the analysis.

Pregnancy was complicated by cerebral hemorrhage in 17 patients; 14 of these hemorrhages took place during gestation. Eleven of the 14 patients who had hemorrhage during gestation had healthy, full-term infants. There was no tendency for hemorrhages to cluster at any point during pregnancy. Of 438 live births, 375 occurred by vaginal delivery. In pregnant women with an unruptured AVM, the hemorrhage rate was .035 per person-year, compared with .031 per person-year in nonpregnant women of childbearing age with an unruptured AVM. The rate of first cerebral hemorrhage from an AVM was not significantly increased by pregnancy. The risk of hemorrhage during pregnancy for women with an AVM was 3.5%.

Women without a previous hemorrhage do not have an increased risk of hemorrhage during pregnancy. If the risk of a fatal outcome after hemorrhage were greater in pregnant than in nonpregnant women, a bias would be introduced into the present study; about 10% of patients die after their first hemorrhage. Based on limited data, the risk of a second hemorrhage occurring during pregnancy is about 5.8%.

▶ This is an important series because it includes a substantial number of patients with AVM and pregnancy. In essence, the results indicate that the risk of hemorrhage during pregnancy is no different from the risk of hemorrhage without pregnancy.

However, there are some drawbacks: This is a highly selected group of patients, and several potential sources of bias are present. Perhaps the most important of these is that the study group could not include patients with an initial fatal intracranial hemorrhage from the AVM. In addition, patients whose hemorrhage was severely disabling would be very unlikely to be referred for proton treatment. Moreover, previous data suggest that for unruptured intracranial AVMs, initial ruptures result in a fatality rate of 25% to 30% (1). If one looks at this particular factor alone, it suggests that in this group of 273 patients with ruptured AVMs, another 80 or so were eliminated from consideration because the initial hemorrhage was fatal. If even only 15 of these patients had hemorrhaged during pregnancy, it would nearly double the rate of first cerebral hemorrhage from an AVM during pregnancy, and the conclusions would be much different.—R.M. Crowell, M.D.

Reference

1. Brown RD Jr, et al: *J Neurosurg* 68:352, 1988.

Intracranial Hemorrhage From Aneurysms and Arteriovenous Malformations During Pregnancy and the Puerperium

Dias MS, Sekhar LN (Univ of Utah; Univ of Pittsburgh)
Neurosurgery 27:855–866, 1990   18–2

Up to 12% of maternal deaths are caused by intracranial hemorrhage (ICH) from an aneurysm or arteriovenous malformation. Data were reviewed on 154 cases of confirmed ICH during pregnancy, including 152 reported in the English language literature.

An aneurysm was implicated in three fourths of the cases. Hemorrhage occurred before delivery in 92% and post partum in 8%. Women bleeding from an angioma were younger than those with aneurysmal bleeding, but they did not differ with regard to parity or gestational age at the time of initial bleeding. One third of the patients had hypertension and/or albuminuria at some time during pregnancy. Operative treatment of aneurysms, not arteriovenous malformations, was associated with lower maternal and fetal mortality rates, independent of other factors. In patients who had not undergone surgery, cesarean delivery was not of apparent advantage.

Neurosurgical considerations should guide the decision on whether to operate for ICH during pregnancy. At the same time, the method of delivery should be based on obstetric considerations. The near-term woman with a viable fetus should be followed perioperatively with continuous fetal monitoring, and emergent operative delivery should be carried out if there is persistent fetal distress.

▶ This is a useful report taken primarily from a literature review on ICH during pregnancy and delivery. The inclusion of cases from many institutions with various operators leads one to exercise some caution when interpreting these results. However, it seems clear that the management of ruptured aneurysms during pregnancies is direct surgical clipping. It is less clear how arteriovenous malformation (AVM) should be managed in this setting. One can interpret the results as supporting a decision to defer surgical correction of the AVM until after delivery. The obstetric approach appears best managed according to obstetric principles without respect to the intracranial problem.—R.M. Crowell, M.D.

Familial Occurrence of Arteriovenous Malformation of the Brain
Yokoyama K, Asano Y, Murakawa T, Takada M, Ando T, Sakai N, Yamada H, Iwata H (Takayama Red Cross Hosp; Gifu Univ, Japan)
J Neurosurg 74:585–589, 1991   18–3

Although arteriovenous malformations (AVMs) of the brain originate from congenital maldevelopment of the brain vessels, reports of familial occurrence are rare. Six affected patients in 3 families were encountered. Data on these 3 families and 10 families reported in the literature were reviewed.

The average age of the patients with familial AVMs was 27 years, which was somewhat younger than the overall age for patients with AVMs. There were 18 males and 11 females, indicating that familial AVM is more frequent in females than would be expected. No specific familial relationship was especially prone to result in AVM, although the disease tended to occur in family members of the same sex. Lesions were supratentorial in 74% of cases, in accordance with the overall population of persons with AVM in a nationwide Japanese survey.

Genetic factors may be involved in the occurrence of AVMs, but the number of cases is too small to draw any conclusions. The presence of a large number of patients with AVM, including those with familial AVM, in a fairly isolated district, suggests the possibility of genetic factors.

▶ This interesting report draws attention to the fact that AVMs may occasionally occur in a familial setting. It is possible that, in certain cases, a genetic basis underlies the development of an AVM. This may also be related to the well-known familial occurrence of intracranial aneurysm in a minority of patients.—R.M. Crowell, M.D.

A Study on the Venous Drainage of 150 Cerebral Arteriovenous Malformations as Related to Haemorrhagic Risks and Size of the Lesion
Albert P, Salgado H, Polaina M, Trujillo F, Ponce de León A, Durand F (Hosp General "Virgen del Rocio," Seville, Spain)
Acta Neurochir (Wien) 103:30–34, 1990   18–4

There appears to be no relationship between risk of bleeding from cerebral arteriovenous malformations (AVMs) and age, sex, or location of the angioma; however, there may be a correlation with the venous drainage of these lesions. The venous drainage of a series of AVMs was studied to correlate the number of efferent veins with the symptoms of clinical onset and size of the lesions.

The study sample comprised 150 patients with cerebral AVMs who had complete serial angiographic studies and reliable clinical records. Data evaluated were age at onset of symptoms, sex, symptoms, size of angioma, and number of drainage veins.

The initial symptoms were meningeal or intraparenchymal hemorrhage in 110 patients; 75% of these had angiomas with only 1 draining vein. Among the 40 patients with other presentations, mainly epilepsy, 70% had a medusa-head angioma drainage system. Thus AVMs with only 1 draining vein had a high probability of bleeding. In addition, angiomas that were less than 2 cm in diameter generally had only 1 draining vein and therefore carried a high risk of hemorrhage. There were no significant correlations between risk of bleeding and age, sex, or location of AVMs.

As the size of AVMs increases, so does the number of drainage veins, thus decreasing the probability of hemorrhage from these lesions. Indications for the various methods of treatment for AVMs are direct excision for small or medium-sized angiomas with 1 or 2 drainage veins in areas of poor functional expressivity; stereotactic radiotherapy for small or medium-sized lesions in functionally important areas; and selective intravascular embolization for large angiomas with a large number of draining veins, especially in older patients.

Functional PET Scanning in the Assessment of Cerebral Arteriovenous Malformations: Case Report
Leblanc R, Meyer E (McGill Univ)
J Neurosurg 73:615–619, 1990   18–5

Functional positron emission tomography (PET) was used successfully in a patient with a cerebral arteriovenous malformation (AVM) to localize the lesion to the precentral gyrus precisely; the PET findings were validated by intraoperative cortical mapping.

Woman, 40, previously healthy, came to the hospital after sustaining a single generalized seizure. Computed tomography, MRI, and cerebral angiography demonstrated a 3-cm AVM in the vicinity of the left central region. The patient underwent PET scanning 7 days before undergoing craniotomy under local anesthesia for intraoperative cortical mapping and intracarotid fluorescein angiography. The surgeon was not informed of the PET findings. Cortical mapping identified the postcentral gyrus behind the AVM. The major arteries supplying the AVM were identified and clipped in series. Fluorescein angiography was used to confirm that the surrounding eloquent cortex did not incur ischemic injury. The patient tolerated the operation well and did not have any neurologic deficits. Stereotactically focused irradiation of the AVM was uneventful. Positron emission tomography was performed twice, first in a baseline setting with the patient lying quietly on a couch, and then in the activation state when the patient's right hand was stimulated by moving a vibrator across the finger tips. In the activation phase, PET produced results identical to those of intraoperative inspection, angiography, and cortical mapping, and it also localized the AVM to the precentral hand region. Computer analysis of the PET scan further supported the findings.

Functional PET scanning may be useful for localizing cortical lesions precisely and helping to plan the optimal approach to AVMs situated in functional important cortex.

▶ This very interesting report confirms that functional PET scanning correlates rather precisely with intraoperative cortical mapping in the case of precentral AVMs. On the other hand, another tack might be taken in this case: Preoperative superselective catheterization of the large middle cerebral artery feeder could be used for selective amytal testing. In the case of a negative test, direct endovascular occlusion of the feeder vessel or vessels might well be accomplished. Further angiographic studies could then delineate the nature of other feeding vessels, which might include vessels of transit to the rolandic cortex. This approach might well delineate the relationship of the lesion to normal vasculature. Depending on the results of such an endovascular diagnostic/therapeutic procedure, further treatment could be carried out. In the case of a favorable result, treatment might include excision of the lesion. In the case of unfavorable results, radiosurgical obliteration might be recommended.

Only further long-term follow-up experience will suffice to demonstrate whether aggressive endovascular and surgical treatment or a physiologically based evaluation with PET scanning produces superior results with such lesions in eloquent areas.— R.M. Crowell, M.D.

Microsurgical Treatment of Arteriovenous Malformations of the Brain in a Defined Population
Hernesniemi J, Keränen T (Univ Central Hosp of Kuopio; Univ of Kuopio, Finland)
Surg Neurol 33:384–390, 1990   18–6

The appropriate treatment of arteriovenous malformations (AVMs) of the brain is still debated. From 1980 to 1989, 90 patients with cerebral AVMs were seen at 1 center. No treatment was possible in 2 patients, who had large hematomas and were moribund at admission. Nine of the remaining 88 patients were treated conservatively, 6 of these because they were too old and debilitated to undergo surgery and 3 because they refused surgery.

Of the 79 patients who had surgery, 4 died (mortality rate, 5%), and another 4 were severely disabled. The remaining 71 patients (90%) were able to function independently postoperatively. The procedures included total excision in 70 cases, subtotal excision in 4, partial excision in 3, and exploration in 2.

The surgical treatment of AVMs remains a challenge for neurosurgeons. In this series, microneurosurgery enabled excision of 90% of

AVMs. A few surgeons specializing in AVM and aneurysm surgery should be available in every country.

▶ This interesting and frank report from Finland indicates that 90% of the AVMs in a defined Finnish population can now be excised with good results. The authors advocate microsurgical excision of small and medium-sized lesions, except in the thalamus and mid-brain. They operated without preoperative embolization. They emphasize the advantages of a team of AVM specialists, even in the smaller countries.— R.M. Crowell, M.D.

Dural AVMs

Management of Dural Arteriovenous Malformations of the Anterior Cranial Fossa
Martin NA, King WA, Wilson CB, Nutik S, Carter LP, Spetzler RF (Univ of California, Los Angeles; Univ of California, San Francisco; Kaiser Permanente Med Ctr, Redwood City, Calif)
J Neurosurg 72:692–697, 1990   18–7

Dural arteriovenous malformations (AVMs) in the anterior cranial fossa have a relatively high rate of bleeding. Eight patients with these lesions were reviewed.

Four patients with apoplexy had CT findings of acute frontal hemorrhage with mass effect. Two others had no evidence of intracranial bleeding. Computed tomography showed an acute hemorrhage within the frontal lobe in 5 patients, with the hematoma involving the anteromedial aspect of the frontal pole and sometimes extending ventrally. In all cases, the primary supply was from the ipsilateral anterior ethmoidal artery. Venous drainage was chiefly into pial veins.

The 5 patients with hemorrhage and 1 with retro-orbital headache underwent surgery. The malformation was approached by a low frontal craniotomy. In no case was extensive excision of dura in the anterior fossa floor required to deal with the AVM. The falx was removed in 1 case. No patient required entry into the orbit. All patients but 1, who ultimately died of pulmonary embolism, recovered neurologically. Postoperative angiograms confirmed complete obliteration of the malformation.

Dural AVMs of the anterior fossa are a cause of spontaneous intracerebral bleeding involving the anteromedial frontal lobe, especially in middle-aged men. The vascular connection between the dura and pial vessels is divided in cases in which bleeding is related to the dural AVM or a venous aneurysm is present.

▶ The authors point out that dural AVMs in the anterior cranial fossa usually present with sudden massive intracerebral hemorrhage. These lesions are supplied consistently by the anterior ethmoidal artery, and a venous aneurysm is the source of hemorrhage. Surgical excision can be carried out with low morbidity and is recommended in the case of hemorrhage or venous aneurysm.— R.M. Crowell, M.D.

A Variant of Arteriovenous Fistulas Within the Wall of Dural Sinuses: Results of Combined Surgical and Endovascular Therapy

Barnwell SL, Halbach VV, Dowd CF, Higashida RT, Hieshima GB, Wilson CB (Univ of California, San Francisco)
J Neurosurg 74:199–204, 1991   18–8

Dural arteriovenous (AV) fistulas can occur in thrombosed areas within a sinus. Drainage is usually through cortical veins or an open sinus. The risk of hemorrhage or neurologic dysfunction is high with venous drainage, and the aim of treatment is to close the fistula and preserve sinus flow.

Variant lesions were found in 7 of 105 patients who were treated for dural AV fistulas during a 5-year period. These fistulas were located within a nonthrombosed major sinus with venous drainage to collateral cortical veins instead of the involved sinus. Two patients had headaches and bruit, 1 had neurologic dysfunction, 1 had seizures, and 3 had intracranial hemorrhage. Craniotomy was performed in 4 patients to correct the fistulas, and the other 3 patients underwent embolization. Angiographic examination 1–3 days after treatment revealed closed AV fistulas in all patients.

This type of variant AV fistula poses a higher risk of neurologic dysfunction and hemorrhage related to the pattern of venous outflow from the fistula. Surgery is usually the safest approach in management of these lesions.

▶ In patients with dural AV fistulas involving drainage to cortical veins, there is a high risk of hemorrhage. Surgery appears to be the best treatment.—R.M. Crowell, M.D.

Cavernous Angiomas and Venous Anomalies

Cavernous Malformations and Capillary Telangiectasia: A Spectrum Within a Single Pathological Entity

Rigamonti D, Johnson PC, Spetzler RF, Hadley MN, Drayer BP (Univ of Maryland, Barrow Neurological Inst, Phoenix; David Grant United States Air Force Med Ctr, Travis Air Force Base, Calif)
Neurosurgery 28:60–64, 1991   18–9

Cerebral vascular malformations have been categorized as arteriovenous, venous, cavernous, and capillary telangiectases. However, there is some question that the latter 2 are separate entities. The histories of 20 patients with cavernous malformations were reviewed and the radiographic, clinical, and surgical/autopsy data related to these lesions were analyzed. Of particular interest in surgical specimens were the appearance of the vascular channels, vessel walls (including the presence of elastic fibers and smooth muscle), and evidence of hemorrhage, hemosiderin, thrombosis, calcification, and ossification associated with vascular lesions. The presence or absence of brain parenchyma between dilated vascular channels was graded for each lesion. Magnetic resonance imaging was performed on a whole-brain autopsy specimen, 15 patients with surgically confirmed cavernous malformations, and 15 relatives of these patients.

The histologic appearance of cavernous malformations consistently revealed contiguous dilated vascular channels. Thin vessel walls of collagen were lined with a single layer of flattened endothelium. None of these specimens contained elastic fibers, and only 2 contained a few smooth muscle fibers. Of 20 specimens, 1 contained brain parenchyma between dilated vascular channels in the center of a lesion; 4 other specimens had brain parenchyma only at the edges of the malformation. Some patients had multiple lesions that included cavernous malformations, capillary telangiectases, and transitions between the 2.

Capillary telangiectasia and cavernous malformations appear to represent 2 pathologic extremes within the same category of vascular malformations. These malformations should be grouped as a single cerebral entity designated cerebral capillary malformations.

▶ The authors present pathologic data supportive of the grouping of cavernous angiomas and capillary telangiectasias as a single entity, but neurosurgical clinical practice dictates that the distinction be maintained: Cavernous angiomas are in some instances dangerous for hemorrhage, are easily diagnosed, and are readily excised surgically. On the other hand, capillary telangiectasias have not shown a significant tendency to hemorrhage, nor is surgical excision necessary. On this practical basis, it seems warranted to maintain the distinction.— R.M. Crowell, M.D.

Vascular Pressures and Cortical Blood Flow in Cavernous Angioma of the Brain
Little JR, Awad IA, Jones SC, Ebrahim ZY (Cleveland Clinic Found)
J Neurosurg 73:555–559, 1990   18–10

The use of MRI has improved the diagnosis of cavernous angiomas. As a result, cavernous angiomas are now recognized as being more common and of greater clinical relevance than was previously believed. Five women (mean age, 31 years) were studied to determine the hemodynamic characteristics of cavernous angiomas of the brain.

Headaches and seizure disorders were the most frequent presenting symptoms. Two patients were found by MRI to have an associated small hematoma. The patients underwent local cortical blood flow studies and vascular pressure measurements during surgery for excision of the cavernous angiomas. Four patients were operated on in the supine position and 1, whose lesion involved the brain stem, in the sitting position.

The cavernous angiomas ranged in size from 2 to 3 cm and had a multilobulated exterior surface. The angiomas were easily removed in 1 piece with minimal bleeding. Direct microscopic observation revealed slow circulation within the angiomas. The mean cortical blood flow adjacent to the lesion was 60.5 mL/100 g/min at a mean $PaCO_2$ of 35 torr. These findings were similar to those in established normal controls. Mean CO_2 reactivity was 1.1 mL/100 g/min/torr. Mean pressures in the cavernous angioma were 7 mm Hg in the seated patient and 38.2 mm Hg in the supine patients.

The findings confirmed MRI as the best diagnostic technique available for demonstrating a cavernous angioma. The hemodynamic features of these lesions suggest that they are relatively passive vascular malformations and are unlikely to produce ischemia in the adjacent brain. As a result of low driving pressures, frank hemorrhage should be self-limiting.

▶ Intraoperative measurements of blood flow and cerebral blood flow physiology indicate normal physiology near cavernous angiomas. The mean pressure of 38.2 mm Hg confirms a low pressure within these lesions. This correlates with the relative ease of removal, without excessive bleeding, and the relatively self-contained local nature of hemorrhage in the untreated state.— R.M. Crowell, M.D.

Surgical Management of Brain Stem Vascular Malformations
Weil SM, Tew JM Jr (Univ of Cincinnati; Mayfield Neurological Inst, Cincinnati)
Acta Neurochir (Wien) 105:14–23, 1990   18–11

Vascular malformations of the brain stem are histologically heterogeneous lesions. They are most commonly seen with sudden, progressive neurologic deficit related to hemorrhage. Eleven patients with these malformations were assessed at 1 center. There were 6 women and 5 men aged 22–43 years. Seven patients had progressive neurologic deterioration caused by recurrent intraparenchymal hemorrhage.

All patients underwent MRI, which documented a consistent morphological appearance, with a central focus of mixed signal intensity representing hemorrhage of various ages. A low signal ring, consistent with hemosiderin deposition from remote hemorrhage, surrounded the nidus. Several MR studies demonstrated a pattern that suggested the presence of multiple vessels containing slow-flowing blood.

Because of their progressive neurologic deficit, 7 patients underwent complete surgical extirpation of the hematoma and malformation. The remaining 4 patients recovered fully and were under observation for signs indicating the need for surgery.

Significant neurologic disability can result from vascular malformations of the brain stem. Magnetic resonance imaging is the definitive diagnostic technique for characterizing these malformations. Total surgical resection of the malformation and hematoma is needed in certain cases to prevent progressive, irreversible neurologic damage.

▶ The authors report 7 cases with complete surgical extirpation of brain stem hematoma and malformation. The indication was progressive neurologic deficit. The histology showed cavernous hemangioma in most of the individuals. The operative morbidity was minimal. The surgical approach was through the inferior vermis for pontomedullary lesions, through the superior vermis for mesencephalic lesions, and, occasionally, subtemporally for lateral mesancephalic lesions. The ND:Yag laser and bipolar cauterization were used for total excision under the operating microscope at all times.—R.M. Crowell, M.D.

Third Ventricle Cavernous Angioma: Report of Two Cases
Ogawa A, Katakura R, Yoshimoto T (Tohoku Univ, Sendai, Japan)
Surg Neurol 34:414–420, 1990   18–12

Cavernous angioma that arises in the third ventricle is extremely rare. The clinical manifestations and surgical approach to third ventricle cavernous angioma were reviewed in 2 patients, as well as in 5 previously reported cases.

Onset of the disease was manifested by hypothalamic symptoms in 3 patients, hydrocephalus caused by compression of the third ventricle in 2, intraventricular hemorrhage in 1, and memory and naming deficits in 1. None had seizures and 6 had signs of a focal mass. Most of the patients showed stepwise aggravation of symptoms. Computed tomography showed high-density areas and enhancement effects. In 1 later patient, MRI was effective in making the differential diagnosis by showing a circumscribed area of low intensity, together with a mixed-intensity mass and irregular high-signal intensity on T2-weighted images.

A bifrontal craniotomy and an interhemispheric translamina terminalis approach were used in the 2 later patients. The falx was cut at the base of the brain. By dissecting both olfactory nerves and a wide area in the interhemispheric fissure, the mobility of both frontal lobes was increased and a wide operative field was obtained with minimal compression of the brain. Both patients recovered, 1 without neurologic deficit and the other with a slight visual disturbance. Postoperative imaging studies showed no signs of tumor shadow.

The bifrontal craniotomy and interhemispheric translamina terminalis approach is a suitable technique for surgery on angiomas of the anterior half of the third ventricle. The procedure allows excision of the entire angioma with minimal damage to the brain.

► This impressive report documents effective removal of anterior third ventricular cavernous angiomas by a bifrontal interhemispheric translaminar approach. The postoperative MRI demonstrated total removal of the lesion. The clinical course was satisfactory in both cases.

The report illustrates the serious deficits that may arise from cavernous angioma bleeding. The effectiveness of MRI diagnosis is again demonstrated. The use of this particular translaminar approach to the third ventricle has recently been mentioned for other pathologies but appears to be useful for such lesions as angioma and aneurysm. Clearly, in such cases the indication of progressive severe neurologic deficit warrants surgery. In patients with milder affliction (e.g., a patient particularly without neurologic deficit or significant bleeding), the indications for surgery or radiosurgery are less clear (1).— R.M. Crowell, M.D.

Reference

1. Lunsford LD, et al: *Neurosurgery* 24:151, 1989.

Cerebellar Venous Angioma Associated With Angiographically Occult Brain Stem Vascular Malformation: Report of Two Cases
Abe M, Asfora WT, DeSalles AAF, Kjellberg RN (Massachusetts Gen Hosp; Harvard Med School, Boston)
Surg Neurol 33:400–403, 1990   18–13

Venous angioma (malformation) is often diagnosed on the basis of angiographic features alone but its clinical significance is controversial. Two patients with angiographically documented cerebellar venous malformation were encountered. Recurrent hemorrhages developed in the pontine tegmentum in the first patient and in the midbrain in the second patient (Fig 18–1). Neither patient had hemorrhage originating from the abnormal cerebellar venous channels.

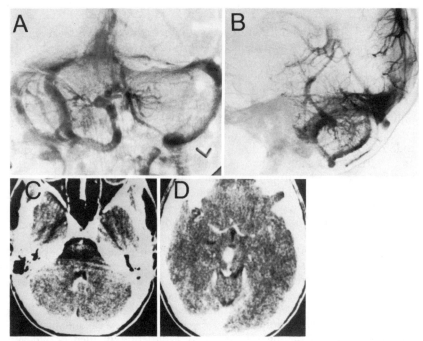

Fig 18–1.—**A,** anteroposterior and (B) lateral views of the left vertebral angiograms in the venous phase demonstrate enlarged veins with numerous dilated medullary veins adjacent to the fourth ventricle. C, CT scan with contrast shows prominence of vein of lateral recess of fourth ventricle and (D) an area of high attenuation with microcalcifications in the right midbrain. (Courtesy of Abe M, Asfora WT, DeSalles AAF, et al: *Surg Neurol* 33:400–403, 1990.)

Vascular malformations of the brain stem are often occult. On the basis of these 2 cases, a review of the literature, and an autopsy study of similar cases, it appears that angiographic venous malformations are benign entities which may support the presence of angiographically occult vascular malformations in proximity to them.

Accurate localization of symptomatic pathologic blood vessels through a combination of CT, MRI, and angiography is important in planning treatment of cerebellar venous angioma. Surgical resection, stereotactic radiation, or particle beam therapy may be used successfully.

▶ This report of 2 cases indicates the definite association of "venous angioma" with occult brain stem vascular malformation of the bleeding type. The report bolsters the notion that "venous angioma" has a very low likelihood of hemorrhage and may well be considered a variant of normal venous anatomy. In that situation, the associated occult malformation would in fact be the lesion responsible for hemorrhage.—R.M. Crowell, M.D.

Cerebral Venous Malformations

Rigamonti D, Spetzler RF, Medina M, Rigamonti K, Geckle DS, Pappas C (Univ of Maryland; Barrow Neurological Inst, Phoenix)
J Neurosurg 73:560–564, 1990   18–14

Cerebral venous malformations are common, but their clinical significance remains controversial. The clinical courses of 14 men and 16 women (mean age, 37 years) were reviewed. Eighteen patients had venous malformations in the supratentorial compartment, 12 had cerebellar lesions, and 1 had both a cerebellar and a pontine venous lesion.

Twenty patients complained of headache, and in 13 patients it was the only complaint. Four patients had nausea and vomiting in addition to headache. Of the 12 patients with cerebellar lesions, 4 had an acute episode of gait ataxia, 3 had diplopia, 2 had numbness, 1 had dysphagia and decreased hearing, 1 had ischemic symptoms, and 1 had epilepsy. Seven patients had multiple symptoms, but 4 of the 12 cerebellar angiomas were associated only with headache. Twenty-five patients underwent angiography, which always showed the typical caput medusae appearance of the lesion. Follow-up periods ranged from 18 to 104 months.

Two patients with cerebellar venous angioma and ataxia were found to have a coexistent cavernous malformation. Both patients were operated on for bleeding presumed to be caused by the cavernous angioma. Neither patient experienced rebleeding or acute episodes of neurologic dysfunction postoperatively. No other patients were operated on. One patient had findings consistent with atherosclerosis and stroke, and 1 patient had a tumor. At follow-up, 23 patients were well and asymptomatic, 2 were still having seizures, and 1 patient remained ataxic and complained of dizziness. One patient continued to experience severe headaches at least once a month, and 1 patient had a carcinoma of the neck. A familial incidence of venous malformation was not established.

The association of venous malformations with cavernous malformations, tumors, or atherosclerosis can easily be overlooked. Symptomatic patients with venous malformations should therefore be further investigated to rule out underlying pathology. If the latter is found, only the underlying pathology should be treated. The venous malformation should be spared, as experience suggests that rebleeding does not occur after treatment of the associated pathology.

▶ This contribution adds support to the contention that venous angiomas, so-called, cause a very low incidence of intracranial bleeding. In this group of 30 cases, only 2 were associated with bleeding, and in both instances an associated cavernous angioma was found surgically. Thus the data add support to the concept advanced by Lasjaunis that "venous angiomas" should instead be regarded as a variant of normal venous anatomy. This view is also consistent with catastrophic venous infarction, which has been observed after removal of such venous channels. If this view is correct, then "venous anomaly" can be anticipated to bleed virtually never mandating a very conservative approach.

I advocate that surgery not be performed on venous anomalies, nor should they be treated with focused radiation for fear of serious vasogenic edema and deterioration. Instead, an intense search for an associated lesion such as a cavernous angioma should be instituted for the potential source of bleeding. (Another 2 case reports from Kjellberg in *Neurosurgery* 1991 also support this view.)—R.M. Crowell, M.D.

Spontaneous Hemorrhage

Spontaneous Cerebellar Hematoma
Gilliard C, Mathurin P, Passagia JG, Kallel S, Thauvoy C, Stroobandt G (Univ Catholique de Louvain, Louvain, Belgium; Univ de Grenoble, Grenoble, France)
Neurochirurgie 36:347–353, 1990   18–15

Spontaneous cerebellar hematoma (SCH) represents 7% to 9% of all cases of cerebral hemorrhage. The earlier challenge of diagnosing SCH was resolved with the introduction of CT and MRI. However, there is still no agreement on the surgical management of SCH.

During a 10-year period, SCH was diagnosed in 21 female and 18 male patients aged 13–82 years. Twenty-six patients were older than age 60 years. One patient had 2 separate SCHs. Twenty-three patients had arterial hypertension as an underlying cause of SCH. Additional causative factors were alcoholism, vascular malformation, anticoagulant therapy, metastatic tumor, and septicemia. In 6 patients a definite etiology was not established. Thirty of the 39 patients were admitted on the day of ictus. Seventeen patients were conscious when admitted, 14 were semiconscious, and 8 were in a coma. One comatose patient died on the way to the hospital.

All patients underwent urgent CT scanning. The SCH was less than 3.5 cm in diameter in 12 patients and larger in 26 patients. In 1 patient the SCH extended to the brain stem. The size of the hematoma was signifi-

cantly associated with the Glasgow Coma Score at admission. Twelve of
15 hematomas in the median-paramedian region, but only 12 of 25 in the
lateral region, showed hydrocephalus on the CT scan. Thus hydrocephalus was significantly associated with median-paramedian localization of
the hematoma. Magnetic resonance imaging was not available, except for
the last 2 patients in this series.

Most patients were treated initially with corticosteroids and observation for 48 hours. However, deterioration of consciousness was an indication for urgent surgery. Nineteen patients had placement of a temporary subcutaneous ventricular drain, and 13 of them subsequently underwent craniotomy for hematoma evacuation. Another 6 patients immediately underwent craniotomy for hematoma evacuation without ventricular drainage previously.

Fourteen patients died (36%), including 6 of 8 who were comatose at
admission, 4 of 14 who were semiconscious, and 4 of 17 who were conscious. The Glasgow Coma Score at admission was an important prognostic indicator of survival. Nineteen of the 25 survivors are living independently and 6 require constant care. One of the 2 initially comatose
survivors remains handicapped and 1 survives without neurologic sequelae.

The Glasgow Coma Score, size of the hematoma, and hematoma location are the 3 most significant prognostic indicators of survival after
SCH. Hematoma size is an important factor in planning surgical treatment.

▶ Once again, the value of CT scanning in management of cerebellar hematoma is demonstrated. In this particular series, lesions smaller than 3.5 cm
in diameter did not require surgical excision unless a primary lesion required
excision.—R.M. Crowell, M.D.

**Experimental Intracerebral Hemorrhage: Early Removal of a Spontaneous
Mass Lesion Improves Late Outcome**
Nehls DG, Mendelow AD, Graham DI, Teasdale GM (Univ of Glasgow; Walter
Reed Army Med Ctr, Washington, DC)
Neurosurgery 27:674–682, 1990   18–16

The sequelae of removing an experimental intracerebral mass were examined in rats implanted with a 50-μL balloon inflated within the right
caudate nucleus. Cerebral blood flow was estimated 24 hours later by autoradiography. Light microscopic study also was carried out. Half of the
animals had the balloon inflated for 10 minutes, half permanently.

Little difference in blood flow was noted between the 2 cerebral hemispheres 24 hours after transient balloon inflation. In contrast, flow was
significantly impaired in the hemisphere ipsilateral to the permanently inflated balloon. Ischemic levels of flow were present in the cortex. Ischemic cell damage was present in all animals even after transient balloon
inflation, but it was more marked after permanent inflation. The neuro-

Score	Neurological Outcome*		
	Neurological Outcome	Group 1 (Transient)	Group 2 (Permanent)
0	No deficit	11	4
1	Mild deficit	4	3
2	Circles with stimula-tion	1	1
3	Spontaneous circling	0	6
4	Brachial monopa-resis	0	2
5	Depressed con-sciousness	0	0

*The neurologic outcome was significantly worse in group 2 (Mann-Whitney U test, P < .02).

(Courtesy of Nehls DG, Mendelow AD, Graham DI, et al: *Neurosurgery* 27:674–682, 1990.)

logic outcome was significantly better after early deflation of the balloon (table).

These findings suggest that early removal of an intracerebral mass lesion may be beneficial. However, the results are not strictly comparable to those that might be obtained by evacuating an intracerebral hematoma surgically.

▶ This interesting experimental study shows that removal of an inflated balloon mass from the brain of a rat leads to improved outcome, suggesting that prompt removal of intracerebral hemorrhage might lead to improved results in human beings. There are a number of issues regarding this study: (1) The model is certainly significantly different from the clinical situation of intracerebral hemorrhage; (2) the damage caused by hemorrhage is not entirely the result of mass effect; (3) no surgical evacuation could be done within 10 minutes after hemorrhage, as was achieved by immediate deflation of the balloon; (4) in patients, the clot is eventually absorbed by the tissues itself; and (5) there is certainly some risk to surgical evacuation of an intracerebral hematoma.—R.M. Crowell, M.D.

19 Ischemia

The Influence of Neutralizing Heparin After Carotid Endarterectomy on Postoperative Stroke and Wound Hematoma
Treiman RL, Cossman DV, Foran RF, Levin PM, Cohen JL, Wagner WH (Cedars-Sinai Med Ctr, Los Angeles)
J Vasc Surg 12:440–446, 1990   19–1

Some surgeons neutralize heparinization after carotid endarterectomy in patients with stroke but others do not. In a 6-year period at 1 center, some surgeons routinely used protamine sulfate to neutralize heparin but others used it only when a synthetic patch was used or wound hemostasis was not readily obtained. To determine the influence of protamine on stroke and wound hematoma, data were reviewed on 697 patients, 159 of whom were operated on more than once.

The mean age was 71 years. In all, 328 patients received protamine and 369 did not; the 2 groups were similar in age and surgical indications, but the group given protamine tended to have more operations for recurrent stenosis and were more likely to be women. All surgeons used the same operative technique except for their use of protamine. The total heparin dose ranged from 6,000 to 10,000 units; the protamine dose ranged from 15 to 75 mg.

The incidence of stroke was 1.8% in the protamine-treated group and 2.7% in those not given protamine, but the difference was not significant, even when 3 strokes unrelated to heparinization were excluded. The incidence of wound hematoma was 1.8% in the group given protamine and 6.5% in those not given protamine—a significant difference. This significance persisted even when 3 hematomas unrelated to protamine were excluded. There was a slightly lower incidence of wound hematoma in patients not given protamine whose wound was drained. In the protamine-treated group there was no difference in incidence of stroke or wound hematoma between patients who received a low dose of heparin and those who received a high dose.

Neutralization of heparin with protamine sulfate after carotid endarterectomy lessens the risk of wound hematoma without increasing the risk of stroke. The risk of wound hematoma is unaffected by the dose of protamine. Wound drainage lessens the risk of hematoma insignificantly in patients who do not receive protamine.

► This study brings out an unexpected and important finding: When protamine was given at the end of the operation to reverse the heparin, the incidence of postoperative stroke was 1.8%; when protamine was not given, the stroke rate was 2.7%, a difference not reaching statistical significance. Existing experimental data would suggest that nonreversal of heparin would be superior, but here are data to the contrary. This is important for the surgeon who may wish to avoid protamine administration. On the other hand, it has been suggested that nonreversal of heparin leads to a lower late risk of restenosis, but the present study does not offer data on that particular issue.

The other point regarding wound hematomas is harder to accept. The 6.5% rate of wound hematoma in the group not given protamine seems inordinately high. If one looks at the number of cases in which there was a hematoma even with a drain in place, this seems rather high (4.4%). Thus one has to question the nature of hemostasis in these procedures. Also, the nature of the drain is not specifically described. We have used the Jackson-Pratt system, connected to 1.5 pounds of wall suction for the last 100 cases, and have experienced wound hematomas in only 2 cases; in each instance a technical defect in the suction system was identified. Thus I question the conclusion that nonreversal with protamine leads to a higher incidence of hematomas.

Another important point is the fact that a severe anaphylactic response to protamine may occur occasionally, most frequently in the setting of insulin-dependent diabetes. Reports suggest that this particular complication has a fatality rate of about 50%. This is not a trivial complication and should be factored into the entire equation.— R.M. Crowell, M.D.

Is Routine Duplex Examination After Carotid Endarterectomy Justified?
Cook JM, Thompson BW, Barnes RW (Univ of Arkansas)
J Vasc Surg 12:334–340, 1990   19–2

Although many surgeons recommend routine noninvasive follow-up of patients undergoing carotid endarterectomy, the role of carotid restenosis in the development of stroke after endarectomy is uncertain. The present authors do not reoperate on asymptomatic patients with recurrent stenosis. The implications of this approach for routine postoperative duplex examination were examined in 120 patients having 143 carotid endarterectomies in a 5-year period. A total of 101 patients with 118 operations were available for clinical follow-up.

Six of the 101 patients had recurrent ipsilateral transient ischemic attacks (TIAs) or stroke. Of the 76 evaluable arteries examined by duplex scanning, 18% had a 50% or greater reduction in luminal diameter. Four of the 14 lesions regressed and 10 remained stable; no vessel became occluded. Two patients with recurrent stenosis had ipsilateral hemispheric TIAs, and 1 of them had a stroke while awaiting surgery. Ipsilateral symptoms developed in 6.5% of arteries without significant recurrent stenosis. Hemispheric symptoms, stroke, and survival did not relate to the presence or absence of hemodynamically significant stenosis.

Recurrent carotid stenosis after endarterectomy is not associated with an increased risk of TIAs, stroke, or death. Routine duplex scanning is not justified postoperatively, and reoperation should be limited to patients who have ipsilateral neurologic symptoms accompanying hemodynamically significant restenosis.

▶ The authors found no increase in TIAs or stroke in patients with recurrent carotid stenosis. They therefore do not suggest routine duplex scanning; rather, they study only patients with symptoms. Nonetheless, it is worthwhile to obtain an ultrasonic study soon after carotid endarterectomy to establish a baseline in case of later symptomatology.—R.M. Crowell, M.D.

Safety and Long-Term Benefit of Carotid Endarterectomy in the Asymptomatic Patient
Park Y, El-Bayar H, Hye RJ, Stabile BE, Freischlag JA (VA Med Ctr, San Diego, Univ of California, San Diego)
Ann Vasc Surg 4:218–222, 1990   19–3

There is controversy as to whether carotid endarterectomy (CEA) can lower the risk of stroke in asymptomatic patients with carotid stenosis. Patients who underwet CEA were followed to document the safety and long-term benefit of this procedure in asymptomatic individuals.

The study sample comprised 53 men and 1 woman who had undergone a total of 60 CEAs during a 6-year period. The mean age was 64 years. The medical records were reviewed for surgical indications and results. Outpatient clinic records and family and patient interviews were reviewed to collect follow-up data, and carotid duplex scans were done in available patients. The mean follow-up was 47 months.

Arteriographic findings were high-grade stenosis of 70% or more in 77% of carotid arteries studied, ulceration in 8%, and both high-grade stenosis and ulceration in 15%. Risk factors identified included coronary artery disease in 60% of patients, smoking in 87%, hypertension in 67%, and diabetes in 22%. Three cranial nerve injuries, 1 myocardial infarction, 1 contralateral stroke, and no deaths occurred in the perioperative period. There were 3 ipsilateral transient ischemic attacks without recurrent stenosis and 1 contralateral attack during the follow-up period. One patient needed reoperation for an ipsilateral stroke after 2 years, and 4 had late contralateral strokes. Four patients died of cardiac problems, 2 of a malignancy, 2 of pulmonary problems, 1 of stroke, and 1 of an unknown cause. On duplex scan evaluation, 87% of patients had less than 50% restenosis, 8.5% had 50% to 75% restenosis, 2% had 80% restenosis, and 2% had 90% restenosis. The ipsilateral stroke-free rate at 5 years and 8 years was 98%.

In asymptomatic patients with carotid stenosis, carotid endarterectomy causes little morbidity and almost no mortality. Late stroke is rare on the ipsilateral side, and significant restenosis occurs in a small percentage of cases. The low rate of restenosis is correlated with the low long-term rate of stroke.

▶ Here is another uncontrolled series of cases subjected to carotid endarterectomy for carotid plaque (usually high-grade stenosis) without symptoms. In general, patients did well with little morbidity and no immediate mortality from endarterectomy. On the other hand, there were numerous myocardial infarctions (sometimes fatal), strokes both ipsilateral and contralateral, pulmonary problems, and death of unknown cause. Four percent of the patients had at least 80% restenosis on follow-up evaluation. The data are interesting, but to establish a beneficial effect for carotid endarterectomy, only controlled randomized studies will suffice. Such a study is underway in the United States under the leadership of Dr. Toole, and we hope that data from this study will help to establish criteria for endarterectomy in asymptomatic patients, if any.—R.M. Crowell, M.D.

Normal Angiograms and Carotid Pathology
Senkowsky J, Bell WH III, Kerstein MD (Tulane Univ)
Am Surg 56:726–729, 1990   19–4

Transient ischemic attacks, amaurosis fugax, and stroke may result from nonstenotic ulcerated atherosclerotic plaques of the carotid arteries. These symptoms have traditionally been investigated by ultrasound and arch aortography angiograms of the area of the carotid bifurcation. It has recently been suggested that ultrasound is the better procedure for detecting and delineating these lesions.

To analyze the ultrasound findings in patients with negative arteriograms, 21 patients with normal angiograms, abnormal findings on real-time B-mode ultrasound examinations, and hemispheric transient ischemic attacks were studied. The 15 men and 6 women had an average age of 66 years. Four had had a cerebrovascular accident and all had a history of ECG evidence of coronary artery disease. The ultrasound determinant of ulceration was irregularity of the carotid wall on B-mode ultrasound; the arteriographic determinant was wall irregularity or loss of contour of the carotid bulb. All patients also had preoperative CT of the head.

Surgical findings confirmed the ultrasound diagnosis of 20% to 50% stenosis and ulcerative plaques. Arteriograms were reevaluated in light of these surgical findings, but only 3 could be read as positive. The results of CT were positive in the 4 patients with a history of cerebrovascular accident and showed old lacunar infarcts in an additional 3 patients. All patients had resolution of symptoms at follow-up of 6 months to 3 years after operation.

Real-time B-mode ultrasound appears to be superior to angiography in detecting nonstenotic lesions of the carotid artery. In patients with appropriate symptoms and ulcerative plaque shown by ultrasound, angiography may not be required before surgery. Surgery should not be done on the basis of angiography alone.

▶ This paper again raises the question of normal angiography in the face of ulcerative plaque in the internal carotid artery. The data suggest that ulcerative plaques can be detected by ultrasound despite apparently normal angiography. There are several problems here. The angiographic studies in Figures 1 and 2 presented in the full-length article as of suboptimal quality, which of course could explain the lack of visualization of the ulcerative plaque. The serial studies again show up holdup of the dye within the ulcer. Criteria for the ultrasound diagnosis of ulceration need to be demonstrated more clearly. The decision to operate in the face of a negative angiogram should be made with great caution, if ever.—R.M. Crowell, M.D.

The Silent Brain Infarct Before and After Carotid Surgery
Habozit B (Clinique Poirier, Chambery, France)
Ann Vasc Surg 4:485–489, 1990   19–5

With the advent of CT scanning, silent cerebral infarctions (SCI) have been found in some patients with carotid artery lesions. To determine the incidence of preoperative and postoperative SCI compared with clinical status, studies were made in 114 homogeneous patients undergoing 131 carotid artery procedures.

Routine CT was performed prospectively before and after surgery. Hemispheric cerebral infarction was detected before surgery in 3 of the 16 hemispheres corresponding to symptomatic lesions, in 18 of 109 hemispheres corresponding to transient ischemic attacks, and in 1 of 4 hemispheres corresponding to lesions responsible for a fixed cerebral vascular accident. Two procedures (1.5%) were complicated by early cerebral infarctions as detected on postoperative CT. In 1 case, these complications resulted in death; the other patient had major sequelae.

Five procedures (3.8%) were complicated by transient ischemic attacks. Three of these were associated with minimal cerebral infarctions visible on CT. Neurologic status was unchanged after 124 procedures (94.6%). Four of these (3.1%) were complicated by silent brain infarctions as seen on postoperative CT.

These findings suggest that existing preoperative and postoperative neurologic classifications are flawed and that surgery is rarely responsible for cerebral infarction. Preoperative and postoperative CT scans should be performed with each carotid procedure.

▶ This interesting study documents that the more you look, the more you see. Postoperative CT scanning shows up cerebral infarction in both symptomatic and asymptomatic cases. Moreover preoperative scanning turns up cerebral infarction in a number of asymptomatic or neurologically normal cases.

The bottom line is that pre- and postoperative CT scanning should be done in patients undergoing carotid endarterectomy.—R.M. Crowell, M.D.

Rupture of Atheromatous Plaque as a Cause of Thrombotic Occlusion of Stenotic Internal Carotid Artery
Ogata J, Masuda J, Yutani C, Yamaguchi T (Natl Cardiovascular Ctr, Osaka, Japan)
Stroke 21:1740–1745, 1990   19–6

The mechanisms of thrombotic occlusion of the internal carotid artery (ICA) in patients who die shortly after the occlusion are seldom studied. The clinical profiles and autopsy findings of 5 patients who died shortly after the onset of cerebral infarction following thrombotic occlusion of the ICA were evaluated.

The 3 men and 2 women were aged 61–78 years and all were hypertensive. The onset of the last stroke was abrupt, with maximal deficit in 3 patients and progressive in 2. None of the patients received anticoagulation or antiplatelet therapy. In all 5 patients histologic specimens from the occluded sites of the ICAs showed tight stenosis caused by atheromatous plaque and rupture of the fibrous lining over the gruel of atheroma as a cause of thrombotic occlusion. The mean shorter luminal diameter of the ICA at the site of occlusion was 1.5 mm, with the plaque occupying a mean of 93% of the original luminal area.

Carotid plaque that contains gruel covered by a thin fibrous lining harbors a risk of rupture that may cause occlusion of a stenotic ICA. In such patients cerebral infarction develops by artery-to-artery embolism or by reduced cerebral perfusion with failure of collateral blood flow.

▶ Among a large number of autopsies done during a decade, ICA occlusion was found in 48 patients, 5 of whom died of the event. All 5 had rupture of the atheromatous plaque as a cause of thrombotic occlusion, suggesting that this is an important and dangerous cause of stroke. It would have been of interest to know the collateral circulatory patterns of these patients, in that when ICA occlusion causes fatality, usually the infarction is very large and comes in relation to poor collateral circulation. The danger of acute carotid occlusion is obvious here and warrants vigorous medical and surgical treatment for its prevention.— R.M. Crowell, M.D.

Effects of STA-MCA Anastomosis for Ischaemic Oculopathy Due to Occlusion of the Internal Carotid Artery
Shibuya M, Suzuki Y, Takayasu M, Sugita K (Nagoya Univ, Japan)
Acta Neurochir (Wien) 103:71–75, 1990   19–7

Occlusion of the internal carotid artery may lead to neovascular glaucoma or other complications. Although photocoagulation of the retina can reduce oxygen demand, increasing the blood supply is more important as a disease cure. In 2 patients with ischemic oculopathy caused by occlusion of the internal carotid artery, superficial temporal artery and middle cerebral artery (STA-MCA) anastomosis was performed.

Both patients improved in visual acuity, central retinal artery pressure, and signs of transient ischemic attack. Postoperative angiography showed a marked decrease in collateral flow with the development of blood flow through the anastomosis (Fig 19–1).

Surgery must be performed in an early disease stage to prevent complications such as venous stasis retinopathy, neovascular glaucoma, or rubeosis iridis. The improvement in visual acuity and increase in pressure

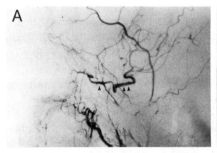 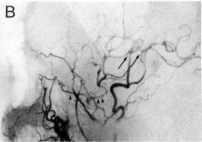

Fig 19–1.—Preoperative and postoperative left carotid angiography. **A,** preoperative angiography shows that internal carotid *(double arrowheads)* and middle cerebral arteries are fed by a reversed flow through the dominant ophthalmic artery *(arrowhead).* **B,** postoperative angiography shows a remarkable decrease in the flow through the ophthalmic artery *(arrowhead)* and internal carotid artery *(double arrowheads)* with formation of blood flow through the STA-MCA double anastomoses *(arrows).* (Courtesy of Shibuya M, Suzuki Y, Takayasu M, et al: *Acta Neurochir (Wien)* 103:71–75, 1990.)

ischemia suggest that ocular ischemia is reduced by STA-MCA anastomosis. An international cooperative study showed negative results of STA-MCA anastomosis for cerebral ischemia, but this surgical procedure improved symptoms of ocular ischemia in 2 patients with occlusion of the internal carotid artery.

▶ In these 2 cases, retinal ischemia declined after STA-MCA bypass. The authors suggest that revascularization at any early stage is valuable in the prevention of eventually universal retinal ischemic complications. Although the report is encouraging, the precise role of such revascularization remains controversial.—R.M. Crowell, M.D.

Comparison of Crystalloids and Colloids for Hemodilution in a Model of Focal Cerebral Ischemia

Korosue K, Heros RC, Ogilvy CS, Hyodo A, Tu Y-K, Graichen R (Univ of Minnesota; Massachusetts Gen Hosp, Boston)
J Neurosurg 73:576–584, 1990
19–8

Hemodilution has been suggested as potential therapy for cerebral ischemia. Colloid solutions have been used as hemodiluting agents in all clinical and experimental studies reported to date. However, colloid solutions are expensive and can cause undesirable side effects. Several studies have suggested that crystalloids are as safe and effective as colloids in the treatment of circulatory shock, but crystalloids have never been used in the treatment of cerebral ischemia.

The feasibility of using crystalloids for hemodilution in focal cerebral ischemia was assessed in 40 dogs subjected to 6 hours of occlusion of the left internal carotid and middle cerebral arteries. Thirty minutes after arterial occlusion, 13 dogs were treated with low-molecular-weight (low-MW) dextran, 13 received lactated Ringer's solution, and 14 were left untreated. All dogs were killed 1 week after arterial occlusion.

Isovolemic hemodilution reduced the hematocrit to 33% or 34% in both treatment groups, and it remained reduced throughout the week. Blood viscosity, plasma total protein levels, and fibrinogen levels were significantly reduced in the acute stage in both treatment groups, but all levels gradually returned to baseline by the end of the week. Hemodilution with lactated Ringer's solution lowered both the osmotic and the oncotic pressures, whereas those pressures remained intact in the other animals. Neurologic conditions in animals treated with lactated Ringer's solution were consistently poorer than those in the other 2 groups. At autopsy, the infarct volume in animals treated with lactated Ringer's solution was significantly larger than that in either untreated controls or in animals treated with low-MW dextran.

In this model of focal cerebral ischemia, hemodilution with colloids was beneficial, whereas hemodilution with lactated Ringer's solution was deleterious. The decrease in oncotic pressure in animals treated with lactated Ringer's solution after hemodilution is probably the main reason for its detrimental effect.

▶ These careful studies indicate that, in a canine model, isovolemic hemodilution with lactated Ringer's solution was deleterious, whereas hemodilution with colloids was beneficial. This may have some bearing on the treatment of focal cerebral ischemia, especially as related to vasospasm, in clinical cases.— R.M. Crowell, M.D.

(S)-Emopamil Protects Against Global Ischemic Brain Injury in Rats

Lin B, Dietrich WD, Busto R, Ginsberg MD (Univ of Miami)
Stroke 21:1734–1739, 1990   19–9

Ischemic cerebrovascular disease is an important cause of death and disability. Treatments to protect the brain from ischemic damage are therefore greatly needed. (S)-Emopamil, a novel phenylalkylamine-class calcium channel blocker, has potent serotonin S_2 antagonist activity. The effects of this agent on the histopathologic consequences of global brain ischemia were studied in anesthetized rats.

Fifteen pretreated rats were given (S)-emopamil, 20 mg/kg intraperitoneally, 30 minutes before and 2 hours after 10 minutes of bilateral common carotid artery occlusion and arterial hypotension. After 3 days, quantitative cell counts showed a marked loss of pyramidal neurons in all subsectors of the hippocampal CA1 region of 15 untreated ischemic rats. In the (S)-emopamil pretreated rats, however, the numbers of normal neurons were significantly higher, by 2.4-fold in the medial subsector, 1.9-fold in the middle subsector, and 1.8-fold in the lateral subsector of the CA1 area. According to semiquantitative grading, (S)-emopamil also reduced ischemic changes in the cerebral cortex. In 10 rats treated beginning 30 minutes after the ischemic insult, no effect on ischemic injury from (S)-emopamil was observed.

(S)-Emopamil pretreatment substantially protects hippocampal neurons from ischemic damage. This finding suggests that *(S)*-emopamil may have a role in the prevention of ischemic neuronal injury in clinical situations in which a global decline in cerebral perfusion is anticipated.

▶ This interesting experimental study demonstrates that pretreatment with the calcium channel blocker (S)-emopamil decreases injury from global brain ischemia in rats but is not effective if given after onset of ischemia.— R.M. Crowell, M.D.

20 Spine

Cervical

Magnetic Resonance Imaging in the Preoperative Evaluation of Cervical Radiculopathy
Wilson DW, Pezzuti RT, Place JN (Maine Med Ctr, Portland)
Neurosurgery 28:175–179, 1991   20–1

Cervical radiculopathy is a significant health problem. For the past 10 years, the preferred initial diagnostic approach to patients with cervical radiculopathy has been CT-myelography. Researchers have now suggested, however, that MRI should be the preferred procedure in patients with suspected cervical radiculopathy.

Forty patients with cervical radiculopathy were assessed preoperatively with MRI. In 27 cases (68%) MRI alone was used. The remainder also underwent CT studies in conjunction with myelography. The primary MRI criterion for a clinically significant lesion was asymmetrical narrowing of the subarachnoid space in the area of the nerve root. Surgery confirmed the abnormality in all 40 cases. The operative findings included a herniated nucleus pulposus in 32 cases, spondylosis in 2, and both in 6. Also, MRI showed a surgical lesion in 92% of the patients (table).

Magnetic resonance imaging with high-resolution axial images may be the procedure of choice in assessment of cervical radiculopathy. Its detection rate is equal to, if not better than, CT-myelography. In addition, MRI has no association with morbidity and costs less than CT-myelography.

▶ This nice surgical-radiologic correlation shows that MRI is very effective in the identification of surgical lesions in the setting of cervical radiculopathy. On

	Correlation of MRI Interpretation With Operative Findings		
Operative Finding	Operative Result (number of patients)	MRI Finding (number of patients)	Findings Correctly Identified by MRI (%)
HNP	38	32[b]	84
Spondylosis alone	2	2	100
HNP and spondylosis	40	37	92

HNP, herniated nucleus pulposus.
*In 6 of 38 patients with a surgically proven HNP, spondylosis was the interpretation by MRI.
(Courtesy of Wilson DW, Pezzuti RT, Place JN: *Neurosurgery* 28:175–179, 1991.)

the other hand, the report does not tell us how often pathology could be missed by MRI. I still believe there is a role for CT with myelography in patients with MRI studies that are negative or equivocal for radiculopathy.—R.M. Crowell, M.D.

Use of MR Imaging-Compatible Halifax Interlaminar Clamps for Posterior Cervical Fusion

Aldrich EF, Crow WN, Weber PB, Spagnolia TN (Univ of Texas, Galveston)
J Neurosurg 74:185–189, 1991   20–2

Posterior cervical fusion can be done using various methods. A recently developed titanium alloy clamp is now available that has the advantages of both interlaminar clamp and MRI compatibility. Halifax interlaminar clamps were used with autogenous iliac crest bone grafting for posterior cervical spine stabilization in 21 patients (Fig 20–1).

The levels involved were the C1–C2 in 8 patients, C4–C5 in 4, C5–C6 in 3, C6–C7 in 3, C4–C6 in 2, and C5–C7 in 1. Unilateral clamps were used in 3 patients and bilateral clamps in 18. All but 1 patient had autogenous iliac bone grafting. The patients were followed for 1–18 months. There were no complications or mechanical failures. Follow-up diagnostic examinations showed rigid fixation and fusion in all patients.

The MR imaging-compatibility of the clamps enables excellent follow-up studies to be done with minimal artifact. The new MR-compatible Halifax interlaminar clamp is safe, easy, and reliable. This procedure

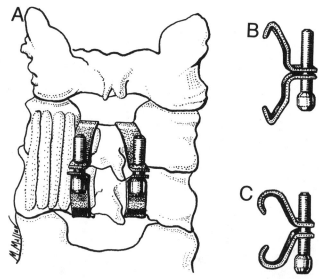

Fig 20–1.—Diagrammatic illustration of Halifax interlaminar clamps. **A,** bilateral Halifax interlaminar clamps with bone grafts (grafting is done bilaterally). **B,** clamp used for all levels except at C1–C2. **C,** clamp used for C1–C2 arthrodesis. (Courtesy of Aldrich EF, Crow WN, Weber PB, et al: *J Neurosurg* 74:185–189, 1991.)

offers an attractive alternative to the conventional use of wire as an internal fixation agent in posterior cervical spine stabilization. The MR compatibility of these clamps permits a noninvasive, life-long follow-up.

▶ Twenty-one patients with posterior cervical fusion were treated with MR-compatible interlaminar Halifax clamps. Solid fusions were recorded in all cases with no mechanical complications. The MR imaging-compatibility allowed excellent studies. This appears to be a very satisfactory way of treating these patients. The results may be compared with the technique described by Dickman et al. (see Abstract 20–3).—R.M. Crowell, M.D.

The Interspinous Method of Posterior Atlantoaxial Arthrodesis
Dickman CA, Sonntag VKH, Papadopoulos SM, Hadley MN (Barrow Neurological Inst, Phoenix; Univ of Michigan; David Grant Med Ctr, Travis Air Force Base, Calif)
J Neurosurg 74:190–198, 1991   20–3

Although a variety of surgical procedures for the treatment of atlantoaxial instability and traumatic C1, C2, or C1–C2 combination fractures are available, the posterior approach using autologous iliac bone grafts is the most popular method of fusion. Previous studies have demonstrated the clinical efficacy of posterior C1–C2 wiring and fusion in selected patients. A modification of this technique was developed.

Between 1984 and 1989, 14 men (mean age, 53 years) and 22 women (mean age, 57.7 years) underwent atlantoaxial arthrodesis. Indications included unstable C2 fractures in 8 patients, unstable atlas-axis combination fractures in 6, rheumatoid C1–C2 instability in 14, os odontoideum in 4, traumatic C1–C2 ligamentous instability in 3, and instability secondary to a C2 tumor in 1 patient.

Technique.—The modified fusion technique used in these patients involves passing a loop of double-twisted no. 24 wire beneath the ring of the atlas in the midline. Notches are placed at the spinolaminar junction of C2 to seat the wire. An iliac crest strut graft, interposed between the posterior arch of C1 and the laminae and spinous process at C2, is held in place by securing the twisted wire around the base of the spinous process of the axis (Fig 20–2). After operation, patients are maintained in a halo brace for 12 weeks. The halo ring is then disconnected from the brace and radiographs are obtained to assess the stability of the fusion. If the fusion mass appears stable, the remainder of the halo device is removed and the patient is instructed to wear a Philadelphia collar for the next 4–6 weeks.

One patient, an 89-year-old woman with long-standing quadriparesis and rheumatoid arthritis, died of hemorrhage at the hip donor site during anticoagulant therapy. Follow-up examination obtained after a mean postoperative period of 33.7 months revealed that 34 (97%) of the 35 surviving patients had a stable C1–C2 postoperative fusion construct.

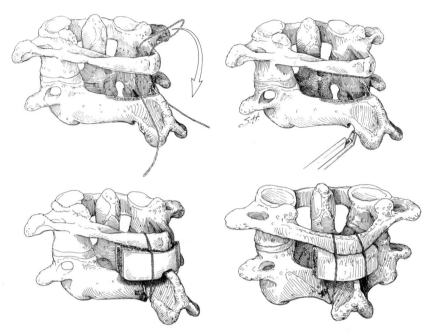

Fig 20–2.—Drawings showing the technique described. **A,** 2 strands of no. 24 wire are twisted (3 turns per cm), and a loop of this double-twisted wire is passed beneath the ring of the atlas in the midline and directed cephalad. **B,** notches are placed at the spinolaminar junction of C2 to seat the wire. **C,** appearance of the final fusion construct. **D,** appearance of the tricortical strut graft initially used with this fusion technique. (Courtesy of Dickman CA, Sonntag VKH, Papadopoulos SM, et al: *J Neurosurg* 74:190–198, 1991.)

There were 30 osseous unions, 1 delayed osseous union, 3 fibrous unions, and 1 nonunion. The only nonunion occurred in a 27-year-old man in whom the bone graft was resorbed after 4 previous failures of posterior cervical fusion. He subsequently underwent successful anterior C1–C2 screw fixation. The interspinous method of posterior atlantoaxial arthrodesis is safe and technically simple; it compares favorably with similar posterior fusion techniques.

▶ Dickman and colleagues at the Barrow Neurological Institute present a series of 36 patients undergoing C1–C2 posterior wiring and fusion, with a remarkable 97% union rate and minimal complications. The authors advocate utilization of no. 24 double-stranded twisted wire with 3 turns per cm in view of reports of its superior tensile strength. Potential disadvantages of this approach in the hands of others have included breakage of wires and injury by the sublaminar wire passage. The Halifax technique avoid both problems, and its effectiveness and safety have also been reported (1). A potential advantage of the Gallie-type fusion is its superiority regarding rotational stability.—R.M. Crowell, M.D.

Reference

1. Cybulski GR, et al: *Neurosurgery* 22:429, 1988.

Anterior Plating of Unstable Cervical Spine Fractures

Mann DC, Bruner BW, Keene JS, Levin AB (Univ of Wisconsin)

Paraplegia 28:564–572, 1990

20–4

Earlier studies have reported that anterior cervical decompression and fusion in treatment of unstable fractures of the cervical spine result in a higher rate of complications than posterior procedures. However, the grafts in these studies had either no or only minimal internal fixation. The quality and maintenance of reductions achievecd with anterior decompression of unstable cervical spinal fractures, using internal plating for stabilization in all cases, were assessed.

A review was made of the medical records and radiographs of 16 patients aged 16–52 years who underwent anterior decompression, bone grafting, and plating of grades III and IV unstable cervical spinal injuries. All patients had at least 3 months of follow-up. Seven had been injured in diving accidents, 6 in motor vehicle accidents, 2 in falls, and 1 in a farm accident. Patients were operated on within 15 days of injury. Autogenous iliac bone grafts were used in all procedures. After operation the patients were immobilized for 2–4 months in a Philadelphia collar and in a soft cervical orthosis for an additional 1–2 months.

At follow-up, 12 of the 16 patients had no complications, and neurologic function had stabilized or improved. One patient had 2 broken screws detected at the 9-month follow-up examination, which did not affect the clinical or radiographic results. Three other patients required reoperation, 1 because of undiagnosed noncontiguous posterior instability and 2 because of broken plates. Plate breakage occurred only in those patients in whom the plate spanned unfused segments of the spine 6–9 months after operation. These problems did not occur when all levels encompassed by the plate were fused. The complications after anterior decompression and plating for stabilization of traumatic injuries of the cervical spine as observed in this study could all have been avoided by not plating unfused segments of the spine.

▶ This communication describes 16 patients with unstable cervical spinal injury treated with anterior cervical plating. Although the anatomical results were satisfactory in the great majority, complications required reoperation in about 20% of the patients.—R.M. Crowell, M.D.

Clinical Long-Term Results of Anterior Discectomy Without Interbody Fusion for Cervical Disc Disease

Yamamoto I, Ikeda A, Shibuya N, Tsugane R, Sato O (Tokai Univ, Isahara, Japan)

Spine 16:272–279, 1991

20–5

The results of anterior cervical diskectomy (ACD) were reviewed in 55 consecutive patients who had surgery for cervical disk disease from 1976 to 1988. Twenty-one patients had a diagnosis of acute soft disk hernia-

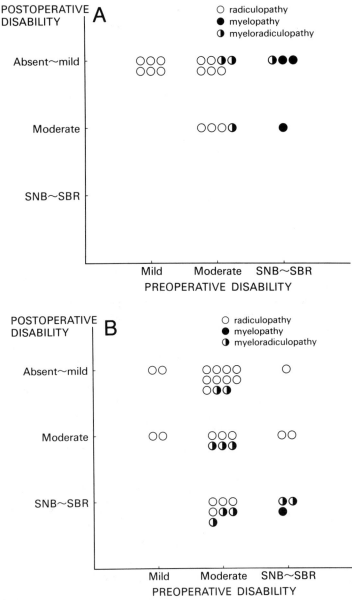

Fig 20–3.—A, comparison of preoperative and postoperative disability of 21 patients with soft disk disease. **B,** 34 patients with spondylosis. *Abbreviations: SNB,* severe nonbedridden; *SBR,* severe bedridden. (Courtesy of Yamamoto I, Ikeda A, Shibuya N, et al: *Spine* 16:272–279, 1991.)

tion and 34 had spondylosis. Surgery was performed with the use of an operating microscope. The disk space was cleared of all disk material without excising the cartilaginous plate.

A satisfactory degree of improvement was noted by 82% of patients with acute soft disk herniation. Forty-seven percent of patients with spondylosis were improved at follow-up (Fig 20–3), but 35% had deterioration. The most troublesome complication was cervical or interscapular pain, or both, which usually developed immediately after surgery and lasted for 1 or 2 months. In 4 patients with spondylosis, pain continued for more than 4 years and finally an interbody fusion was added. Two patients had recurrent nerve palsy and 2 had worse radicular symptoms after operation.

Anterior cervical diskectomy with the use of an operating microscope is an effective and safe approach to soft disk herniation. Diskectomy with interbody fusion remains the preferred operation for patients with advanced spondylosis.

▶ The authors present 55 patients with anterior diskectomy without fusion for cervical disk disease. Their results indicate a good outcome for patients with soft disks but a number of less satisfactory responses in patients with spondylosis. This leads the authors to recommend diskectomy without fusion for the soft disk patients but fusion for those with spondylosis.— R.M. Crowell, M.D.

Ten-Year Results of Operations for Rheumatoid Cervical Spine Disorders
Santavirta S, Konttinen YT, Laasonen E, Honkanen V, Antti-Poika I, Kauppi M (Orthop Hosp of the Invalid Found, Helsinki; Hosp of Joint Diseases Orthop Inst, New York; Univ Central Hosp, Helsinki; Rheumatism Found Hosp, Heinola, Finland)
J Bone Joint Surg 73–B:116–120, 1991   20–6

The short-term results of surgical treatment of rheumatoid disorders of the cervical spine have been published previously. The long-term outcomes in these patients were reviewed.

Between 1972 and 1978, 30 women and 8 men with rheumatoid disorders aged 35–77 years underwent operation of the cervical spine in treatment of painful subluxations. Thirty-two patients had seropositive rheumatoid polyarthritis, 3 had seronegative disease, 2 had juvenile rheumatoid arthritis, and 1 had ankylosing spondylitis. The mean disease duration before operation was 17 years, and the average duration of cervical spinal symptoms was 6.4 years. Of the patients, 27 had painful anterior atlantoaxial subluxation, 9 had subaxial subluxation, and 2 had severe cranial subluxation of the odontoid, 1 of whom had concomitant subaxial subluxation. Twenty-seven patients had previous joint operations and 21 had more than 4 such operations. All patients had at least 10 years of follow-up after operation.

Four patients had postoperative complications. One patient died 8 weeks after operation from staphylococcal septicemia and pneumonia. Another 18 patients died during follow-up of causes unrelated to cervical spine involvement or its surgical treatment. The interval from operation to death averaged 4.2 years and ranged from 2 months to 11 years. Mortality was increased among patients with coincident cardiac or other diseases and among those with cranial odontoid subluxation of more than 3 mm.

Operation relieved the occipitocervical pain in 30 patients and cured dysesthesia of the hands in 21 of 29 patients who had this symptom. Of 24 Gallie fusions performed, 12 were solidly united, 4 had united with fibrous union, and 8 were associated with pseudarthroses. The clinical outcome did not correlate with radiographic results. Four patients required further operations to treat subluxation that occurred below the fused segments. Because cervical subluxations are usually late developments in the aggressive forms of rheumatoid disease, patients with severe rheumatoid disease should be examined frequently for neck symptoms so that they can be treated before irreparable lesions develop.

▶ The most interesting aspect of this report is the 10-year follow-up. The results indicate that posterior fusion for C1–C2 instability is usually successful in relieving pain and medullary compression where that exists. On the other hand, only half of the standard Gallie fusions were united, with no correlation between the clinical and radiologic outcome. Complications from the operations were uncommon, but almost half of the patients died during the follow-up period. These results suggest that posterior fusions are often worthwhile, but improved technique (perhaps with the Halifax instrumentation) might improve the overall results.—R.M. Crowell, M.D.

Surgical Decompressive Procedures for Cervical Spondylotic Myelopathy: A Study Using Magnetic Resonance Imaging
Batzdorf U, Flannigan BD (Univ of California, Los Angeles; Valley Presbyterian Hosp, Van Nuys, Calif)
Spine 16:123–127, 1991   20–7

Spinal cord decompression for cervical spondylotic myelopathy (CSM) is based on the premise that compression is a major cause of the condition, although it is recognized that many other factors may contribute. An MRI study was done to establish whether the goals of surgery were achieved, as assessed by the adequacy of decompression rather than neurologic status.

The study sample was a series of 22 patients with CSM and confirmed spondylotic cervical spinal cord compression. Sixteen patients had posterior decompression alone, 5 had anterior decompression alone, and 1 had both. All had significant osteophyte formation, sometimes with fragments of disk material. Magnetic resonance imaging was done in all patients at postoperative intervals ranging from 2 weeks to 11 years. If axial and sagittal T1- and T2-weighted MRI scans showed that the cord was free of any impingement or effacement, decompression was judged to be complete.

Decompression was judged to be adequate in 12 cases. Residual cord indentation was present in the remaining 10 patients. Cord atrophy was seen in 6 patients, an abnormal increase in cord signal suggesting gliosis or intrinsic cord damage was seen in 11, and abnormal spinal curvature was seen in 15 patients. These factors were thought to have contributed to residual deficit in several patients. A second decompressive procedure was done in 1 patient who had residual cord indentation; a second follow-up MRI scan showed that this procedure was successful.

Magnetic resonance imaging can distinguish mechanical problems from intrinsic spinal cord damage or atrophy. Patients who have residual deficit after spinal decompression for CSM should have MRI to help determine whether they should have a second operation.

▶ This report emphasizes the utility of postoperative MRI to detect persistent cord compression, which may be amenable to a secondary procedure. This also emphasizes the utility of MRI-compatible fixation devices for fusion of the spine (compare with Abstract 20–2).—R.M. Crowell, M.D.

Lumbar

Microsurgery Versus Standard Removal of the Herniated Lumbar Disc: A 3-Year Comparison in 150 Patients

Barrios C, Ahmed M, Arrótegui J, Björnsson A, Gillström P (Karolinska Hosp, Stockholm)

Acta Orthop Scand 61:399–403, 1990   20–8

Microsurgical techniques have been employed in the removal of herniated lumbar disks for about 15 years, with a success rate ranging from 75% to 90%. In a study of patients with classic sciatica caused by herniated lumbar disks results after microsurgery and standard diskectomy were compared.

Two groups of 75 patients each were followed for an average of 3 years after surgery. With the microsurgical technique, a needle indicator was used with an image intensifier to locate the intervertebral space. Standard surgery consisted of unilateral partial hemilaminectomy with removal of a variable amount of the medial facet and routine nucleotomy. The patients underwent standard postoperative physiotherapy after both procedures.

Both techniques resulted in a good or excellent outcome in 85% of patients. Blood loss was less with microsurgery, but the duration of surgery was similar for the 2 techniques. Hospitalization was shorter and recuperation more rapid with microsurgery. Though 3 patients in the microsurgery group required reoperation because of incomplete disk removal, all 3 achieved excellent results after the second operation. Microsurgery was associated with a higher rate of recurrent disk prolapse.

Overall, microsurgery was slightly more successful than the standard operation. To avoid recurrence of disk prolapse, the surgeon should remove as much as possible from the entire disk space. Earlier hospital discharge and a shorter period of convalescence are the major advantages of microsurgery.

Automated Percutaneous Discectomy
Davis GW, Onik G, Helms C (Allegheny Gen Hosp, Pittsburgh; Univ of California, San Francisco)
Spine 16:359–363, 1991   20–9

Automated percutaneous diskectomy is a new technique for treating herniated lumbar disks that are still contained by the annulus or posterior longitudinal ligament. A total of 518 patients seen consecutively were treated with this method. The series included 240 women and 278 men aged 20–76 years. Follow-up for at least 1 year.

Treatment was successful in 85% and failed in 15% (table). Of 427 noncompensation patients, 87% were treated successfully. Of 91 compensation patients, 74% had successful treatment. The 79 patients in whom treatment failed were subsequently studied more extensively with myelography, CT, or MRI. Thirty-three of the patients had extruded disk fragments outside the interspace. In all of these patients, microdiskectomy was successful. Thirty-six patients older than 60 years were assessed separately; the procedure was successful in 70% of this group. Seventy percent of successfully treated patients were able to return to work in less than 2 weeks. There were no intraoperative or postoperative complications.

Automated percutaneous diskectomy should play a valuable role in the treatment of primary and recurrent disk herniation. More research is needed, especially concerning patient selection and exclusion of patients with free fragments, to better determine who will benefit from the procedure.

▶ The authors present results in 518 patients treated with automated percutaneous diskectomy. They record 85% success (moderate to complete pain relief without narcotics, return to preinjury functional status, and patient satisfaction with results). Interestingly, a high rate of good response was achieved in the compensated cases (74%), those with previous operations (91%), and patients

Results at 1-Year or Longer Follow-Up		
	N	*(%)*
Overall	518	
Successes	439	(85)
Failures	79	(15)
Noncompensated cases		
Number of cases	427	
Successful	371	(87)
Failures	56	(13)
Compensated cases		
Number of cases	91	
Successful	68	(74)
Failures	23	(26)

(Courtesy of Davis GW, Onik G, Helms C: *Spine* 16:359–363, 1991.)

older than 60 years (70%). This method should be considered for certain patients with lumbar disk disease.— R.M. Crowell, M.D.

Percutaneous Automated Lumbar Nucleotomy
Gobin P, Theron J, Courtheoux F, Huet H, Chos D, Loyau G (Centre Hosp Univ, Caen, France)
J Radiol 71:401–406, 1990   20–10

Percutaneous automated lumbar diskectomy is a means of treating a herniated lumbar disk. The technique involves mechanical fragmentation and extraction with suction of the fragmented disk material, using a newly designed aspiration probe. Decompression of a herniated intervertebral lumbar disk can be accomplished without total disk excision. Aspiration of the disk material takes about 20–40 minutes. The procedure is usually performed with the use of neuroleptanalgesia.

Between February and August 1988, 40 patients aged 23–58 years were treated. Thirty-nine patients were available for follow-up, which ranged from 3 to 10 months. All 39 patients had experienced sciatic pain for at least 1 month; none had responded to medical treatment. One patient, a professional soccer player, was treated 7 days after experiencing incapcitating sciatic pain. Patients previously operated on, those with bone compression, or patients with significant neurologic involvement were excluded. Nine patients with pain in the lumbar region had conclusive radiographic evidence of nuclear herniation. Eleven patients had radiographic evidence of extrusion. Four patients had previously undergone chemonucleolysis at the same level. Patients whose findings on scanning corresponded to clinical findings did not undergo further exploration. Treated were 1 lumbar disk at L3–L4, 15 disks at L4–L5, and 23 disks at L5–S1.

Twenty-one patients (70%) had very good or good relief of sciatic pain, 2 (7%) had moderate pain relief but still required sedentary work and frequent use of analgesics, 5 (17%) had minimal or no pain relief, and 2 had initial pain relief but of very short duration. When the 2 patients who had previously undergone chemonucleolysis were excluded in the tabulation, the overall success rate reached 77% for patients with sciatic pain. Of the 9 patients with lumbar pain, 5 had very good or good pain relief and 4 had moderate pain relief.

Percutaneous automated lumbar diskectomy is well tolerated. It should be considered as first-line therapy in the treatment of single, radiographically well-documented herniated lumbar disks.

▶ The authors report a 77% success rate for patients with sciatic pain (and no previous chemonucleolysis). There were no significant complications. This adds, therefore, to the significant numbers of reports suggesting good results from this form of treatment.

Percutaneous lumbar nucleotomy has been debunked by many neurosurgeons. Part of this has undoubtedly been related to fear of economic loss. Another part is surely the result of the widespread marketing of the procedure by its originators and manufacturers of the equipment. Nonetheless, the reported good results bear attention. The issue can be resolved only by appropriate well-designed, controlled scientific studies of the benefits and risks of this form of treatment.—R.M. Crowell, M.D.

Percutaneous Nucleotomy: An Anatomic Study of the Risks of Root Injury
Patsiaouras T, Bulstrode C, Cook P, Wilson D (Oxford Univ, Nuffield Orthopaedic Centre, Headington, Oxford)
Spine 16:39–42, 1991   20–11

Percutaneous nucleotomy for a prolapsed intervertebral disk was first developed 13 years ago. A 2.8-mm cannula is commonly used today. Computed tomography scanning can be used to determine the optimal position for the skin portal and the correct angle for the approach to the center of the disk. Correct positioning of the guidewire, over which the definitive instrument is passed, is essential. Referred pain can result if the original guidewire transfixes a nerve root in its course to the annulus of the disk. Any subsequent instrument of larger diameters will compound the injury. The variability and position of the lumbar roots in the lumbar plexus were studied.

Fifteen cadaver dissections were performed. All 44 guidewires inserted were in contact with at least 1 nerve root; 8 transfixed a root. Guidewires

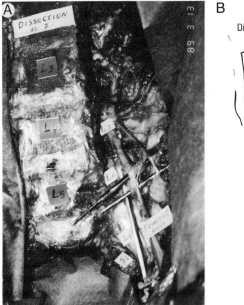
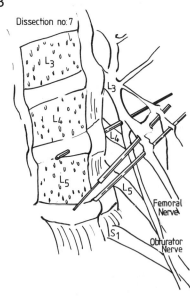

Fig 20–4.—A, B, guidewires passing anterior to or transfixing nerve roots. These wires lie anterior to the center of the disk. (Courtesy of Patsiaouras T, Bulstrode C, Cook P, et al: *Spine* 16:39–42, 1991.)

that passed anterior to nerve roots always passed anterior to the disk's center. Safe entry to the center of the disk was not possible when lateral displacement of the skin entry point occurred. Entry to the center of the disk avoiding the nerve root was easiest when the skin entry was as close as possible to the midline (Fig 20–4).

The variability of position of the lumbar roots passing from their foramen to the lumbar plexus complicates percutaneous posterolateral access to the L4–L5–S1 disks. Attempts to enter the intervertebral disk from a lateral portal are associated with an increased risk of nerve root transfixation and come too close to the contents of the paracolic gutter and major vessels. Although an entry that is too close to the midline prevents entry to the disk lateral to the facet joint, entry should be made as medially as is safe, with the guidewire passing posteromedial to the nerve roots. Such entry reduces the risk of transfixation of the nerve roots and perforation of the peritoneum or large vessels.

▶ This anatomical study indicates that nerve root transfixation is likely to be a significant complication in percutaneous nucleotomy. Although this complication has not been emphasized in the literature, certainly those involved in this type of treatment should be careful to avoid it. The authors suggest that entry as near the midline as possible is helpful in this respect.—R.M. Crowell, M.D.

Dorsal Root Ganglionectomy for Failed Back Surgery Syndrome: A 5-Year Follow-up Study
North RB, Kidd DH, Campbell JN, Long DM (Johns Hopkins Univ)
J Neurosurg 74:236–242, 1991   20–12

Dorsal rhizotomy in treatment of chronic intractable radicular pain after lumbosacral spine surgery has been disappointing. Anatomical studies have identified numerous ventral root afferents with cell bodies in the dorsal root ganglia, suggesting that dorsal root ganglionectomy should be more effective. Initial trials of dorsal root ganglionectomy have been inconclusive. The long-term results in patients who underwent dorsal root ganglionectomy for lumbar postlaminectomy syndrome were assessed.

During an 8-year period, 9 women and 4 men aged 30–68 years underwent dorsal root ganglionectomy for failed back surgery syndrome. These 13 patients had undergone a total of 48 operations previously (an average of 3.7 operations per patient). Twelve patients underwent preoperative diagnostic paravertebral nerve root blocks with small volumes of local anesthetic under fluoroscopic guidance at the levels to be subjected to ganglionectomy. At a mean of 5.5 years after dorsal root ganglionectomy, follow-up interviews were conducted by a disinterested third party who had not been involved with the patients' treatment.

Treatment success was defined as at least 50% sustained pain relief and patient satisfaction with the results. Two years after operation, 2 patients (15%) met these criteria, but 5.5 years after operation, none of the patients met these criteria. The results were equivocal in 1 patient who had at least 50% sustained pain relief but without clear-cut satisfaction. A few patients had improvements in activities of daily living and a few reported loss of function. Sixty-nine percent of the patients reported loss of touch sensation in the segments operated on, 46% reported a decrease in muscle strength or control, and 23% reported a decrease in bladder or bowel control. None of the patients reported improvement in any of these functions. Dorsal root ganglionectomy would appear to have a limited role in the management of failed back surgery syndrome. Alternate approaches should be considered.

▶ This carefully studied series of 13 patients provides useful data on the failed back surgery syndrome treated by dorsal root ganglionectomy. In essence, treatment success was not obtained at 5 years in any case, with only 1 equivocal success. Sensory motor function was impaired in a number of patients. The results indicate that this approach should be used sparingly, if at all.—R.M. Crowell, M.D.

MRI in Failed Back Surgery Syndrome: Comparison to Computed Tomography
Trattnig VS, Stiglbauer R, Ungersböck K, Cech Th, Schindler E, Imhof H (Universität Wien, Vienna)
Fortschr Röntgenstr 152:369–373, 1990   20–13

Failed back surgery syndrome (FBSS) is characterized by recurrent treatment-resistant lumbosciatic pain, with or without sensory or motor radicular symptoms of varying degrees after lumbar disk surgery. Previous studies have estimated the incidence of FBSS to range from 10% to 40%. The most frequent causes of FBSS are lateral and central stenosis of the spinal canal, arachnoiditis, and epidural fibrosis. Because epidural fibrosis has a poor prognosis for successful reoperation, an accurate preoperative differential diagnosis before planning reoperation is essential. The diagnostic accuracy of CT and MRI was assessed by comparing the findings with intraoperative findings.

Ten men and 8 women aged 19–71 years underwent reoperation for FBSS. The interval between the last operation and CT and MRI ranged from 3 months to 23 years. The average interval was 3½ years. Fifteen patients had 1 previous operation and 3 had been operated on twice. The involved disk was L5–S1 in 9 patients, L4–L5 in 8 patients, and L3–L4 in 1 patient.

The diagnoses at reoperation were disk herniation in 4 cases, epidural fibrosis from scar formation in 2, and mixed forms of herniated disk, fibrosis, and epidural fibrosis in 12. Computed tomography with intravenous contrast medium agreed with intraoperative findings for 13 of the 18 patients. All incorrect CT diagnosis involved patients with mixed findings. Misdiagnosis was in part attributable to misinterpretation of the CT scans and in part to incomplete visualization of the abnormalities on CT. Findings on MRI agreed with intraoperative findings in 17 patients. Additional intraoperative findings included a prominent venous plexus combined with recurrent disk herniation in 7 patients and spondyloarthrosis deformans with unilateral spinal canal stenosis in 7 patients. Two patients had evidence of a pseudomeningocele. Magnetic resonance imaging with intravenous gadolinium diethylenetriamine pentaacetic acid is the technique of choice for preoperative differential diagnosis of FBSS as it is far more accurate than CT with intravenous contrast medium.

▶ This report confirms that MRI, without or with gadolinium, is the study of choice in the postoperative spine. Undoubtedly, this is attributable in large measure to the ability of the technique to discriminate between a herniated intervertebral disk and epidural fibrosis.—R.M. Crowell, M.D.

Expansive Laminoplasty for Lumbar Spinal Stenosis
Tsuji H, Itoh T, Sekido H, Yamada H, Katoh Y, Makiyama N, Yamagami T
(Toyama Med and Pharmaceutical Univ Hosp, Toyama, Japan)
Int Orthop 14:309–314, 1990   20–14

A number of procedures are available for treating patients with degenerative spinal stenosis. Expansive laminoplasty, an operation that decompresses the canal and reinforces spinal stability, is indicated for patients with developmental stenosis or intraspinal ossified masses, or for relatively young patients who require reinforcement of stability.

The technique of expansive laminoplasty is similar to that of laminoplasty for cervical myelopathy. The spinal processes are removed and used as a bone graft (Fig 20–5). Two weeks after the operation, the patient is allowed to walk with a short cast or a Williams flexion orthosis.

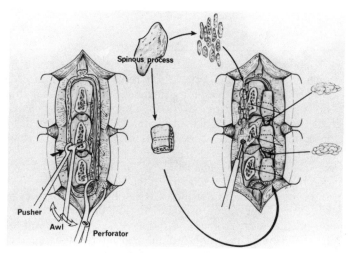

Fig 20–5.—Diagram showing technique of expansive laminoplasty. (Courtesy of Tsuji H, Itoh T, Sekido H, et al: *Int Orthop* 14:309–314, 1990.)

Bony union of the transposed laminae usually occurs within 3–4 months.

Man, 37, had severe low back and leg pain that restricted his walking. As a heavy worker, the patient had experienced attacks for 10 years. The pain was such that flexion and extension of the spine were impossible. Radiographs showed narrowing of the disks at many levels, with ossification of the ligamentum flavum at L3, L4, and L5. Expansive laminoplasty was carried out from L2 to L5. The patient had an excellent outcome, with full function and only a slightly limited range of movement.

Of 141 patients with degenerative spinal stenosis who were operated on at the study institution from 1908 through 1987, 4 underwent expansive laminoplasty. These patients were younger (average age, 38 years) than the group as a whole (average age, 62 years). The outcome was satisfactory in all 4 patients. Expansive laminoplasty is suitable for active patients with multisegmental degenerative lumbar spinal stenosis.

▶ This is another description of expanding the spinal canal by unroofing the posterior spinal arch. The technique depends on the use of high-speed drills (such as the Midas Rex). The clinical improvement observed in 4 of 4 cases is impressive. Certainly, further experience is required to establish the place of this form of treatment. It is hoped that investigators other than the Japanese will participate in this investigation to obtain the widest application.—R.M. Crowell, M.D.

Biomechanical Evaluation of Lumbar Spinal Stability After Graded Facetectomies
Abumi K, Panjabi MM, Kramer KM, Duranceau J, Oxland T, Crisco JJ (Hokkaido Univ, Sapporo, Japan; Yale Univ)
Spine 15:1142–1147, 1990   20–15

Facetectomy often is done to decompress spinal nerve roots or to excise a herniated disk or spinal tumor. The results of graded facetectomies were examined in an in vitro study using fresh human lumbar functional spinal units. The supraspinous and interspinous ligaments were transected, and unilateral medial to bilateral total facetectomies carried out before kinematic testing of the 3-dimensional stability of the lumbar spine.

Flexion was significantly increased by unilateral medial facetectomy and markedly increased after bilateral total facetectomy (Fig 20–6). Extension range of motion did not increase significantly even after bilateral total facetectomy. The range of axial motion did not increase significantly after medial facetectomies but did increase after bilateral total facetectomies. Division of the supraspinous and interspinous ligaments did not alter the range of motion for any loading mode.

Total facetectomy makes the lumbar spinal segment unstable in axial

EXTENSION

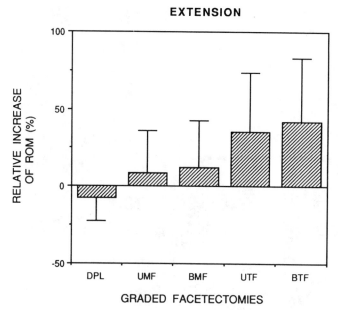

Fig 20–6.—Extension loading. Each *bar* represents a mean relative increase of range of motion with 1 SD after each injury with respect to the intact functional spinal unit. (Courtesy of Abumi K, Panjabi MM, Kramer KM, et al: *Spine* 15:1142–1147, 1990.)

rotation and flexion. It therefore calls for spinal fusion from the viewpoint of optimal biomechanical stability.

▶ In this autopsy study, medial facetectomy did not create instability, but unilateral total facetectomy did.—R.M. Crowell, M.D.

Other

Total Sacrectomy and Reconstruction for Huge Sacral Tumors

Tomita K, Tsuchiya H (Kanazawa Univ, Kanazawa, Japan)
Spine 15:1223–1227, 1990
20–16

Total sacrectomy is a challenging procedure. An intraperitoneal operation is done first to ligate the chief tumor vessels and excise the anterior ligaments and intervertebral disk. A posterior approach then is used to broadly expose the entire sacrum and divide all ligaments connected to it. The sacrum with tumor then is removed en bloc, and continuity of the spine and pelvic ring is restored using sacral rods or AO plates and, when necessary, a plate on the public symphysis. Autogenous bone is grafted between the iliac wings and the posterolateral side of the spine.

Man, 36, with coccygodynia and constipation, was found to have a giant cell tumor of the sacrum that necessitated symphysiotomy for adequate access (Fig 20–7). Part of the bony structure of S1 was removed with the tumor and rein-

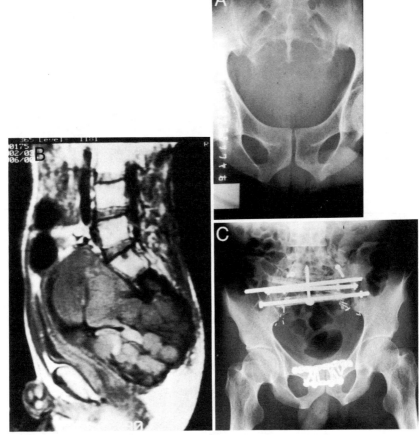

Fig 20–7.—**A,** anteroposterior view of a plain radiograph before surgery. **B,** MRI before surgery (lateral view). **C,** reconstruction by autogenous autoclaved bone and sacral rods. (Courtesy of Tomita K, Tsuchiya H: *Spine* 15:1223–1227, 1990.)

serted as an autograft between the iliac wings. The sacrum and L5 body were fixed with AO cancellous screws. Three sacral rods and a plate on the pubic symphysis provided further stability. A graft also was placed between the autoclaved bone, the iliac wing, and the L5 body. The patient walked with crutches 12 weeks postoperatively. At 33 months he required catheterization only intermittently and could walk with a cane, but he sometimes preferred a wheelchair. The autoclaved bone was revascularized.

Total sacrectomy can be a rewarding operation for those having a huge sacral tumor, despite the significant structural and neurologic damage it causes. It is critical to restore the continuity of the pelvic ring and spinal column.

▶ For chordoma or giant cell tumors of the sacrum, total sacral removal may be carried out en bloc, with reconstruction of the pelvic spinal axis using special instrumentation. This is mega-surgery, and teams of surgeons are needed to obtain good results.—R.M. Crowell, M.D.

Circumspinal Decompression for Thoracic Myelopathy Due to Combined Ossification of the Posterior Longitudinal Ligament and Ligamentum Flavum

Tomita K, Kawahara N, Baba H, Kikuchi Y, Nishimura H (Kanazawa Univ, Kanazawa, Japan)
Spine 15:1114–1120, 1990

20–17

In the thoracic spine, ossification of the posterior longitudinal ligament (OPLL) combined with ossification of the ligamentum flavum (OLF) can cause severe myelopathy. In the more advanced stages of the disease the OPLL and OLF can fuse and cause circumferential compression of the spinal cord. Ten patients with combined OPLL and OLF underwent circumferential decompression of the spinal cord, also called circumspinal decompression. The average follow-up period was 3.4 years (range, 1–6 years).

Technique.—Circumspinal decompression involves 2 steps: posterior and lateral decompression of the spinal cord by removal of the OLF (first step) and anterior removal of the OPLL for anterior decompression (second step), followed by interbody fusion. In the first step 2 deep parallel gutters that cover the extent of the OPLL to be removed anteriorly are drilled down from the rear into the vertebral body along both sides of the dura to safely and easily remove the OPLL anteriorly in the next step. Depending on the affected level, the second step of anterior decompression requires a standard thoracotomy in the middle or lower thoracic spine and costotransversectomy in the upper thoracic spine.

According to the evaluation system for cervical myelopathy of the Japanese Orthopedic Association (JOA), 9 patients improved after operation. Except for 1 patient whose neurologic deficit worsened, the recovery ratio after circumspinal decompression ranged from 56% to 100%. Most patients had a satisfactory neurologic recovery and walked without a cane within a year. The mean duration of operations was 9.7 hours (range, 6.8–12.5 hours) and the average blood loss was 3,190 mL. Surgical complications included a tear in the dura in 1 patient, fracture of the grafted iliac bone in 1, transient increase in liver enzymes in 2, and transfusion hepatitis in 1.

In patients with thoracic myelopathy caused by OPLL and OLF, circumspinal decompression is absolutely indicated for those whose JOA score is below 6 points and relatively indicated for those whose JOA score is 6 points or higher. Although this radical procedure is time consuming and demands meticulous preparation and utmost care during the operation, it has brought more satisfactory neurologic recovery in most patients with combined OPLL and OLF than either anterior or posterior decompression.

▶ This interesting report describes radical decompressive anterior and posterior surgery for combined OPLL and OLF. This is very major surgery requiring about 10 hours and 3,000 cc of blood transfusion. However, 9 of 10 patients improved soon after surgery in this series, and it is said that most had a satisfactory neurologic recovery.

Certainly, further experience with this extremely aggressive approach is needed to judge the indications. A graded approach with posterior decompression as a first stage might be adequate to alleviate the patient's neurologic condition.—R.M. Crowell, M.D.

Vertebral Hemangiomas: Fat Content as a Sign of Aggressiveness
Laredo J-D, Assouline E, Gelbert F, Wybier M, Merland J-J, Tubiana J-M (Saint-Antoine Hosp, Paris; Lariboisière Hosp, Paris)
Radiology 177:467–472, 1990   20–18

Some vertebral hemangiomas (VHs) that compress the spinal cord or nerve root must be treated aggressively. The radiologic appearance of a VH plain radiography and CT reliably demonstrates its aggressiveness. Data were reviewed on 32 VHs to determine whether the appearance of the stroma between the osseous trabeculae on CT scans and MRI is related to lesion aggressiveness and hypervascularization.

Thirty VHs were assessed with nonenhanced CT–19 with T1-weighted MRI, 21 with CT enhanced with contrast material; 15 VHs were assessed with selective spinal arteriography. The stroma between the osseous trabeculae corresponded with fatty tissue and/or soft tissue. Eleven asymptomatic VHs demonstrated complete fatty stroma on CT and increased signal intensity on MRI. All 4 compressive VHs showed soft tissue attenuation on CT. Three compressive lesions had low signal intensity on MRI. Primarily fatty stroma at CT and increased spinal intensity on MRI were associated with normal or only slightly increased vascularization at selective spinal arteriography or contrast-enhanced CT. Soft tissue stroma on CT and low signal intensity on MRI were associated with distinct hypervascularization.

Fatty VHs may represent inactive forms of VH, whereas soft tissue content on CT and low signal intensity on MRI may suggest a more active vascular lesion that has the potential to compress the spinal cord. Both CT and MRI may be particularly useful for assessing patients with clinical signs or symptoms of uncertain origin and findings compatible with VH on plain radiography.

▶ This interesting study suggests that lack of fat content indicates hypervascularity and aggressiveness in VHs. Further data are needed to confirm this interesting correlation.—R.M. Crowell, M.D.

Eosinophilic Granuloma of the Cervical Spine: A Case Report and Review of the Literature

Dickinson LD, Farhat SM (Univ of Michigan; St Joseph Mercy Hosp, Ann Arbor)
Surg Neurol 35:57–63, 1991   20–19

Eosinophilic granuloma is a rare focal, granulomatous bone disorder usually seen in children. One woman had a solitary granuloma that involved the second cervical vertebra.

Woman, 33, had progressive pain in the neck and occipital region for 8 weeks, and cervical motion was noted to be limited. Torticollis was present, with rotation of the head to the right. Computed tomography showed an expansile soft tissue lesion in the right pedicle of C2 (Fig 20–8). A CT-guided needle biopsy yielded only inflammatory tissue and was reported to be nondiagnostic. An MRI study confirmed a soft tissue mass in the medullary cavity of C2. A skeletal survey revealed no other bone lesions. A biopsy specimen yielded eosinophilic granuloma. After curettage of the involved bone, a fusion was performed using an iliac bone graft. The patient received radiation therapy after operation and was free of symptoms at 4 months, when a CT scan showed resolution of the C2 lesion.

Only 4 other cases of cervical eosinophilic granuloma have been reported in adults. Twenty-eight other lesions occurred in children. Neck

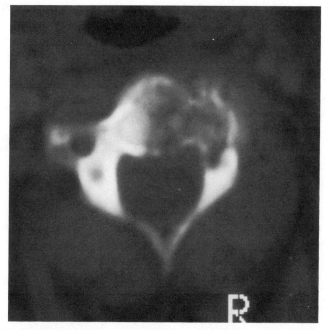

Fig 20–8.—Computed tomography scan through C2 vertebra shows expansile mass in right pedicle and body. Superior images (not shown) showed involvement of odontoid process. (Courtesy of Dickinson LD, Farhat SM: *Surg Neurol* 35:57–63, 1991.)

pain was the most frequent presenting complaint. Usually, the cervical lesion was the only 1 described. In most cases an osteolytic lesion was present without collapse, in contrast to thoracic lesions.

Immobilization lessens symptoms in these cases. Surgery is indicated if there is evidence of instability or impending neurologic compromise. There is no clear evidence that radiation therapy is beneficial.

Treatment of Spinal Metastases From Kidney Cancer by Presurgical Embolization and Resection

Sundaresan N, Choi IS, Hughes JEO, Sachdev VP, Berenstein A (Mt Sinai Hosp and Med School, New York; Univ; St Luke's/Roosevelt Hosp Ctr, New York)
J Neurosurg 73:548–554, 1990   20–20

Profuse blood loss often complicates the surgical treatment of bone metastases of kidney cancer. Data were reviewed on 30 consecutive patients undergoing surgery for spinal metastases of kidney cancer from 1983 through 1988. Three fourths of the patients had undergone nephrectomy. Embolization used ethyl alcohol when a feeding pedicle was superselectively catheterized. The goal of surgery was total resection.

Twenty-five embolization procedures were carried out preoperatively in 17 patients, most of whom had highly vascular metastases with arteriovenous shunting. The neurologic deficit and pain lessened postoperatively in 90% of the 30 patients, but a second operation often was necessary. Fifty-two operations in all were done. Operative mortality was 6%. The median survival time was 16 months, with actuarial 2- and 5-year survival rates of 33% and 15%, respectively. Patients with spinal metastases of kidney cancer should undergo spinal angiography and embolization before resection of the tumor and before external radiotherapy.

▶ This report emphasizes the helpful effects of presurgical embolization before spinal surgery for kidney cancer metastasis. In our institution, we have also found this approach remarkably helpful to prevent the massive hemorrhage that can occur intraoperatively during spinal removal of these tumors. This seems to be well on its way toward standard therapy, opening the door to more aggressive utilization of surgery in these patients.—R.M. Crowell, M.D.

Intraoperative Sonography of Cervical Spinal Cord Injury: Results in 30 Patients

Mirvis SE, Geisler FH (Maryland Inst for Emergency Med Services Systems, Baltimore)
AJR 155:603–609, 1990   20–21

There are a variety of uses for intraoperative spinal sonography (IOSS), but its value in demonstrating, characterizing, and grading the type, severity, and outcome of acute cervical spinal cord parenchymal injuries has not been discussed. Intraoperative spinal sonography was performed in 30 patients with cervical spinal injuries associated with neurologic deficits.

Twenty-five patients underwent laminectomy and 5 underwent anterior corpectomy; these procedures provided the IOSS imaging window. Surgery was performed a mean 12 days after injury as part of initial treatment for either spinal decompression or fixation. A sonographic injury score was developed based on the size and sonographic character of the lesions. This score was compared with initial and subsequent motor neurologic deficits and with cervical spine MR studies done in 12 patients.

The IOSS revealed 32 spinal lesions in 29 patients; 3 patients had 2 lesions each. Results were not interpretable in 1 patient. The IOSS detected parenchymal spinal cord lesions at the level of cervical fracture or stenosis that were compatible with initial neurologic deficits in 28 patients. One patient had a grade 0 IOSS score, 2 had grade I, 11 had grade II, 11 had grade III, and 4 had grade IV scores. Initial American Spinal Injury Association (ASIA) motor scores correlated well with IOSS scores, indicating that IOSS echogenicity is related to the extent of initial clinical motor deficit. Both the IOSS injury grade and initial ASIA scores correlated with follow-up ASIA scores, but the addition of the IOSS injury grade did not enhance the predictive quality of the follow-up ASIA motor score, possibly because it provided little new information that was not already included in the initial ASIA score.

In the comparison of IOSS and cervical spine MR imaging, IOSS confirmed parenchymal lesions demonstrated by MR in 5 patients and revealed cord lesions not found by suboptimal MR studies in 3 patients. It also better characterized lesions with early cyst formation in 2 patients. Because of the limited field of view, IOSS failed to detect possibly significant herniated intervertebral disks in 2 patients.

Intraoperative spinal sonography is a highly sensitive method of detecting and confirming the presence or absence of spinal cord injury after trauma. The extent and character of IOSS-detected cervical spinal cord lesions correlates with the extent of neurologic motor deficit, but IOSS studies add little to the predictive value for recovery of motor function. Investigation with IOSS appears to be at least as sensitive as MR for detecting spinal cord injury, and it can be used when MR is suboptimal or cannot be performed at all. The IOSS technique is limited by its restriction to surgically managed patients and its circumscribed field of view.

▶ This report suggests that IOSS for cervical spine injury reveals about the same amount of information on pathology as high-quality MR. When MR is suboptimal or impossible, this method may be of great utility.— R.M. Crowell, M.D.

Rerouting Peripheral Nerves for Spinal Cord Lesions
Romano VM, Blair SJ, Wurster RD (Loyola Univ, Maywood, Ill; Hines VA Med Ctr, Hines, Ill)
J Orthop Res 9:54–60, 1991   20–22

Various attempts to "bridge" the spinal cord above and below lesions to restore function to paralyzed limb muscles have met with limited suc-

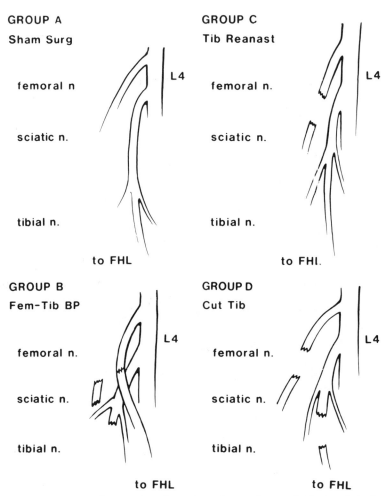

Fig 20–9.—Diagrams of surgery for each experimental group. In group A *(sham surg)*, the femoral and tibial nerves were exposed on 1 side but left intact. In 3 other groups, these 2 nerves were transected. In group B *(fem-tib BP)*, the distal tibial nerve was anastomosed to the proximal femoral nerve. In group C *(tib reanast)*, the tibial nerve was repaired. In group D *(cut tib)*, the nerves were left divided. (Courtesy of Romano VM, Blair BJ, Wurster RD: *J Orthop Res* 9:54–60, 1991.)

cess. Another possibility, that of rerouting an intact peripheral nerve innervated above the lesion to a peripheral nerve innervated below the lesion, was examined in an animal model.

Forty-eight rats were divided into 4 treatment groups of 12 animals each. In a sham surgical group (group A), 2 exposed nerves were left intact. The tibial nerve in the 3 other groups was transected proximally and the femoral nerve transected just before entering the quadriceps femoris. In group B, a femoral-to-tibial anastomosis or bypass was formed. The animals in group C had the tibial nerve reanastomosed to itself. In group D the tibial nerves were left cut (Fig 20–9).

Assessment of lower hind limb motor function throughout the recovery period was accomplished with a twitch tension device. Toe flexion of the control side in the sham surgery group was similar to that of the sham-operated side. Toe flexion was approximately 80% of the control side in group C and 50% of the control side in group B. In group D, only a small toe flexion response was recorded on the experimental side. At 4- to 6-month follow-up, 54% of motor function had returned in the experimental animals.

Six months after surgery, when nerve regeneration was completed, an L4 spinal transection was performed. Twitch tension responses to spinal cord outlet stimulation persisted only in the experimental groups.

It is possible to reinnervate the lower hindlimb of a rat by a peripheral nerve receiving innervation from higher spinal cord levels that normally innervates the upper portion of the hindlimb. Direct clinical applications may be limited, but the model demonstrates that spinal cord lesions can be partially bypassed by rerouting peripheral nerves.

▶ This interesting report indicates that femoral to tibial anastomosis after spinal cord interruption can maintain neural function in the tibial nerve innervated motor segment. Whether this interesting concept can be translated to clinical usage remains to be seen.—R.M. Crowell, M.D.

21 Trauma

Clinical Studies

Acute Regional Cerebral Blood Flow Changes Caused by Severe Head Injuries

Marion DW, Darby J, Yonas H (Univ of Pittsburgh)
J Neurosurg 74:407–414, 1991
21–1

Derangements in cerebral blood flow (CBF) after head injury may result in ischemia or hyperemia. Acute regional CBF changes after severe head injury, especially during the first day after injury, were evaluated using stable xenon/CT (Xe/CT) CBF measurement technique. The CBF in various types of traumatic lesions and the prognostic value of blood flow studies were also explored.

Sixty-one CBF studies were obtained in 32 adults with severe head injuries. Forty-three percent of the studies were made in the first 24 hours, with the remainder made up to 7 days after injury. Mass lesions were associated with a high global CBF and bihemispheric contusions with the lowest flow (Fig 21–1). The patients without surgical mass lesions who died had a lower global CBF than patients with a better outcome. Within 24 hours after injury, the high or low CBF values seen initially had stabilized to between 32 and 55 cc/100 g/min within 36–48 hours. Lobar, basal ganglion, and brain stem blood flow values frequently differed by 25% or more from global averages. Vasoresponsivity to CO_2 increased in the 4 patients with acute subdural hematomas, particularly on the side of the lesion. A reduction in CO_2 responsivity has been associated with low CBF.

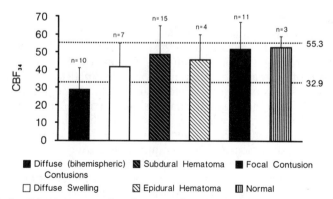

Fig 21–1.—*Abbreviation: n*, number of patients. Effect of type of posttraumatic injury on cerebral blood flow normalized to a pco_2 of 34 mm Hg (CBF_{34}). Patients with bihemispheric contusions had significantly lower flows than those with any other lesion except diffuse swelling ($P < .05$, Duncan's multiple range test). (Courtesy of Marion DW, Darby J, Yonas H: *J Neurosurg* 74:407–414, 1991.)

Because critically low CBF or abnormal CO_2 vasoresponsivity is not possible to predict on the basis of clinical examinations or CT findings, an individual management plan should be formulated for each patient. The severity of the neurologic injury, direct measurements of intracranial pressure, CT findings, and serial measurements of regional CBF should be used to determine treatment. Early CBF information can be used to control decreased or elevated CBF, reducing the incidence of regional ischemia and leading to an improved outcome.

► This careful study of 32 severely head-injured adults using Xe/CT technique comes up with some interesting observations. The investigators show that in some of the cases substantial ischemia was present that could not be predicted from the CT scan. In view of the fact that patients with ischemia may respond adversely to hyperventilation, it is suggested that direct CBF measurement by this technique may be an important adjunct in the treatment of this difficult group of patients. More clinical experience is required to establish the best method of treatment.— R.M. Crowell, M.D.

Diffuse Axonal Injury: Analysis of 100 Patients With Radiological Signs
Levi L, Guilburd JN, Lemberger A, Soustiel JF, Feinsod M (Rambam Med Ctr, Haifa, Israel)
Neurosurgery 27:429–432, 1990   21–2

Differential acceleration of parts of the brain on impact can produce shearing forces at the gray-white matter junction, in the brain stem, or in the corpus callosum. Axons and small vessels tear as a result, producing a picture of diffuse axonal injury (DAI). One hundred consecutive cases of DAI diagnosed between 1983 and 1988 were reviewed. The diagnosis was based on the presence of small, nonexpansive hemorrhagic lesions at the corticomedullary and nuclear-medullary junctions, corpus callosum, or cerebellum.

Road accidents were the chief cause of injury, followed by falls from a height. Eighty-two of the patients had a Glasgow Coma Scale score of 8 or less. Seventy patients had "deep" CT lesions that most often were single and located in the corticomedullary region. Adults had multiple lesions more often than did children. Twenty-five patients had signs suggestive of DAI, usually generalized brain swelling and intraventricular hemorrhage. Forty-eight patients had a skull fracture. After 3 months, 28 patients had recovered well, 13 had moderate disability, 34 had severe disability, and 5 remained in a vegetative state. Most of the 20 patients who died had an associated intracranial lesion. Age was an important prognostic factor. Patients with "deep" lesions had a poorer outcome than did those with peripheral lesions. Computed tomography will detect DAI in some patients with seemingly mild head injury.

► The authors present an interesting series of patients of all ages with DAI, defined by small hemorrhagic lesions or interventricular blood with generalized brain swelling. Those patients who did well generally emerged from coma within 24 hours. Patients who postured with or without pupillary abnormalities at 24 hours had extremely poor outcomes.

With improved CT images, it is common to see small petechial hemorrhages consistent with DAI, and therefore it is possible to make this diagnosis in patients who have moderate or minor head injuries (Glasgow Coma Scale scores 9 to 12 and 13 to 15, respectively). Overall, DAI has correlated with poor outcome in the past. It is likely that the milder forms were overlooked previously, and this study brings out this point. Diffuse axonal injury is an important diagnosis, and its outcome can be classified by knowing the scores after 24 hours, using the proposed grading scheme. It should prove a useful guide for clinicians in discussions of individual patient outcome.—R.M. Crowell, M.D.

Penetrating Head Injuries

Wartime Neurosurgical Experience in Lebanon, 1982–85. I: Penetrating Craniocerebral Injuries
Levi L, Borovich B, Guilburd JN, Grushkiewicz I, Lemberger A, Linn S, Schachter I, Zaaroor M, Braun J, Feinsod M (Rambam Med Ctr, Haifa, Israel; Technion-Israel Inst of Technology, Haifa)
Isr J Med Sci 26:548–554, 1990   21–3

The lethality of modern weapons has led to increased mortality during warfare, despite advances in transport and medical care. Among the most devastating injuries of warfare are penetrating wounds of the brain. A new approach to the treatment of intracranial bone fragments is possible with CT scanning.

During warfare in Lebanon from June 1982 through June 1985, 116 penetrating wounds of the brain were treated at the Rambam Medical Center. Patients were examined with CT on admission and throughout their treatment. The 2 main causes of injury were high-velocity bullets (13%) and shrapnel (75%) and stones (2.5%) from explosive devices. Nearly half of the patients had multisystem injury.

The damaged brain and skull, the missile tract, different types of projectiles, and the presence and types of mass lesions were revealed by CT. Surgery was performed in 83% of the patients. Although mass lesions were excised, only indriven fragments that were easily accessible were removed. The median duration of hospitalization was 13 days. Using the Glasgow Outcome Scale, at hospital discharge 49 patients had a good recovery, 24 had moderate disability, 7 had severe disability, 6 were in a coma, and 30 died. Outcome was directly related to the patients' admission Glasgow Coma Score. Mechanisms of injury also influenced the mortality rate, which was 80% for gunshot wounds but 19% for shrapnel injuries.

By using CT, neurosurgeons were able to detect small intracranial foreign bodies undetected by conventional radiography, estimate the extent of damage in penetrating craniocerebral injury, and disclose associated lesions. In some cases, foreign bodies were present even when there was no external scalp wound. The findings of CT studies had an immediate influence on the method of treatment.

▶ This sobering communication from Lebanon demonstrates how CT scanning helps to direct the treatment of patients with penetrating cerebrocranial injuries. Not only metallic fragments, but also in-driven bone fragments, hematomas, and edema are detected by CT. Interestingly, the policy of leaving untouched bone fragments in deep locations, necessitating brain resection, did not lead to brain abscess or uncontrolled epilepsy in any of the 24 cases so treated.—R.M. Crowell, M.D.

Wartime Neurosurgical Experience in Lebanon, 1982–85. II: Closed Craniocerebral Injuries
Levi L, Borovich B, Guilburd JN, Grushkiewicz I, Lemberger A, Linn S, Schachter I, Zaaroor M, Braun J, Feinsod M (Rambam Med Ctr, Haifa, Israel; Technion-Israel Inst of Technology, Haifa)
Isr J Med Sci 26:555–558, 1990   21–4

During warfare, nonpenetrating craniocerebral injuries are less common than penetrating craniocerebral injuries; nevertheless, about one third of the head injuries during the Lebanon conflict of 1982–1985 were of the former type. The nature of the nonpenetrating craniocerebral injuries, methods of diagnosis and treatment, and outcome in 64 patients brought to the Rambam Medical Center were reviewed, and these military-related injuries were compared with closed head injuries sustained by 251 civilians during 1985.

Each patient had a brain CT scan as part of the initial evaluation. Neurosurgery was performed in 38 patients and craniotomies in 21. A pathologic lesion other than fracture was revealed by CT in 68% of the military patients and in 42% of the civilian group. Surgery was required in 59% of the military patients. The mean duration of hospitalization was 8 days.

Among the military patients, the outcome on discharge (using the Glasgow Outcome Scale) was good recovery in 39, moderate disability in 5, severe disability in 3, and death in 12. Mortality was affected by the mechanism and severity of injury and the presence of multiple trauma.

In a follow-up of the 37 Israeli military survivors, all showed a steady improvement; 10, however, had some degree of mental and cognitive disability. When compared with the civilian cases of nonpenetrating injury, there were major differences in proportion and severity in the military cases. A high proportion of diffuse brain injuries was noted in the military, a result of blasts caused by side mines. Such injuries were detected with the early and liberal use of CT.

▶ Ordinarily, one thinks of penetrating brain injury in relation to combat experience. On the other hand, a very substantial number of nonpenetrating craniocerebral injuries are also experienced in wartime. Many of these are related to a last mechanism. This leads to an unusually high incidence of diffuse brain injury. This is well detected by CT scanning, which is very valuable in the management of these cases.—R.M. Crowell, M.D.

Civilian Gunshot Wounds to the Head: A Prospective Study
Grahm TW, Williams FC Jr, Harrington T, Spetzler RF (Barrow Neurological Inst, Phoenix)
Neurosurgery 27:696–700, 1990   21–5

It is not established that aggressive resuscitative attempts in the field, triage to a neurosurgical center, and early surgery can improve the outcome for victims of cranial gunshot injury. Studies were made in 100 consecutive prospective patients admitted in an 18-month period with gunshot wounds to the head.

If 2 or more neurologic signs persisted after aggressive field treatment and intubation, CT was carried out. Rapid surgical débridement was the rule unless the patient was clinically brain dead. The Glasgow Coma

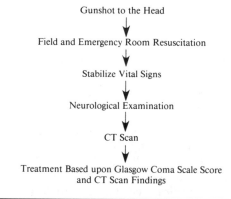

Gunshot to the Head
↓
Field and Emergency Room Resuscitation
↓
Stabilize Vital Signs
↓
Neurological Examination
↓
CT Scan
↓
Treatment Based upon Glasgow Coma Scale Score
and CT Scan Findings

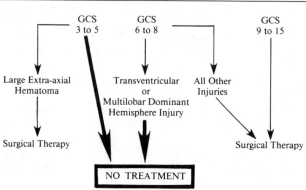

Fig 21–2.—Algorithm for the treatment of patients with gunshot wounds. (Courtesy of Grahm TW, Willims FC Jr, Harrington T, et al: *Neurosurgery* 27:696–700, 1990.)

Scale (GCS) score following resuscitation was 3 to 5 in 58 patients, 6 to 8 in 8, 9 to 12 in 12, and 13 to 15 in 22. Seventy-six patients had CT studies and 43 underwent craniotomy.

Sixty patients in this series died, 2 remained in a vegetative state, and 6 were severely disabled. Thirteen patients had a good outcome. There were 10 postoperative deaths. No patient with a GCS score of 3 to 5 had a satisfactory outcome, but the outcome improved progressively with increasing GCS scores at admission.

All gunshot head wound victims should receive aggressive field resuscitation (Fig 21–2). If the GCS score is 3 to 5 after full resuscitation and a large hematoma is excluded, further treatment should be withheld. Aggressive surgical treatment is warranted for patients with a GCS score above 8 and for those with scores of 6 to 8 who have a large mass lesion.

▶ This carefully studied series of 100 consecutive patients indicates that the GCS can be used to guide treatment. If the GCS is 5 or less with no operable hematoma, then no further therapy is recommended. All patients with a GCS of more than 5 are recommended for aggressive surgical treatment.—R.M. Crowell, M.D.

Motorcycle Injuries

Motorcycle Helmets—Medical Costs and the Law
McSwain NE Jr, Belles A (Tulane Univ; South West Texas State Univ, San Antonio)
J Trauma 30:1189–1199, 1990   21–6

In 1966, the federal government began withholding highway safety development funds to states lacking mandatory motorcycle helmet legislation. By the mid–1970s, nearly all states had complied, but after 1975, a dramatic rise in motorcycle deaths occurred as many states repealed these laws (Fig 21–3). The medical and financial effects of repeal in Kansas, and of reinstatement of legislation in Louisiana following its repeal, were examined.

Rates of helmet use fell from 99% to 50% in the absence of legislation and rose to more than 95% when laws requiring helmet use were reinstated. Nonhelmeted riders required twice as long an average hospital stay, and their fatality rate was about fourfold greater than that of riders wearing helmets. Rates of accidents and of fatal accidents were lower in states with active helmet laws. Medical costs declined by nearly half after reinstatement of legislation. The average disability was about halved.

Based on 1989 dollars, $121 million of additional medical care and rehabilitation costs per year were ascribed directly to the nonuse of helmets. Surely, legislation requiring the use of protective helmets by motorcyclists is a viable alternative to raising taxes. Voluntary efforts and educational programs are ineffective.

Motorcycle Fatality Rate
USA

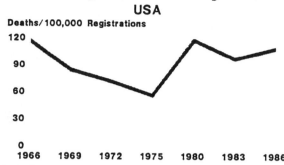

Fig 21–3.—With the institution of mandatory helmet laws in 1966, fatality rates dropped significantly until 1975 when Congress allowed states to repeal motorcycle helmet legislation. The fatality rates have risen significantly since that time. (Courtesy of McSwain NE Jr, Belles A: *J Trauma* 30:1189–1199, 1990.)

▶ These interesting data underline the obvious: Use of motorcycle helmets protects against severe brain injury and fatality. With helmet legislation, helmet utilization rises sharply; therefore, helmet legislation decreases injuries, costs, and fatalities from motorcycle use. This type of report provides the data that cry out for helmet legislation. All physicians should vigorously support this endeavor.—R.M. Crowell, M.D.

Head Injury Associated Deaths From Motorcycle Crashes: Relationship to Helmet-Use Laws
Sosin DM, Sacks JJ, Holmgreen P (Ctrs for Disease Control, Atlanta)
JAMA 264:2395–2399, 1990

21–7

Approximately 12% of motor vehicle deaths occur in motorcycle riders. Head injuries are a leading cause of death from motorcycle accidents, but evidence indicates that safety helmets can reduce the incidence and severity of head injuries. The descriptive epidemiology, time trends, and association between deaths and motorcycle helmet use laws in patients involved in motorcycle crashes were reviewed.

Death certificate data were collected from the National Center for Health Statistics for the period from 1979 to 1986. Motorized scooters, mopeds, and tricycles were included as motorcycles, and both passengers and drivers were classified as motorcyclists. Persons were considered to have died of head injuries if fracture of the vault or base of the skull, unqualified and multiple fractures of the skull, intracranial injury, late effects of skull and face fracture, or late effects of intracranial injury without skull fracture were listed in part I of the death certificate. To compensate for underreporting of head injuries, 500 randomly selected cases with nonspecific diagnoses also were included. Information on motorcycle helmet use laws was obtained from the Motorcycle Industry Council.

During the 8-year study period, 28,749 motorcyclists died of motorcycle-related injuries. Head injury was involved in 53% of deaths. More than 90% of decedents were white males; 69% were white males aged 15–34 years. Fifty-two percent of head-injury–related deaths were caused by collision with another motor vehicle and 40% resulted from loss of control of the motorcycle. Fourteen percent of head-injured decedents were passengers. For deaths associated with head injuries, the annualized death rate was 5.5 fatalities per million residents in states with full helmet use laws, 10.2 in states with partial laws, and 10.4 in states with no laws. In 3 states that changed from full to partial helmet use laws during the study period, death rates went up after laws were liberalized. Conversely, in 1 state that strengthened its law, death rates declined. The rate of motorcycle-related deaths associated with head injuries declined slightly during the study period and was lowest in states with the most comprehensive helmet use laws.

Efforts should be expanded to reduce the number of head-injury–related deaths in motorcycle accidents. Helmet use laws appear to be effective in helping to reduce such deaths. The adoption and enforcement of comprehensive motorcycle helmet use legislation are recommended.

▶ Statistical studies of this type from epidemiologic centers give us the big picture: Without doubt, helmet use reduces the number of deaths from motorcycle crashes. Just as surely, helmet use laws increase helmet use and thus reduce motorcycle deaths. All physicians should work to implement helmet use laws.—R.M. Crowell, M.D.

Treatment

Dimethyl Sulfoxide in the Management of Patients With Brain Swelling and Increased Intracranial Pressure After Severe Closed Head Injury

Kulali A, Akar M, Baykut L (Dicle-Univ School of Medicine, Diyarbakir, Turkey)
Neurochirurgia 33:177–180, 1990   21–8

The prognosis after severe head injury remains poor. Brain swelling can increase intracranial pressure (ICP), resulting in cerebral hypoxia and further brain edema. Many treatment strategies involve a combination of therapies aimed at preventing elevated ICP or normalizing it. The efficacy of dimethyl sulfoxide was assessed in the treatment of 10 patients with brain swelling and elevated ICP. Glasgow coma scale scores and severity of edema were carefully determined in all cases.

Patients received an intravenous bolus infusion of dimethyl sulfoxide, 50 cc in 5% dextrose, when the ICP was 25 mm Hg or more until it was lowered to 15 mm Hg or less. Three patients died of their head injuries. In most cases, the ICP dropped markedly within 10 minutes of initiation of infusion. Continuous dimethyl sulfoxide administration did not prevent ICPs from returning to their initial elevated levels.

Dimethyl sulfoxide rapidly reduces raised ICP, increases cerebral perfusion pressure, and improves the neurologic outcome of severely head-injured patients. It does not affect the systemic blood pressure or responsiveness in most cases. The rebound effect did not occur with dimethyl sulfoxide administration in this series.

▶ There are only limited data available from this study, but it suggests that dimethy sulfoxide may have a useful clinical role in the control of intractable increased intracranial tension.— R.M. Crowell, M.D.

Recovery From Vegetative State of Six Months' Duration Associated With Sinemet (Levodopa/Carbidopa)
Haig AJ, Ruess JM (Univ of Vermont, Burlington)
Arch Phys Med Rehabil 71:1081–1083, 1990   21–9

A number of medications offer promise of improving the function of head-injured patients. Treatment with Sinemet (levodopa/carbidopa) resulted in cognitive and physical progress in a patient who had been unresponsive for 6 months.

Man, 24, sustained a closed head injury in a motor vehicle accident. Sixteen weeks after the injury, the patient showed a response to pain, reflex grasp, and severe spasticity, but no clear response to commands. Nine weeks of intensive therapy had not improved his cognitive status. Sinemet treatment was started in week 28. The patient's level of consciousness rose within 3 days and speech started to return. Sinemet was discontinued over 2 weeks beginning at week 40 with no change in the patient's mental status. He had improved from level II on the Rancho Los Amigos Head Injury Scale before Sinemet to level VI at completion of Sinemet therapy. Although the patient continues to have memory deficits and decreased attention, he is making small improvements and is able to live at home with his family. Contractures and spasticity, which developed during the early period of hospitalization, contributed to some of his most severe functional problems.

Pharmacologic rehabilitation in such cases appears to depend on affecting the dopaminergic pathway. Even with long-standing lesions, drug intervention may significantly improve neurologic function. Although Sinemet should probably not be used in all patients with traumatic head injuries, the drug may benefit those who have no signs of spontaneous recovery. The drug should be discontinued after a few weeks if no changes are apparent.

▶ The remarkable recovery of a young man after closed head injury was associated with Sinemet therapy. The prompt improvement appeared within 3 days of onset of treatment. Of course, it is possible that the patient would have improved without this form of treatment. Nonetheless, the possibility that pharmacologic manipulation may assist recovery after injury deserves further careful clinical evaluations.— R.M. Crowell, M.D.

Laboratory Studies

Ischemic Brain Damage in a Model of Acute Subdural Hematoma

Miller JD, Bullock R, Graham DI, Min-Hsiung-Chen, Teasdale GM (Univ of Mississippi; Univ of Glasgow; Young-Ming Med College, Taipei, Taiwan)
Neurosurgery) 27:433–439, 1990   21–10

The fact that many patients with acute subdural hematoma caused by head injury have a conscious interval suggests that much of the ischemic damage results from secondary, potentially treatable mechanisms. Hemispheric ischemic damage was characterized in a rat model of acute subdural hematoma, produced by injecting 400 μL of autologous blood (about one fifth of the intracranial volume) into the subdural space.

The hematomas typically were .5–1.5-mm thick and largest over the

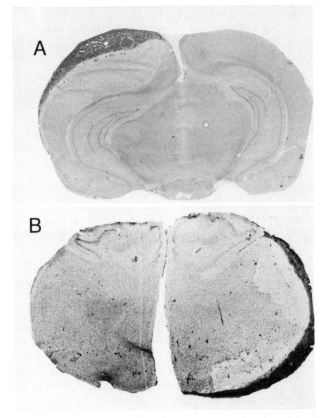

Fig 21–4.—Coronal sections stained with hematoxylin and eosin after acute subdural hematoma in the rat. **A,** section at the level of the hippocampus in a rat that was perfusion fixed 4 hours after induction of acute subdural hematoma. Note the region of pallor with a clearly defined margin beneath the subdural hematoma. **B,** section at the level of the frontal cortex in a rat perfusion fixed 4 hours after hematoma induction. (Courtesy of Miller JD, Bullock R, Graham DI, et al: *Neurosurgery* 27:433–439, 1990.)

midparietal convexity, extending for 8–10 mm. Several animals had small hematomas in the subcortical area underlying the subdural hematoma. Ischemic damage (Fig 21–4) within 4–24 hours after lesion production involved 14% to 16% of the hemispheric volume. Intracranial pressure peaked at 51 mm Hg and remained elevated to 3 times normal for 3 hours. The damage chiefly affected the frontal cortex. This appears to be a useful model with which to investigate the pathogenesis of the ischemic damage produced by acute subdural hematoma.

▶ The authors have developed a clinically relevant model of subdural hematoma in the experimental animal. Using this model, the report notes important consequences of the hematoma. Under the acute clot in the rat model, the brain became ischemic. The authors intend to use this model to elucidate the pathogenesis of this process, which may well underlie the appallingly high morbidity and mortality of diffuse brain injury associated with these lesions in patients.—R.M. Crowell, M.D.

Mass Concentration Measurements of Creatine Kinase BB Isoenzyme as an Index of Brain Tissue Damage
Delanghe JR, De Winter HA, De Buyzere ML, Camaert JJ, Martens FE, De Praeter C (Univ Hosp, Gent, Belgium)
Clin Chim Acta 193:125–136, 1990   21–11

Measurements of the creatine kinase isoenzyme BB (CK-BB) in serum and CSF have proved useful as a tumor marker and for assessing the extent of brain lesions. Because CK-BB is unstable, mass concentration measurements, which are insensitive to changes in catalytic enzyme properties, are preferable. A 2-site immunoenzymometric method of estimating CK-BB mass concentration in the CSF was developed based on 2 monoclonal antibodies directed against the CK-B subunit.

The assay was evaluated in 10 patients hospitalized for acute head trauma, 20 adults with headache, and 186 neonates having varying indications for lumbar puncture. Within-assay and between-assay coefficients of variation ranged from 6% to 9%. The assay findings were unaffected by the presence of sulfate and sialic acid groups on the enzyme. Specific enzyme activity declined steadily after acute head trauma (Fig 21–5). Repeated measurements in the first 24 hours after injury allowed the size of brain lesions to be estimated. In both head trauma victims and neonates, the CSF values of CK-BB correlated well with the clinical findings.

This immunoenzymometric assay is a sensitive and reproducible means of estimating mass concentrations of CK-BB in the CSF. The sharp and continuous rise in CK-BB activation energy seen after the onset of brain damage accords with the general concept of tissue enzyme denaturation after enzyme release. The cumulative release of CK-BB after acute head trauma provides a better prognostic measure than the admitting Glasgow Coma Scale score. In addition, the measurement is a good predictor of

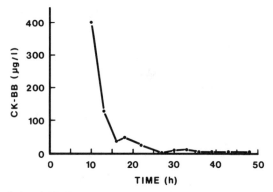

Fig 21–5.—Evolution of CK-BB mass concentration in the CSF of a patient with acute head trauma during the first 2 days of hospitalization. (Courtesy of Delanghe JR, De Winter HA, De Buyzere ML, et al: *Clin Chim Acta* 193:125–136, 1990.)

the severity of brain lesions in neonates with various acute neurologic disorders.

▶ This creative study indicates that the CK-BB isoenzyme may be used as an index of brain tissue damage in trauma patients. In essence, CSF from a ventricular drain was sampled for enzymatic evidence of brain damage. The magnitude of the isoenzyme correlated with the Glasgow Outcome Scale score. Further data are required to learn whether this type of determination, in concert with clinical and CT findings, will improve prognostication. It is also possible that this approach might be used to grade brain damage from other sources, e.g., cerebral ischemia and stroke.—R.M. Crowell, M.D.

22 Pediatrics

Intracranial Germ-Cell Tumors in Children
Hoffman HJ, Otsubo H, Hendrick EB, Humphreys RP, Drake JM, Becker LE,
Greenberg M, Jenkin D (The Hosp for Sick Children, Toronto; Univ of Toronto)
J Neurosurg 74:545–551, 1991   22–1

Germ cell tumors arise in the midline of the brain and are most frequently encountered in childhood. They are more commonly located in
the pineal region than in the suprasellar region. The outcome of 51 patients treated for germ cell tumors was analyzed to assess preferred methods of management.

Of 51 tumors reviewed, 32 were in the pineal region, 16 in the suprasellar region, and 3 in both the pineal and suprasellar regions. Forty-nine
patients underwent surgical resection. The operating microscope, ultrasonic surgical aspirator, or laser beam was used to remove deep-seated
tumors in the pineal region (Fig 22–1). Twenty-five patients with germinomas who received radiotherapy had a 5-year survival rate of 85%.
Thirteen patients with non–germinoma germ cell tumors had a 5-year
survival rate of 45.5% after radiotherapy.

Resection of pineal or suprasellar germ cell tumors is recommended
for an accurate histologic diagnosis to guide adjuvant therapy. Adjuvant
local radiotherapy is adequate for pure germinoma with no dissemination. In cases of malignant nongerminoma germ cell tumors, adjuvant

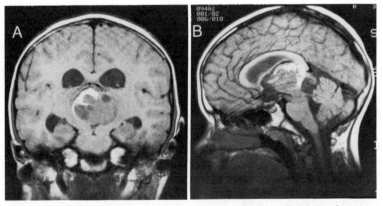

Fig 22–1.—T1-weighted MR images, anteroposterior view (**A**) and lateral view (**B**), of a patient with
mixed germinoma, endodermal sinus tumor, and teratoma in the pineal region. Mixed densities are seen
in this tumor. (Courtesy of Hoffman HJ, Otsubo H, Hendrick EB, et al: *J Neurosurg* 74:545–551,
1991.)

therapy should include chemotherapy and craniospinal axis radiotherapy.

▶ This contribution from the Hospital for Sick Children in Toronto provides an extensive experience on intracranial germ cell tumors in children. The authors demonstrate that surgery of these lesions in the pineal and suprasellar areas can be accomplished safely. They argue persuasively that the treatment of choice is local radiation for germinomas, which will often be cured by this approach. On the other hand, about a third of all their tumors were non-germinoma germ cell tumors, and much more extensive treatment was required, including an effort at removal as well as whole-axis radiation and, in some cases, chemotherapy including cisplatin. The results in this category are much less favorable. It is interesting that in this highly experienced center, the use of tumor markers was only rarely helpful, and biopsy was the keystone of diagnosis.—R.M. Crowell, M.D.

Craniopharyngiomas in Children: Long-Term Effects of Conservative Surgical Procedures Combined With Radiation Therapy
Fischer EG, Welch K, Shillito J Jr, Winston KR, Tarbell NJ (Children's Hosp, Boston; Joint Ctr for Radiation Therapy, Boston; Harvard Med School)
J Neurosurg 73:534–540, 1990   22–2

The radical excision of craniopharyngiomas in children is not without risk. As they grow up, many survivors of such surgery experience intellectual and psychosocial deficits. Conservative surgical procedures combined with radiation therapy seem to offer a more favorable outlook. Follow-up was made of 37 children for at least 10 years to determine the relationship between various tumor treatments and successful independent adult living.

In 8 patients (group I), complete tumor resection was thought to have been accomplished. Some received radiation therapy for possible microscopic residual tumor. The 6 patients in group II underwent partial resection of the tumor followed by radiation therapy. The remaining 21 patients (group III) were treated with radiation therapy alone, or with conservative surgical procedures followed by radiation therapy.

Three patients died, 1 in each treatment group. Of the 34 survivors, 32 were available for evaluation. Tumor recurrence or regrowth occurred in 5 patients—4 in group I and 1 in group III. Thus treatment was successful (no recurrence or death) in 37.5% of patients having radical excision and in 89% of those who underwent more conservative surgery and irradiation.

The highest level of functioning was attained by 76% of the group III survivors. Approximately half of these patients could function competitively, whereas none of the 4 patients in group I who had reached the age of high school graduation could work independently. Yet, patients in all 3 treatment groups had psychological problems, e.g., immature behavior, irritability, and depression. Diabetes insipidus developed in all but 1 of those who underwent radical resection or attempted radical resection. A patient whose tumor was not attached to either the pituitary stalk or the hypothalamus had no endocrine deficit.

Because of the problems resulting from hypothalamic injury, surgical procedures that minimize such injury are preferable for treating childhood craniopharyngioma. Radiation therapy, although not without its own risks, seems to be the best method of control for tumor remaining in situ.

▶ This report provides data suggesting superior results with conservative surgery and radiation for pediatric craniopharyngiomas. Several questions remain, however: In the total removal cases, how many were operated on with the surgical operating microscope? How does this compare with the Toronto series (29 patients, total removal in 25, 4 recurrences, mean follow-up 2.6 years)? (1) What is the role of intracavitary P32 for cystic lesions?

There seems to be a role for conservative surgery and radiation, but technological advances will continue to modify the approach.—R.M. Crowell, M.D.

Reference

1. Hoffman HJ: *Can J Neurol Sci* 12:348, 1985.

Cerebral Blood Flow in Moyamoya Disease. Part 2: Autoregulation and CO₂ Response

Ogawa A, Nakamura N, Yoshimoto T, Suzuki J (Tohoku Univ, Sendai, Japan)
Acta Neurochir (Wien) 105:107–111, 1990   22–3

In moyamoya disease, an abnormal vascular network develops as a result of the gradual occlusion of both internal carotid arteries. The cause of the condition is unknown. To determine the cerebrovascular response in moyamoya disease, autoregulation and carbon dioxide (CO_2) responses in 16 patients were investigated. The krypton-81m continuous cerebral blood flow (CBF) measurement technique was used to make 32 measurements over the anterior and posterior circulation. The CBF measurements were made during loading trials in hypertension, hypotension, CO_2 inhalation, and hyperventilation. The vascular response of the frontal lobe perfused by the internal carotid artery (ICA) and the occipital lobe and cerebellum perfused by the vertebral artery also were studied.

The study group included 7 adults and 9 children. All but 1 patient had transient ischemic attacks. In pediatric patients, autoregulation deficits were more severe in response to hypotension than to hypertension in regions of both ICAs and vertebral arteries. However, the deficits were mild. Both adults and children had deficits in the ICA region in response to hyperventilation, and in both groups some responses were paradoxical. In general, children had more severely deficient responses than did adults. There were also significant regional differences in deficits.

Vascular responses in patients with moyamoya disease vary with age and regions of perfusion of the ICA and the vertebral artery. Several surgical treatments for moyamoya disease have been reported, including superior cervical ganglionectomy and vascular reconstruction, but these procedures require further evaluation.

▶ In this useful study, 16 patients with moyamoya disease and transient ischemic attacks were studied with the intra-arterial krypton washout CBF technique. Autoregulation deficits were demonstrated in these patients that were more severe in response to hypotension than to hypertension, a circumstance not unexpected in relation to the occlusive nature of the cerebrovascular process. Although the data remain anecdotal, this sort of information may be helpful in understanding more precisely the pathophysiology of moyamoya disease and in tailoring treatment to the individual patient. This may also help us to more satisfactorily recommend revascularization in appropriate cases.—R.M. Crowell, M.D.

Encephalo-Duro-Arterio-Synangiosis in Children With Moyamoya Disease
Matsushima T, Fukui M, Kitamura K, Hasuo K, Kuwabara Y, Kurokawa T (Kyushu Univ, Fukuoka, Japan)
Acta Neurochir (Wien) 104:96–102, 1990   22–4

In 1980, encephalo-duro-arterio-synangiosis (EDAS) for treatment of patients with moyamoya disease was first reported. The EDAS is a nonanastomotic method that results in new collateral formation. Good results have been reported, although some cases have been refractory (Fig 22–2).

The EDAS procedure was performed in 16 Japanese children with moyamoya disease on 22 sides. The results were evaluated clinically, angiographically, and by positron emission CT (PET). In 72% of the patients, good collateral circulation was demonstrated on the postoperative angiograms. After 6 months, symptoms had disappeared in 31% of patients and were partially resolved in 44%.

Postoperative collateral circulation was sometimes insufficient with this indirect bypass procedure. In some cases, there was good new collateral formation in the middle cerebral arterial area but insufficient formation in other areas. The EDAS procedure was particularly appropriate and effective in children with the ischemic type of moyamoya disease.

▶ This communication from a very experienced group in the moyamoya area again emphasizes the suitability of EDAS for children with ischemic moyamoya disease. However, many questions remain regarding the approach.—R.M. Crowell, M.D.

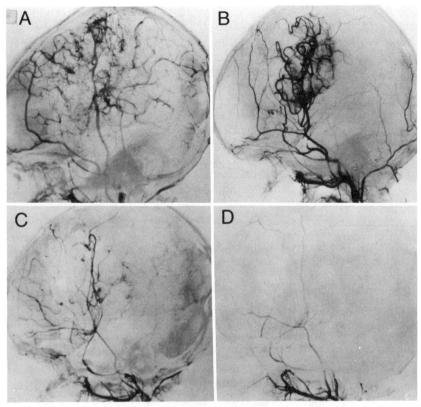

Fig 22–2.—Classification of development of collateral vessel formation on the postoperative external carotid angiograms. **A,** good development. The area fed by EDAS is larger than one third of the middle cerebral artery (MCA) distribution. **B,** fair development. The area is smaller than one third of the MCA distribution but more than 2 cortical branches of the MCA distribution were supplied through EDAS. **C,** poor development. Only 1 cortical branch of the MCA is visualized through EDAS. **D,** no development. No collateral circulation. (Courtesy of Matsushima T, Fukui M, Kitamura K, et al: *Acta Neurochir (Wien)* 104:96–102, 1990.)

Intracranial Arachnoid Cysts in Children: A Comparison of the Effects of Fenestration and Shunting

Ciricillo SF, Cogen PH, Harsh GR, Edwards MSB (Univ of California, San Francisco)
J Neurosurg 74:230–235, 1991   22–5

There is still controversy over the best surgical approach to congenital intracranial arachnoid cysts in children. Options include needle aspiration, cyst-peritoneal shunting, ventriculocystostomy, and craniotomy for fenestration of the cyst. The effectiveness of fenestration and of shunting in the treatment of children with intracranial arachnoid cysts was compared.

Twenty-six boys and 14 girls with ages from newborn to 15 years at the time of referral were studied. Seventeen children had symptoms and signs of elevated intracranial pressure, 15 had craniomegaly, 12 had developmental delay, 11 had seizure disorders, and 10 had headaches. Computed tomography or MRI revealed intracranial cystic masses containing fluid of CSF density. Thirty-five children had evidence of compressed surrounding neural or ventricular structures, and 5 had cysts smaller than 5 cm in diameter and no compression of surrounding structures. These 5 children did not require operation. Fifteen children were treated initially by craniotomy in which the cyst cavity was fenestrated into the subarachnoid space. Three of these children had previously undergone ventriculoperitoneal (VP) shunting for hydrocephalus. The other 20 children underwent shunting initially.

After follow-up of 3 months to 12 years, 5 of the 15 children whose cysts were treated initially by fenestration had a reduction in the size of the cyst and at least some clinical improvement. The other 10 children had no clinical or radiographic improvement. Eight children have since undergone cyst-peritoneal shunting, 1 had VP shunting, and 1 child had revision of a VP shunt placed for hydrocephalus before cyst fenestration. Two children with existing VP shunts required no further treatment. After a median follow-up period of 8 years, only 3 of the 15 children initially treated by fenestration remained shunt-independent. All 20 children initially treated by cyst shunting were improved by this operation (Fig 22–3). Six of these 20 children have since required shunt revision because of cyst recurrence. Shunting of cysts in most locations is more suc-

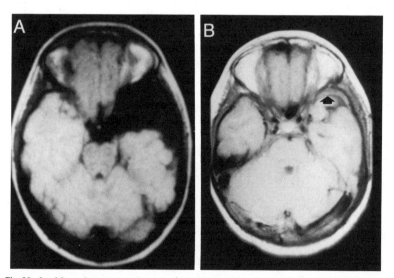

Fig 22–3.—Magnetic resonance images of an 11-year-old girl with partial complex seizures and headaches. **A,** initial study demonstrates a large left middle cranial fossa arachnoid cyst (TR 800 msec, TE 20 msec). **B,** follow-up image obtained 1 year post shunting shows the cyst catheter (*arrow*) lying along the anterior wall of the middle fossa. The temporal lobe completely reexpanded to fill the middle fossa. (TR 800 msec, TE 20 msec). (Courtesy of Ciricillo SF, Cogen PH, Harsh GR, et al: *J Neurosurg* 74:230–235, 1991.)

cessful than fenestration and should therefore be considered as the initial surgical procedure for most intracranial arachnoid cysts.

▶ This helpful report from the University of California at San Francisco provides data to guide the surgeon faced with an intracranial arachnoid cyst in a child. Of a substantial number of patients, a small minority were made shunt independent after treatment by fenestration. In all locations, shunting was more successful than fenestration. It is concluded that, for the majority of patients, cyst-peritoneal or cyst-VP shunting is the procedure of choice.— R.M. Crowell, M.D.

Clinical and Pathological Analysis of Spinal Cord Astrocytomas in Children
Rossitch E Jr, Zeidman SM, Burger PC, Curnes JT, Harsh C, Anscher M, Oakes WJ (Duke Univ)
Neurosurgery 27:193–196, 1990   22–6

Spinal cord astrocytomas comprise only 4% of CNS tumors in children. A review was made of the findings in 12 children aged 4–17 years who had pathologically confirmed cord astrocytomas. These patients were seen at Duke University Medical Center beginning in 1952. The mean follow-up was 10½ years.

Weakness, scoliosis, and gait disorder were the most frequent presenting features. Six tumors were primarily in the cervical cord and 6 others were chiefly thoracic in location. Myelography showed cord widening in all cases. Contrast MRI in 1 case demonstrated a discrete enhancing mass. Six patients received radiotherapy; 4 had clinical recurrences, and 2 died of disease. Eight patients survived for a mean of nearly 9 years without symptoms of recurrence. Three of 8 patients who underwent biopsy or subtotal resection had recurrences, compared with 1 of 4 patients who underwent "total" resection. All of the tumors were well-differentiated astrocytomas lacking mitotic activity and necrosis.

Magnetic resonance imaging may be very helpful in the surgical management of spinal cord astrocytomas. Surgery is desirable, but its extent should be considered carefully in view of the generally good course observed for well-differentiated tumors. This is particularly true of infiltrating fibrillary lesions, the total removal of which might necessitate an unacceptable degree of cord dysfunction.

▶ In this series of 12 cases, the authors confirm Epstein's contention that almost all of the spinal cord astrocytomas in children are grade I or II. The study shows that MRI, particularly with gadolinium, is highly sensitive and precise in the localization of these lesions. The results suggest the utility of surgical resection, but the numbers are too small and the growth rates too slow to permit conclusions regarding the importance of total resection. Likewise, the value of postoperative irradiation cannot be assessed properly with this particular study.— R.M. Crowell, M.D.

Cesarean Section Before the Onset of Labor and Subsequent Motor Function in Infants With Meningomyelocele Diagnosed Antenatally
Luthy DA, Wardinsky T, Shurtleff DB, Hollenbach KA, Hickok DE, Nyberg DA, Benedetti TJ (Swedish Hosp Med Ctr, Seattle; Univ Hosp Med Ctr, Seattle)
N Engl J Med 324:662–666, 1991   22–7

The best management of antenatally detected meningomyelocele is unknown. Labor and vaginal delivery may cause pressure on exposed nerve roots, thereby causing additional loss of neural function. The level of motor function in infants with meningomyelocele who were delivered by cesarean section was compared with that of infants whose condition was detected at birth.

The 2 groups were identified in a 10-year study period and accounted for 95% of cases in the state of Washington during that period. There were 81 antenatally detected cases and 119 discovered at the time of delivery. Of these, 47 infants were delivered by cesarean section before labor began, 35 were delivered by cesarean section after labor had begun, and 78 were delivered vaginally; an additional 40 pregnancies were excluded for various reasons. When meningomyelocele without severe hydrocephalus was detected antenatally, cesarean section was done before the onset of labor; these infants were compared with those delivered vaginally and those delivered by cesarean section after a period of labor. Infants were reexamined at 2 years of age.

At follow-up, the 2 groups of children who underwent labor were 2.2 times more likely to have severe paralysis than those delivered by cesarean section before labor. The mean level of paralysis in the latter group was 3.3 segments below the level of the spinal lesion, compared with a level of 1.1 for vaginally delivered infants and .9 for those delivered by cesarean section after the onset of labor. Other factors (e.g., maternal age and the infant's sex) did not affect those differences. The experience of labor had no effect on the frequency of neonatal complications or intellectual performance.

Cesarean delivery before the onset of labor may result in better motor function than cesarean delivery after the onset of labor or vaginal delivery for fetuses with uncomplicated meningomyelocele. Planned cesarean section allows rapid back closure and precludes trauma to the exposed nerves. Larger studies are needed to determine whether cesarean section after the onset of labor offers any benefits in motor function.

▶ The outcomes of 82 patients delivered by cesarean section and 78 delivered vaginally were compared. Delivery by cesarean section before the onset of labor resulted in better subsequent motor function.— R.M. Crowell, M.D.

23 Infection

Chronic Neurologic Manifestations of Lyme Disease
Logigian EL, Kaplan RF, Steere AC (Tufts Univ)
N Engl J Med 323:1438–1444, 1990   23–1

Lyme disease is associated with a wide range of neurologic abnormalities, both acute and chronic. The chronic abnormalities were investigated in a series of 27 patients with chronic neurologic symptoms after an episode of Lyme disease. All patients had current evidence of immunity to *Borrelia burgdorferi,* the tickborne spirochete that causes Lyme disease and lacked evidence of other causes for their symptoms. Eight patients were followed prospectively for 8–12 years after onset of infection.

About 40% of patients had severe headache, mild neck stiffness, or spinal pain during the acute illness. Symptoms of chronic peripheral neurologic disorder developed a median of 16 months after the onset of infection, and CNS involvement began after a median of 26 months. Twenty-four patients had mild encephalopathy, usually manifested by memory loss. Nineteen patients had polyneuropathy, which nearly always included sensory symptoms. One patient had evidence of leukoencephalitis 6 years after the onset of Lyme disease.

All 27 patients received 2 g of intravenous ceftriaxone each day for 14 days. Improvement often did not begin until several months after completion of ceftriaxone therapy. Nerve conduction and neuropsychological function tended to improve, but serum and CSF antibody responses often were unchanged. Five patients with abnormal cerebral MR images improved clinically despite a lack of change in the lesions. Seventeen of the 27 patients were improved when last seen. Six others had improved but later relapsed, and 4 were no better.

The response to antibiotic therapy supports a role for spirochetal infection in the pathogenesis of chronic neurologic syndromes. The results, however, were not as good as those in previous reports. Some nonresponders may have irreversible nervous system damage.

▶ This careful investigation of 27 patients with chronic neurologic symptoms gives insight into the CNS manifestations of Lyme disease. Of particular note is that about 40% of the patients had severe headache, mild neck stiffness, and spinal pain. The chronic neurologic disorder was characterized by memory loss and peripheral neuropathy. After 2 weeks of intravenous ceftriaxone, 17 of the 27 patients had improved, but a number were unchanged or had relapsed. Evidently, antispirochetal therapy is helpful in many patients, but in others there may be permanent CNS damage that resists treatment.—R.M. Crowell, M.D.

Definition of the Role of Contemporary Surgical Management in Cisternal and Parenchymatous Cysticercosis Cerebri

Couldwell WT, Zee C-S, Apuzzo MLJ (Univ of Southern California)
Neurosurgery 28:231–237, 1991
23–2

Increasing immigration to North America has increased the incidence of neurocysticercosis. A retrospective study was done to assess the role of surgery in 237 patients (mean age, 31 years) with large cystic parenchymal and cisternal lesions seen during a 5-year period.

Of those with cystic mass lesions primarily affecting the brain parenchyma and cisternal spaces, 8.4% with large cystic lesions underwent surgery. Surgical intervention was indicated in these 20 patients because of emergent presentation or because the lesions were refractory to medical treatment. Clinical manifestations included elevated intracranial pressure (ICP), focal neurologic deficit, and seizure. Computed tomography and/or MRI showed cisternal lesions in 12 patients, parenchymal lesions in 7, and in both compartments in 1. Based on imaging guidelines, 30 operative procedures were done. There were 14 craniotomies, 8 CSF diversions, 7 stereotactic procedures, and 1 burr hole drainage. Seventy-five percent of the patients improved neurologically or symptomatically during a median 36.4-month follow-up. Three surgery-related complications occurred. None of the patients died.

Large cysts in patients with cisternal and parenchymatous cysticercosis may be amenable to surgery if they are rapidly progressive or refractory to medical treatment. Symptomatic intraparenchymal cysts are best treated with stereotactic techniques, with placement of cyst catheter-reservoirs to permit serial aspiration during a treatment course with praziquantel or albendazole. Open craniotomy and excision is the best management for large basilar cisternal cysts in the absence of radiographically discernible basilar arachnoiditis that would preclude their removal.

▶ Praziquantel and albendazole have had a major impact on the treatment of CNS cysticercosis. In this report, the authors make a logical case for aspirations of intraparenchymal cysts refractory to medical therapy. A catheter-reservoir system appears to be a reasonable technique. The efficacy of open excision for cisternal disease is also reasonably documented.— R.M. Crowell, M.D.

Albendazole Therapy for Subarachnoid and Ventricular Cysticercosis: Case Report

del Brutto OH, Sotelo J (Natl Inst of Neurology and Neurosurgery, Mexico City)
J Neurosurg 72:816–817, 1990
23–3

Albendazole is an imidazole drug that is active in neurocysticercosis and at present is considered superior to praziquantel in the treatment of parenchymal cerebral cysticercosis. A patient was seen with both intraventricular and subarachnoid involvement. She responded adequately to treatment with albendazole.

Woman, 19, complained of 10 months of headaches and vomiting. She had increased muscle-stretch reflexes but otherwise normal neurologic findings. In childhood she had been treated for intestinal taeniasis. An enzyme-linked immunosorbent assay for anticysticercus antibody was positive, and cranial CT showed multiple nonenhancing parenchymal cysts in the brain, as well as subarachnoid cysts in the quadrigeminal and ambient cisterns. A large cysticercus was seen in the occipital horn of the right lateral ventricle. Albendazole was given in a dose of 15 mg/kg daily for 8 days. Three months later, CT showed no intracranial lesions, and the patient was without symptoms.

Medical treatment may be an effective nonoperative approach to cysticercosis involving the subarachnoid space or ventricles. A trial of albendazole is suggested before surgical removal is attempted when a cyst is present in the lateral cerebral ventricle.

▶ Albendazole at a daily dose of 15 mg/kg for 8 days is the treatment of choice for neurocysticercosis. It is effective in the treatment of 85% of parenchymal cysts. For a cyst in the lateral ventricles, a trial of albendazole therapy may obviate the need for surgical extirpation; however, a controlled study will be needed to prove this point. At present, removal of the fourth ventricular cyst is probably still warranted because of increased intracranial pressure.—R.M. Crowell, M.D.

Spinal Epidural Abscess: A Ten-Year Perspective
Hlavin ML, Kaminski HJ, Ross JS, Ganz E (Case Western Reserve Univ)
Neurosurgery 27:177–184, 1990   23–4

Spinal epidural abscess reportedly is increasing in frequency. Recently, some have recommended nonoperative management for selected patients. Data were reviewed on 40 patients seen between 1980 and 1989 with nontuberculous spinal epidural abscesses. The incidence during this period exceeded that of previous years. Twenty-six patients had chronic disease and 9 had nonpenetrating back trauma. Two patients had osteoarthritis and 1 was pregnant. A probable source of infection was identified in 31 cases.

Back pain was the most common presenting symptom, and three fourths of the patients had fever, sweats, or rigors. Thirteen patients described radicular sensory disturbance. Both the acuteness of presentation and the rate of neurologic deterioration varied. In most cases, the CSF findings reflected parameningeal infection. Two thirds of the patients had bone changes suggesting a destructive process. In some cases, MRI was superior to CT myelography (Fig 23–1).

All patients but 1 were operated on and received prolonged antibiotic treatment postoperatively. Mortality was 23%; the patients who died tended to be older and to be paralyzed before surgery. All but 2 patients who survived after operation improved, but not always fully. Of 11 pa-

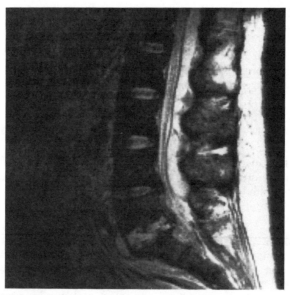

Fig 23–1.—T2-weighted MRI scan shows a mass of high signal intensity. Diskitis can be seen as increased signal intensity and absence of the intranuclear cleft. There is also vertebral osteomyelitis, which exhibits a higher signal intensity than normal bone. (Courtesy of Hlavin ML, Kaminski HJ, Ross JS, et al: *Neurosurgery* 27:177–184, 1990.)

tients who initially were neurologically normal but deteriorated before surgery, only 3 recovered fully; 2 of these became paralyzed.

Immediate decompression and antibiotic therapy remain the best measures for treating spinal epidural abscess. The key to lowering mortality is early diagnosis using modern imaging methods.

▶ The authors address an important clinical problem, the diagnosis of which may be overlooked easily, with resultant poor outcome. The duration and type of antimicrobial therapy remain matters of some controversy. Many patients, particularly those without significant cord compression, can be managed successfully with appropriate antibiotic therapy if the causative organism is cultured. Percutaneous biopsy and culture, leading to appropriate antibiotic treatment, often will be sufficient in patients without cord compression. There is no solid evidence that nonoperative management requires longer courses of antibiotics and protracted hospitalization. Indications for surgical management include compression of neural elements, spinal instability, and failure to obtain a satisfactory culture of the organisms.—R.M. Crowell, M.D.

Magnetic Resonance Imaging and the Nonoperative Treatment of Spinal Epidural Abscess
Hanigan WC, Asner NG, Elwood PW (Univ of Illinois, Peoria)
Surg Neurol 34:408–413, 1990   23–5

The use of MRI has greatly aided in the evaluation and treatment of patients with spinal epidural abscess (SEA) under optimal conditions. In 3 cases of SEA the diagnosis was established and the nonoperative treatment was monitored by MRI.

All 3 patients had fever, localized and often severe back pain, and an elevated sedimentation rate. One patient was neurologically intact, another had moderate neurologic deficit, and the third was severely paraparetic with loss of bladder and bowel control.

Magnetic resonance imaging showed the extent of the abscess and cord compression and was effective in demonstrating the formation of an abscess adjacent to the vertebral osteomyelitis in 1 patient. The pathogenic organism was identified through a CT-guided biopsy of the paraspinal mass in 2 patients and blood cultures in 1. Antibiotic therapy was continued until the patients improved clinically and radiographically. In all patients MRI demonstrated resolution of the abscess as treatment progressed. All patients remained neurologically stable or improved.

This study shows the ease and specificity of MRI in the evaluation and nonoperative treatment of SEA. A review of 33 previously reported cases and the present 3 suggests that nonoperative treatment may be a reasonable alternative for SEA under certain clinical conditions, including identification of the pathogenic organism, a stable neurologic condition, access to MRI or CT for potentially rapid reevaluation, and appropriate neurosurgical consultation and nursing care. Nonoperative treatment may be also a reasonable alternative for patients with severe concomitant medical illness or for children who require extensive multilevel laminectomy.

▶ This nice report demonstrates the effectiveness of MRI in following the course of spinal epidural abscess during antibiotic treatment. All 3 of these cases were treated successfully. Of great importance is identification of the offending organism by CT-guided biopsy or blood cultures. Obviously, if the patients have significant neurologic signs in relation to the abscess, surgical evacuation is mandatory.—R.M. Crowell, M.D.

24 Functional

Epilepsy

Presurgical Evaluation for Partial Epilepsy: Relative Contributions of Chronic Depth-Electrode Recordings Versus FDG-PET and Scalp-Sphenoidal Ictal EEG

Engel J Jr, Henry TR, Risinger MW, Mazziotta JC, Sutherling WW, Levesque MF, Phelps ME (Univ of California, Los Angeles)

Neurology 40:1670–1677, 1990

24–1

The effective and safe surgical treatment of refractory partial epilepsy depends on accurate identification of epileptogenic brain tissue. A series of 153 medically resistant patients were examined by the chronic stereotactic depth-electrode EEG (SEEG) technique after positron emission tomography (PET) using ^{18}F-fluorodeoxyglucose (FDG). In addition, scalp-sphenoidal EEG telemetry was carried out. The findings from the scalp-sphenoidal EEG and metabolic studies were reviewed to determine when the SEEG recordings provided further useful information.

In only 3 instances was FDG-PET localization misleading. In these patients, with a temporal lobe SEEG ictal onset, extratemporal or contralateral hypometabolism was ascribed to nonepileptic structural defects. The

Sensitivity and Specificity of EEG, FDG-PET, and SEEG Studies in Patients Studied With Depth Electrodes Who Had Epileptiform Regions Localized by Some Method

	Scalp sphenoidal ictal onsets	PET	SEEG ictal onsets
Lateralization			
True	58 (49%)	76 (64%)	114 (93%)
False	3 (3%)	2* (2%)	2 (2%)
Localization			
True	56 (47%)	71 (60%)	114 (93%)
False	5 (4%)	7*† (6%)	2 (2%)
No information	58 (49%)	41 (34%)	6 (5%)
Total	119	119	122

*Includes 2 patients with contralateral hypometabolism caused by depth electrode artifacts.

†Includes 1 patient with occipital hypometabolism caused by previous suboccipital surgery, 2 patients with hemispheric hypometabolism, and 2 patients for whom localization of the epileptogenic region remains in doubt.

(Courtesy of Engel J Jr, Henry TR, Risinger MW, et al: *Neurology* 40:1670–1677, 1990.)

scalp-sphenoidal ictal onset was misleading in 5 patients. Three others had nondiagnostic SEEG studies, and at least 1 of them may have been denied beneficial surgery as a result. SEEG recordings were by far the most accurate form of study (table).

Anterior temporal lobectomy may be carried out without chronic intracranial recording as long as specific criteria for a focal scalp-sphenoidal ictal EEG onset are met and hypometabolism is predominantly localized to the same temporal lobe. Nearly 25% of the present patients could have gone without the SEEG study. More quantitative PET analysis and better spatial tomographic resolution enhance the results of metabolic study.

▶ The UCLA group presents evidence that use of noninvasive PET and EEG may be used to select patients for anterior temporal lobectomy in certain instances. The results are interesting and appear to support this approach, but it should be pointed out that PET has not been widely used in other centers, and confirmatory data would be helpful here. In other centers, chronic depth electrode recordings will probably continue to be used for selection of patients for epilepsy surgery.—R.M. Crowell, M.D.

Anterior Temporal Lobectomy and Medically Refractory Temporal Lobe Epilepsy of Childhood
Mizrahi EM, Kellaway P, Grossman RG, Rutecki PA, Armstrong D, Rettig G, Loewen S (Baylor College of Medicine; The Methodist Hosp, Houston; Texas Children's Hosp, Houston)
Epilepsia 31:302–312, 1990   24–2

When medical treatment fails to control complex partial seizures (CPS) of temporal lobe origin, anterior temporal lobectomy may be considered. Surgery performed soon after it is determined that temporal lobe epilepsy is refractory to antiepileptic drugs may limit deterioration of quality of life in some cases. The value of early surgery was explored, and factors that may deter referral of children for early assessment of surgical control of epilepsy were investigated in 22 patients.

All had CPS with onset in childhood that proved refractory to drug treatment and arose from a temporal lobe. No clearly defined structural abnormalities were shown by CT or MRI in any of the patients. All 22 underwent anterior temporal lobectomy, with improvement in seizure control. Most (82%) had a reduction in seizure frequency of 95% or greater. Many patients had problems adjusting to a seizure-free life, with patients whose surgery was delayed until adulthood having a higher frequency of psychosocial, behavioral, and educational problems.

Although early surgery does not ensure a good outcome in all patients, anterior temporal lobectomy is an important, underused treatment for control of medically refractory temporal lobe epilepsy in children. Surgery done soon after medical intractability becomes evident may limit the problems associated with prolonged, uncontrolled seizures.

▶ This communication emphasizes once again that anterior temporal lobectomy should be offered promptly when medical treatment is ineffective in the treatment of temporal lobe epilepsy in childhood.—R.M. Crowell, M.D.

Language Function Following Anterior Temporal Lobectomy
Hermann BP, Wyler AR, Somes G (Baptist Mem Hosp, Memphis; Univ of Tennessee, Memphis; Semmes-Murphey Clinic, Memphis)
J Neurosurg 74:560–566, 1991   24–3

Functional mapping of cortical language ability is used in patients undergoing anterior temporal lobectomy for complex partial seizures of temporal lobe origin; however, not all patients can tolerate such surgery. To determine whether patients who do not have functional cortical mapping have postoperative language deficits, a prospective study was done using patients who underwent nondominant temporal lobectomy as controls.

The study sample comprised 64 consecutively treated patients who underwent partial resection of the anterior temporal lobe without functional mapping. Twenty-nine resections were in the dominant lobe and 35 in the nondominant lobe. Resection of the lateral temporal cortex was conservative, but that of the medial temporal cortex was aggressive. The Multilingual Aphasia Examination was done before surgery and 6 months postoperatively to assess the patients' language ability.

Patients who underwent dominant anterior temporal lobectomy had no significant losses of language function compared with patients who underwent nondominant lobectomy—reading comprehension was the only comparison that reached significance, with the dominant group scoring lower. Patients who underwent dominant lobectomy had significantly more improvement in complex receptive language comprehension than those who underwent nondominant lobectomy. Variables associated with postoperative language change were visual naming in the dominant lobectomy group, and oral fluency and token test in both groups.

Conservative resection of the lateral temporal cortex without language mapping appears to be an option for patients with complex partial seizures of medial temporal lobe origin. There is little risk to language function and an excellent surgical outcome. Presence of a lesion in the dominant lobe is not a contraindication to surgery.

▶ This series of 29 cases suggests that anterior temporal lobectomy in the dominant hemisphere for epilepsy can be carried out safely and effectively under general anesthesia. In fact, the authors suggest that the results are better than with language-mapping and local anesthesia, in that microdissection of mesial structures can be carried out with greater precision. This approach is counter to the experience of Ojemann and colleagues at the University of Washington, but further experience (with follow-up including MRI) is needed to establish the best technique here.—R.M. Crowell, M.D.

Magnetoencephalographic Localization of Interictal Spike Sources: Case Report

Eisenberg HM, Papanicolaou AC, Baumann SB, Rogers RL, Brown LM (Univ of Texas, Galveston; Transitional Learning Community, Galveston)
J Neurosurg 74:660–664, 1991   24–4

Magnetoencephalography (MEG) is more accurate than EEG in estimating the location, strength, and orientation of interictal spike sources. Magnetoencephalography was used to localize interictal spike sources in a patient with focal temporal epilepsy.

Man, 27, had a history of seizures since childhood that were uncontrolled with a variety of drugs. He had 5 or 6 partial complex seizures per month in the 6 months before operation. He had a T4 spike and slow-wave epileptiform discharge on routine surface EEG and high-amplitude spikes and spike and slow-wave discharges localized to SP2 and T4 on EEG monitoring with sphenoidal electrodes. The patient underwent right temporal lobectomy with electrocorticography performed from the exposed cortex. He underwent 2 preoperative MEG examinations 1 month apart in a magnetically shielded room. The estimated sources were projected onto MR images of the patient's brain and were found to lie within 1 cm of each other within the resected area. Intraoperative cortical findings correlated well with the MEG localization. The patient was free of seizures 7 months postoperatively.

Magnetoencephalography can be a reliable technique for localizing interictal spike sources in patients with epilepsy. Estimated sources fall in the area indicated by preoperative and intraoperative EEG.

▶ This sample case report supports the reliability of spike localization by MEG in focal epilepsy. Further experience is needed to establish this technique as superior to other methods.— R.M. Crowell, M.D.

Influence of Intraoperative Antibiotic Choice on the Incidence of Early Postcraniotomy Seizures

Michenfelder JD, Cucchiara RF, Sundt TM Jr (Mayo Clin and Found, Rochester, Minn)
J Neurosurg 72:703–705, 1990   24–5

There is concern that the intraoperative administration of penicillin might cause early postoperative seizures in patients undergoing craniotomy. For this reason, an attempt was begun in 1987 at the Mayo Clinic to use nonpenicillin antibiotics in this setting. Records were reviewed for a total of 1,316 procedures. A penicillin, usually nafcillin, was the primary antibiotic used in 518 procedures done between 1984 and 1985 and in 101 of the 658 done between 1987 and 1988.

None of 323 patients experienced seizures after suboccipital craniectomy. Among 993 patients undergoing supratentorial procedures were 30 who had seizures within 6 hours of surgery; 19 of them had generalized seizures. Early seizures occurred in 4.7% of patients given penicillins and in 1.8% of the others, a significant difference. The relationship between penicillin and early seizures persisted after patients operated on for intractable seizures were excluded. One nafcillin-treated patient with intractable seizures had generalized convulsions postoperatively and died. Penicillins should be avoided, if possible, during and soon after craniotomy in patients operated on for supratentorial pathology.

▶ This study convincingly demonstrates an increase in seizures in patients given penicillin antibiotics in relation to craniotomy for supratentorial pathology. Nonpenicillin antibiotics (e.g., vancomycin) are recommended instead of penicillin in these patients. The report illustrates how a hunch can be substantiated by careful statistical analysis of a problem.—R.M. Crowell, M.D.

Other

Fetal Homotransplants (Ventral Mesencephalon and Adrenal Tissue) to the Striatum of Parkinsonian Subjects

Madrazo I, Franco-Bourland R, Ostrosky-Solis F, Aguilera M, Cuevas C, Zamorano C, Morelos A, Magallon E, Guizar-Sahagun G (Inst Mexicano del Seguro Social, Mexico City; Inst Nacional de la Nutricion Salvador Zubiran, Mexico City; Univ Nacional Autonoma de Mexico, Mexico City)
Arch Neurol 47:1281–1285, 1990   24–6

Adrenal medullary autografts are beneficial to young patients with mild Parkinson's disease, but they are less helpful and more dangerous in severely ill or elderly patients. Animal experiments indicate that implantation of fetal tissue can ameliorate altered motor function and improve biochemical, behavioral, and histologic parameters.

Six men and 1 woman with idiopathic Parkinson's disease received fetal homotransplants. The mean age was 48.4 years and the mean duration of illness was 8.9 years. The mean dose of levodopa was 946.4 mg/day, but the beneficial effects were gradually decreasing. Fetal ventral mesencephalon was used in 4 patients and fetal adrenal tissue was used in 3, with grafting to the caudate nucleus. The donor tissue came from spontaneous abortions of healthy fetuses certified as dead by 2 pediatricians unrelated to the transplant group. All recipients received immunosuppression therapy with cyclosporine A before and after surgery.

In the 4 patients who received ventral mesencephalon grafts, rigidity, bradykinesia, postural imbalance, gait disturbance, and facial expression were significantly ameliorated, although tremor remained. Three of these patients were able to return to work. In the 3 patients who received adrenal tissue grafts improvements were less dramatic, with amelioration in only rigidity and bradykinesia. All were able to resume their basic daily activities and 1 was able to resume her household tasks, but the other 2 could not return to work. There were no surgical problems, although 1 patient contracted an infection of the bone flap and had a brain abscess related to the immunosuppression and another had a deep vein thrombosis of the leg.

Results of early experiments with fetal brain tissue transplantation for Parkinson's disease are encouraging, but much further study is required. The mechanism of action of brain grafts is unknown. The better results achieved with ventral mesencephalon grafting may have been related to the heterogeneity of the disease or type of graft, or both.

▶ In this report, encouraging results are reported for transplantation of fetal brain tissue to the striatum of parkinsonian subjects. It is to be noted that this is the same Mexican group that reported with such enthusiasm positive results for adrenal-to-intracranial transplantation several years ago. It is also important to note that further careful studies have failed to bear out a substantial beneficial effect for standard adrenal-to-intracranial grafting in Parkinson's disease. Thus extreme caution is advisable in interpretation of the present studies. Certainly, much more work will be required by other workers to confirm or disprove the validity of these results.— R.M. Crowell, M.D.

Continuous Infusion of Intrathecal Baclofen: Long-Term Effects on Spasticity in Spinal Cord Injury
Loubser PG, Narayan RK, Sandin KJ, Donovan WH, Russell KD (Baylor College of Medicine, Houston)
Paraplegia 29:48–64, 1991   24–7

Previous studies reported encouraging results with the use of intrathecal baclofen for the treatment of intractable spasticity in spinal cord injury patients. A 2-stage, placebo-controlled trial of intrathecal baclofen was performed in 9 men with traumatic, nonprogressive spinal cord injury whose spasticity had been refractory to conventional treatment, including oral baclofen.

Stage 1 consisted of a 5-day dose-finding phase during which either baclofen or placebo was infused percutaneously via an external pump. Clinical evaluations included measurement of spasticity using the Ashworth and neurologic reflex scales, assessment of functional abilities and personal independence, and a global assessment scale. All data were obtained at the start of the trial, after infusion of the amount of baclofen that provided optimal control of spasticity, and after intrathecal placebo infusion. In stage 2 of the study, 7 patients underwent implantation of a permanent programmable infusion pump. The other 2 patients did not want to undergo follow-up laboratory testing or permanent infusion pump implantation.

Neurophysiologic testing before and after intrathecal baclofen administration showed multiple changes, including decreased or absent withdrawal from plantar stimulation in 4 patients, higher thresholds for triggering spasms in 2, and decrease of minimal voluntary motor control in 2. One patient had no changes on any of the parameters tested. Electromyographic examination of the lower extremity musculature confirmed diminished reflex motor activity in 5 patients. Isokinetic dynamometry showed evidence of narrowing of the hysteresis loop after baclofen infu-

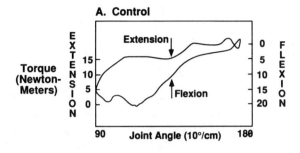

A. Control

Torque
(Newton-
Meters)

EXTENSION

15
10
5
0

Extension

Flexion

90   Joint Angle (10°/cm)   180

0
5
10
15
20

FLEXION

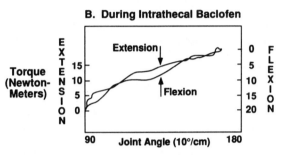

B. During Intrathecal Baclofen

Torque
(Newton-
Meters)

EXTENSION

15
10
5
0

Extension

Flexion

90   Joint Angle (10°/cm)   180

0
5
10
15
20

FLEXION

Fig 24–1.—Representative change in isokinetic dynamometry, obtained by moving the right knee (angular velocity—120 degrees per second) through 90–180 degrees passively. The force produced in hamstrings (extension) and quadriceps (flexion), before (**A**) and during intrathecal baclofen (**B**) is demonstrated. (Courtesy of Loubser PG, Narayan RK, Sandin KJ, et al: *Paraplegia* 29:48–64, 1991.)

sion in 4 patients, indicative of a decreased tone in response to stretch (Fig 24–1). Complications were minor, and pump-related infections did not occur. There was no clinical evidence of any significant neurotoxicity in either stage of the study, but the only ambulatory patient in this study experienced marked lower extremity weakness during stage 1 and was temporarily unable to walk. Intrathecally administered baclofen is effective and safe for the control of spasticity in spinal cord injury patients who are refractory to conventional oral medications.

▶ This careful and intensive study of 9 spinal cord injury patients confirms the effectiveness and safety of intrathecal baclofen in the treatment of refractory spasticity (1).—R.M. Crowell, M.D.

Reference

1. Penn RD, et al: *N Engl J Med* 320:1517, 1989.

Idiopathic (Vago)-Glossopharyngeal Neuralgia: Analysis of 14 Personal Cases and Literature Review
Sindou M, Henry JF, Blanchard P (Univ de Lyon; Hôp Jules-Courmont, Pierre-Benite, France)
Neurochirurgie 37:18–25, 1991   24–8

Idiopathic neuralgia of the ninth nerve, also known as glossopharyn-geal neuralgia, may involve both the throat and the ear, or the throat or the ear independently. Neuralgia of the ninth nerve is rare compared to neuralgia of the fifth nerve or trigeminal neuralgia, representing only .75% to 1% of all cases of trigeminal neuralgia.

During a 12-year period 7 men and 7 women aged 32–81 years had surgery for idiopathic glossopharyngeal neuralgia. Thirteen of the 14 had left-sided involvement. Four patients had concomitant ipsilateral trigemi-nal neuralgia. In all cases, medical treatment was ineffective or patients had become resistant to drug therapy. All patients underwent extensive evaluation before operation to eliminate other etiologies for their pain.

Most patients could not accurately depict their pain, but 3 described it as a burning sensation and 2 as an electric discharge. Pain episodes lasted from 10 seconds to 3 minutes, followed by pain-free periods. Two pa-tients regularly fainted during pain.

Surgical treatment consisted of percutaneous thermocoagulation of the Andersh ganglion in 3 patients; microsurgical vascular decompression at the level of the ninth and tenth nerves in 9 patients, 1 of whom also un-derwent rhizotomy of the ninth nerve; and simple rhizotomy in 2 patients because no neurovascular abnormalities were found at operation. Ther-mocoagulation had to be discontinued in the first patient because of cor-onary pain. The procedure was then done under general anesthesia in the next 2 patients.

Total relief of pain was achieved in 2 of the 3 thermocoagulated pa-tients and in all of those having microvascular decompression. During a follow-up of 2 months to 10 years, all 13 patients remained free of neu-ralgia. Complications of thermocoagulation included permanent hypoes-thesia in the area of the ninth and tenth nerves, difficulty in swallowing, and large hematomas at the puncture sites. The patients treated by rhizo-tomy also had some permanent neurologic deficits. In contrast, 2 of the 9 patients who underwent microvascular decompression had no complica-tions, and the others had varying degrees of mild, transitory neurologic sequelae. Microvascular decompression via a direct approach is the rec-ommended treatment for idiopathic glossopharyngeal neuralgia. It pro-vides uniformly good results with the fewest complications.

▶ The authors report 14 cases of glossopharyngeal neuralgia treated surgically. They achieved total pain relief in 13 cases. Surgery consisted of percutaneous thermal coagulation in 3 cases, microvascular decompression in 9, and root section in 2. Surgical treatment should be strongly considered in these pa-tients, who require the most delicate evaluation and preoperative imaging.— R.M. Crowell, M.D.

25 Nerve

Surgical Decompression Without Transposition for Ulnar Neuropathy: Factors Determining Outcome
LeRoux PD, Ensign TD, Burchiel KJ (Seattle VA Med Ctr; Univ of Washington)
Neurosurgery 27:709–714, 1990   25–1

There is still disagreement on the correct surgical treatment of ulnar neuropathy. Given the pathophysiologic evidence of involvement of the cubital tunnel in ulnar neuropathy, simple decompression has become the authors' standard procedure for the treatment of this disorder. To assess which factors correlate with outcome, 51 surgical decompressions without nerve transposition for ulnar neuropathy in 46 patients were studied retrospectively. The disease was bilateral in 5 patients and involved the nondominant arm in 24. The average follow-up period was 17.8 months (range, 5–32 months).

Decompression was performed under local anesthesia, and the nerve remained undisturbed in the cubital tunnel (Fig 25–1). Operative findings included compression of the nerve predominantly in the epicondylar groove in all cases, narrowing of the nerve in 28 (55%), dense scar tissue adherent to the nerve in 21 (41%), and 2 pseudoneuromas (4%).

Symptomatic improvement was achieved in 41 (80%) surgical decompressions, mostly within the first month after surgery. Patients with pain,

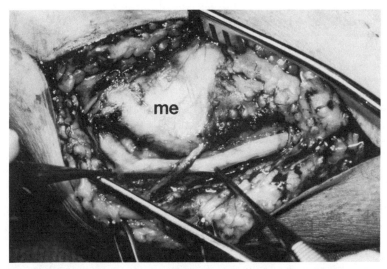

Fig 25–1.—Intraoperative photograph at completion of decompression of the ulnar nerve in the cubital tunnel. The nerve remains undisturbed in the cubital tunnel behind the medial epicondyle *(me)*. (Courtesy of LeRoux PD, Ensign TD, Burchiel KJ: *Neurosurgery* 27:709–714, 1990.)

paresthesias, and sensory impairments responded better to surgery than did those with muscular atrophy. Similarly, patients with symptoms of less than 1 year's duration were helped more by surgery than those with symptoms of longer duration. The combination of muscle wasting and symptoms of more than 1 year's duration was an adverse prognostic factor. The relative magnitude of the slowing of the ulnar nerve conduction velocity across the elbow and the operative findings did not correlate with outcome.

Simple decompression without transposition of the ulnar nerve may be an effective treatment for selected cases of ulnar neuropathy. Patients with progressive and intractable pain and sensory impairment should undergo surgery before the development of muscular atrophy, because both a long duration of symptoms and the presence of atrophy are predictive of a poor response to surgery.

▶ This carefully described series demonstrates that simple decompression without transposition of the ulnar nerve is an effective treatment for ulnar compressive neuropathy. Simple decompression is quicker, easier, and safer than transposition. It can be done under local anesthesia with minimal sedation. Complications of nerve kinking, ischemia, and fibrosis can be avoided. This would appear to be the treatment of choice for compressive ulnar neuropathy at the elbow.—R.M. Crowell, M.D.

Morphofunctional Evaluation of Fibrin Glue Versus Microsuture Nerve Repairs
Maragh H, Meyer BS, Davenport D, Gould JD, Terzis JK (Eastern Virginia Med School, Norfolk; Microsurgical Research Ctr, Norfolk)
J Reconstr Microsurg 6:331–337, 1990   25–2

Microsuture repair of peripheral nerves is subject to a range of complications, and in some situations (e.g., limited exposure or very fine structures) suture repair is virtually impossible. A study was done in rats to test the efficacy of fibrin glue repair versus microsuture coaptation.

The study animals were 25 male Sprague-Dawley rats whose left and right sciatic nerves were exposed, sectioned, and repaired by either tissue glue coaptation or standard microsuture nerve repair techniques. The fibrinogen-based tissue glue mixture Tisseel was used on 1 side and 3 equidistant 10–0 monofilament nylon sutures were used on the contralateral side. The repairs were tested for tensile strength, compound action potential (CAP) recordings (Fig 25–2) and quantitative morphometry.

There were no significant differences in tensile strength between the 2 types of repairs at 2, 4, and 8 weeks after surgery, although the microsuture repairs tended to have a stronger hold. On CAP recordings microsuture repairs were found to have significantly faster conduction velocities at onset, larger areas under the curve, and higher peak amplitudes. There were no significant differences in onset and peak latencies. Histologic studies showed no significant difference in axonal counts proximal and

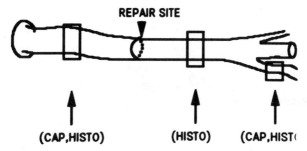

Fig 25–2.—Biopsy sites. *Abbreviation: HISTO,* histologic evaluation. (Courtesy of Maragh H, Meyer BS, Davenport D, et al: *J Reconstr Microsurg* 6:331–337, 1990.)

distal to the repair; however, suture repairs seemed to have more myelinated axons. Fibrin glue failed to maintain coaptation in 13% of repairs.

Although sutureless repairs hold great promise in the future of microneurovascular surgery, the use of tissue glue is associated with some undesirable effects. With tissue glue repairs a somewhat smaller population of regenerating axons reach the distal nerve branches and the conductive properties of these axons appear to be compromised. Future research may include preparations of glues that use the patient's own serum.

▶ These studies argue for the superiority of microsuture repair as compared with fibrin glue repair.— R.M. Crowell, M.D.

Posterior Interosseous Nerve Palsies
Cravens G, Kline DG (Louisiana State Univ; Charity Hosp, New Orleans)
Neurosurgery 27:397–402, 1990   25–3

Isolated weakness of muscles innervated by the posterior interosseous nerve is rare, and the diagnosis may be missed because wrist drop does not occur. Traumatic paralysis of this nerve can occur with open injuries to the proximal forearm. Closed injuries caused by radial fracture also can produce paralysis. Nontraumatic progressive paralysis may result from inflammatory states (e.g., rheumatoid arthritis) or compression by a local mass (Fig 25–3).

Of 170 patients seen in a 15-year period with radial nerve disorders, 32 had involvement only of the posterior interosseous nerve. Weak wrist extension with a radial drift and difficulty extending the fingers characterized these cases. Thumb extension was paralyzed and thumb abduction was weak. The most frequent causes were entrapment at the arcade of Froshe, laceration, and fracture.

Twenty-six patients were operated on, 2 for bilateral lesions. All operated-on nerves had function of grade 3 or more of a possible 5 after 4 years of follow-up, and 7 had normal function. Twenty-three nerves were in continuity, often conducting action potentials of low amplitude across the lesion. Four nerves underwent neurolysis and 4 were managed by

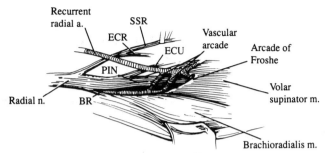

Fig 25–3.—Drawing of the relationship of anatomical structures at the level of the elbow. *ECR* = extensor carpi radialis branch; *ECU* = extensor carpi ulnaris branch; *PIN* = posterior interosseous nerve; *SSR* = superficial sensory radial nerve; *BR* = brachioradialis branch. (Courtesy of Cravens G, Kline DG: *Neurosurgery* 27:397–402, 1990.)

graft or suture repair. Three of 5 nerves not in continuity required graft repair.

Lesions of the posterior interosseous nerve may simulate more proximal nerve injuries clinically. Surgery should be considered if function does not return within 3 months. Good results can be expected from neurolysis or repair by direct suture or an interfascicular graft.

▶ This important article documents the experience in Dr. Kline's unit at Louisiana State University. In a 15-year period, 170 patients with radial nerve disorders were seen, 32 of whom had selective involvement of the posterior interosseous nerve.

Lesions involving this nerve may present with a picture simulating more proximal radial nerve entry, especially in the setting of injury at the elbow and forearm. Patients without return of function clinically or electrically after 3 months may be candidates for surgical exploration. Neurolysis, direct suture, or interfascicular grafts have provided good to excellent results in almost all cases.—R.M. Crowell, M.D.

Progress in Peripheral Nerve Reconstruction
Millesi H (Univ of Vienna, Austria)
World J Surg 14:733–747, 1990   25–4

The advent of microsurgical techniques and optical magnification in the 1970s laid the groundwork for modern neurolysis, neurorrhaphy, and nerve grafting. External neurolysis has always been an effective approach to peripheral nerve reconstruction. One goal is to free the nerve from adhesions to surrounding tissue. Whether internal neurolysis is a useful technique remains controversial; many have had adverse experiences with the procedure. Any operation that transects the epifascicular epineurium to open up the nerve trunk may be considered internal neurolysis. The goal is to decompress the trunk, fascicle groups, and, eventually, individual nerve fascicles. The limit of the procedure is when the nerve trunk is totally fibrotic, or when the fascicles are fibrotic and the fascicular structure of the nerve is lost.

End-to-end nerve repair is the best way of restoring continuity to a transected nerve, but it is not always feasible. In a clean transection without loss of neural tissue, the gap between the stumps can easily be overcome by applying a small force to elongate nerve tissue on either side. The merits of epineural versus fascicular nerve repair are still debated.

Methods of differentiating between motor and sensory fibers will make neurorrhaphy more functionally effective. Possible approaches to managing a nerve defect include shortening the distance between the nerve stumps (as by resecting a bone segment), elongating nerve tissue through implantation of a tissue expander, and adding new tissue, through either grafting or the spontaneous outgrowth of nerve tissue in a predefined direction.

Several different nerve grafting methods are available. Only a free nerve graft having a large surface in relation to its diameter has a chance of totally surviving without becoming fibrotic. Some nerves can be transferred as island flaps to preserve existing vascularization. Microvascular techniques make it possible to transplant a nerve on its vascular pedicle through microvascular anastomosis.

▶ This article reviews the current status of nerve reconstruction as described by the world leader in the field. The present approach emphasizes microsurgical techniques with precise microsuture and grafting where necessary. The success and failure of this approach is outlined nicely, emphasizing the relatively poor results in the severe injuries, despite modern technique.—R.M. Crowell, M.D.

26 Miscellany

North American Symptomatic Carotid Endarterectomy Trial: Methods, Patient Characteristics, and Progress
Barnett HJM, for the North American Symptomatic Carotid Endarterectomy Trial (NASCET) Steering Committee (The John P. Robarts Research Inst, London, Ont)
Stroke 22:711–720, 1991   26–1

Fifty North American centers have attempted to determine the benefit of carotid endarterectomy to patients who have symptoms caused by arteriosclerotic carotid stenosis. Patients younger than 80 years of age were entered into the trial within 4 months of a hemispheric transient ischemic attack or nondisabling stroke. All had angiographic evidence of at least 30% stenosis in the appropriate carotid vessel. Between 1988 and 1990, 596 patients were randomized to receive optimal medical care, including antiplatelet drugs, and 616 to undergo carotid endarterectomy.

Survivors were followed for an average of 18 months. Perioperative stroke morbidity and mortality totalled 5%; 3% of medically treated patients had stroke morbidity or mortality during a similar 1-month period. The risk of any stroke or death from any cause was reduced by endarterectomy in patients with 70% or greater carotid stenosis. The absolute risk reduction exceeded 7%. Benefit was apparent within 3 months of surgery. Crossover from the medical to the surgical arm of the study was 4.2%.

The trial was stopped subsequently for patients with 70% or greater carotid stenosis. Whether symptomatic patients with moderate carotid stenosis or asymptomatic patients will benefit from endarterectomy remains to be determined.

▶ This is probably the most important investigation in clinical neuroscience reported in 1991. At last, reliable controlled data have demonstrated the superiority of carotid endarterectomy over medical treatment for patients with internal carotid artery stenosis of 70% to 99%. The numbers are substantial, the statistical methods powerful, and the results irrefutable. Moreover, the tighter the stenosis, the greater the benefit. It is interesting to note that the 70% stenosis is just about equivalent to the 2-mm stenosis suggested by Dr. Fisher years ago as appropriate for endarterectomy. It should be emphasized, however, that further studies of lesser degrees of stenosis are required to determine the anticipated threshold stenotic value below which endarterectomy is no longer superior to medical treatment. The study again emphasizes the great importance of controlled randomized investigation with proper statistical validation for the establishment of indications for clinical treatment methodologies.

Hats off to Dr. Barnett and his group for a spectacular study! Carotid endarterectomy makes a stunning comeback.—R.M. Crowell, M.D.

State of the Art in Perioperative Prophylaxis of Thrombo-Embolism in Neurosurgery

Moskopp D, Popov-Cenič S (Rheinische Friedrich Wilhelms-Univ Bonn, Germany)

Neurochirurgia 33:137–145, 1990   26–2

The efficacy of prophylactic low-molecular-weight heparin therapy in the prevention of thromboembolic complications in the non-neurosurgical specialties has been well documented. Neurosurgery is in a unique position in that none of the drugs used prophylactically in general surgery are currently recommended for use in neurosurgery. One of the problems in evaluating the efficacy of prophylactic drugs for neurosurgical use is that none of the available studies has included a sufficient number of neurosurgical patients to support statistically valid conclusions.

Although no specific drugs are recommended, thromboembolism prophylaxis is used in neurosurgery, but each center follows its own guidelines. Most centers currently base their decision to use prophylactic drug therapy on individual assessment of risk factors in a given patient. Some centers do not use prophylactic drug therapy in any of their patients, relying only on mechanical measures (e.g., early mobilization and physical therapy), whereas others use drug therapy in almost all of their patients with the exception of those with subarachnoid hemorrhage.

An additional problem in arriving at statistically valid recommendations for prophylactic drug therapy in neurosurgery is the fact that there is no international consensus on how to design controlled, prospective, clinical trials. In France and Germany, low-molecular-weight heparin cannot be compared with placebo for ethical reasons, and only conventional heparinization may be used for comparison. In contrast, the use of placebo is allowed in North America and Canada.

A review of the literature shows a multitude of available diagnostic and therapeutic regimens, many of which give contradictory results. There is not even agreement on whether the use of prophylactic drug therapy is ultimately cost saving; some reports state that the general use of thromboembolism prophylaxis is more expensive than individual treatment of thrombosis once it has occurred, whereas others report the opposite. However, the additional cost of prophylaxis would be justifiable economically if it could be shown that prophylaxis improves the quality of life, a fact that remains to be established for neurosurgical patients. The current status of the perioperative use of prophylactic drug treatment in the prevention of thromboembolism in neurosurgical patients suggests the need for a large, prospective, controlled, multicenter clinical trial among neurosurgical centers.

▶ This communication reviews a large number of studies on the prophylaxis of thromboembolic complications in neurosurgery. Although prophylaxis in many branches of surgery is currently recommended, this is not the case in neurosurgery because of fear of intracranial hemorrhage. After a study of these various investigations, the authors suggest that a controlled, multicenter, randomized trial be undertaken to establish a more scientifically valid approach to the prevention of these devastating complications.—R.M. Crowell, M.D.

Outcomes Management
Langfitt TW (Glenmede Trust Co, Philadelphia)
Surg Neurol 35:111–115, 1991   26–3

The goal of outcomes management is to help patients, care providers, and payers to make rational care-related choices by assessing how these choices will affect the patient's life. Greater reliance is placed on standards and guidelines than physicians are able to use in selective interventions. There are systematic estimates of general well-being and functioning, as well as measurements of disease-specific clinical outcomes. Clinical data are pooled on a very large scale so that results can be compared for similar types of patients. Results of analyzing each segment of the database are conveyed to the appropriate decision-makers (patients and third-party payers).

Through outcomes management, physicians will have ready access to information on clinical outcomes for patients in each disease category with which they deal. Physicians cannot clearly appreciate their clinical experience without the means of accurately and quantitatively analyzing their practices. All results are available for all to see. Busy physicians may find the system overly time consuming and cumbersome, which leads to questions of whether they will learn to practice outcomes management.

First-year medical students should begin their education in outcomes management, learning the concepts involved and how to enter clinical data into the database. In year 2, they learn how to compare groups of patients having the same disorder. Outcomes management will encourage continuity of care in the later school years and in postgraduate training.

Through outcomes management, physicians will better understand their long-term patient responsibilities and the nature of their practices. They can improve management practices on a continuing basis; in a sense, each practitioner will become a clinical investigator.

▶ Dr. Langfitt provides yet another interesting insight into the complexities of modern medical practice. In this contribution, he describes outcomes management, a technology utilizing definition of interventions, measurement of patient functioning, pooling of clinical data, and results analysis according to treatment modalities and providers. The essence of the approach is assessment of quality of care. This issue is of paramount importance to all interested in health care, and it carries some threat to individual practitioners. Nonetheless, Langfitt stresses the utility of the method and the value of accepting and promulgating this approach in the practice of medicine and in medical education.—R.M. Crowell, M.D.

Gene Mapping and Other Tools for Discovery

Leppert MF (Univ of Utah)
Epilepsia 31:S11–S18, 1990
26–4

Gene mapping studies can assist in understanding the molecular basis of inherited diseases for which the biochemical basis is unknown. For these studies each family member must submit sufficient peripheral blood to obtain enough DNA substrate for genotypic characterization. The typical amount of DNA substrate needed is .3–1 mg. Mapping studies may be done in a single, large pedigree for studies of dominant inheritance. The number of affected individuals sampled should be as large as possible to obtain the best estimate of gene recombination. Nuclear families with more than 1 affected sibling may provide the best information for studies of recessive inheritance. The recent development of more than 1,000 polymorphic DNA markers for the genome is the basis for the success of genetic mapping; in a family that is segregating a disease allele, there is a good probability that at least 1 marker will be linked to the disease marker.

Restriction fragment length polymorphisms (RFLPs) make up most of the markers in current use. The RFLPs, which result from single-base-pair-substitutions or from the presence of a variable number of tandemly repeated oligonucleotide units at a locus (VNTRs), are recognized by digesting DNA with restriction enzymes and separating the fragments according to size on an electrophoretic gel. The VNTRs provide more linkage information than single-site polymorphisms because family members are more likely to be heterozygous. Using linkage data relating marker loci to each other in normal families, genetic maps can be constructed to facilitate the search for disease genes. Once a disease gene has been localized to a specific chromosomal region, cytogenetic or molecular rearrangements in affected individuals and candidate genes known to be in the region can be used to identify the gene. The same clinical phenotype may be caused by more than 1 gene and families may have nongenetic phenotypes, both of which may obscure genetic linkage findings.

Gene mapping is an effective means of localizing and identifying genes in inherited disease, despite its limitations. It is hoped that this technique will aid in understanding of the inherited forms of epilepsy.

▶ All clinicians should be aware of the enormous strides being made by neuro-genetics. Correlation of extensive pedigree data with gene mapping studies has led to important advances in a number of areas, e.g., identification of the neurofibromatosis gene and the gene for benign familial neonatal convulsions (described in this article). It is likely that other genes will be identified that control the development of intracranial gliomas and other tumors, and it is possible that other neurologic conditions (e.g., intracranial aneurysm) will also be found to have a neurogenetic basis.—R.M. Crowell, M.D.

New Triple Coaxial Catheter System for Carotid Angioplasty With Cerebral Protection

Theron J, Courtheoux P, Alachkar F, Bouvard G, Maiza D (Ctr Hosp Univ de Caen, France)
Am J Neuroradiol 11:869–874, 1990   26–5

The fear of dislodging an embolus from an ulcerative plaque in patients undergoing percutaneous transluminal angioplasty (PTA) of a stenotic carotid artery has led to the development of a catheter system designed to protect the cerebral circulation during PTA. With this technique, the flow within the internal carotid artery is temporarily arrested during manipulation of the ulcerated plaques. A new triple coaxial catheter system was developed that simplifies the technique.

Thirteen patients aged 55–77 years with stenosis of a carotid artery ranging from 70% to more than 95% underwent PTA with the complete triple coaxial system. In 5 patients, obviously ulcerated plaque was observed angiographically. All patients underwent Doppler studies before and after treatment. The mean follow-up period was 8½ months.

In 10 patients a normal or subnormal diameter of the dilated carotid artery was obtained. The aspirated blood was analyzed for 6 patients. Four blood samples contained large cholesterol crystals with sizes ranging from 600 to 1200 μm. Of the 3 patients in whom a normal or subnormal diameter was not obtained, 1 had a 30% residual stenosis on the immediate post-angioplasty angiogram, but the arterial wall had a smooth appearance and there was no residual hemodynamic modification on Doppler examination. The second patient had a persistent 50% stenosis of the internal carotid that was hemodynamically significant on Doppler study. The third patient had a 20% residual stenosis that was not significant on Doppler examination. None of the patients experienced local or neurologic complications during or after angioplasty, and none has had further symptoms since undergoing the procedure. The new triple coaxial catheter system for carotid angioplasty that incorporates cerebral protection appears to prevent iatrogenic emboli from reaching the cerebral circulation.

▶ This communication describes a new triple-lumen catheter system for carotid angioplasty together with initial results in 13 cases. This ingenious device permits balloon angioplasty of the carotid, with a distal balloon acting as an umbrella to catch the debris. A third lumen is used to withdraw the debris from the trapped proximal internal carotid artery (ICA) by irrigation-suction. In essence, this system answers the persistent critique that ICA angioplasty will lead to embolic stroke.

Results in 13 cases have been encouraging, with technical success in the great majority and no new deficits after angioplasty. The report is extremely promising. Nonetheless, establishment of indications for the method must await controlled clinical trials. It is worth noting that the results of surgery are so good in symptomatic patients with tight stenosis that demonstration of superior results will take a truly remarkable track record.—R.M. Crowell, M.D.

Subject Index

A

Abscess
  spinal epidural
    MRI and nonoperative treatment,
      370
    ten-year perspective, 369
Acquired immunodeficiency syndrome
  in child, stroke in, 87
Adenosine
  for hypotension during cerebral
    aneurysm surgery, 221
Adolescence
  dyslexia during, MRI of planum
    temporale in, 30
Adrenal
  tissue fetal homotransplant in
    Parkinson's disease, 377
Adrenoleukodystrophy
  X-linked, of marrow transplant, 190
Aged
  anesthesia and superior brain functions,
    172
  brain tumors, malignant, increasing
    incidence, 248
  cerebrovascular disease, silent, 54
  dementia, general practitioners'
    detection of, 113
  depression, general practitioners'
    detection of, 113
  influenza vaccine for, adverse reactions
    to, 163
Agenesis
  callosal, stereo perception in, 36
Aging
  coronary artery disease in Alzheimer's
    disease, 48
AIDS
  in child, stroke in, 87
Albendazole
  in cisticercosis, subarachnoid and
    ventricular, 368
Alcohol
  excessive drinkers with peripheral
    neuropathy, thiamine in, 140
Alzheimer's disease
  coronary artery disease and aging, 48
  familial, amyloid precursor protein gene
    mutation in, 46
  genetic linkage studies in, 45
  myoclonus in, 49
  paratonia in, 49
  seizures in, 49
Amnesia
  memory for temporal order of events in,
    34

transient
  global, case review and follow-up,
    169
  syndromes, toward a classification of,
    170
Amyloid protein (*see* Protein, amyloid)
Amyotrophic
  lateral sclerosis, lymphoma and motor
    neuron disease, 147
Analgesic
  effects of caffeine in headache, 109
Anastomosis
  STA-MCA, for ischemic oculopathy,
    316
Anesthesia
  brain functions and, superior, in aged,
    172
  spinal, continuous, cauda equina
    syndrome after, 154
Aneurysm(s)
  basilar artery
    bifurcation and trunk, 214
    temporary balloon occlusion of,
      227
  basilar-vertebro systems, MRI of, 287
  carotid
    artery, bifurcation, direct surgery,
      271
    artery, temporary balloon occlusion
      of, 227
    giant, rupture after bypass, 277
    -ophthalmic artery, giant, clipping,
      274
  cerebellar artery
    endovascular coil, embolization of,
      226
    trigeminal sensory loss secondary to,
      276
  of cerebellar artery-vertebral artery
    complex, 275
  cerebral
    angiography (in primate), 263
    artery, saccular, 272
    blood flow patterns in (in rat), 264
    intracranial, elastic skeleton (in rat),
      265
    ruptured, angiography missing, 269
    surgery, hypotension control with
      adenosine or nitroprusside during,
      221
  Hunt and Hess grades IV and V, case
    review, 280
  intracavernous giant, carotid saphenous
    vein graft for, 217
  intracranial
    cerebral, elastic skeleton (in rat), 265
    endovascular treatment, 223

Author Index

A

Abe, M., 305
Abumi, K., 336
Adams, H.P., Jr., 56
Adams, R.D., 295
Adour, K.K., 192
Agnew, R.A.L., 139
Aguilera, M., 377
Ahmed, M., 329
Akamatsu, H., 206
Akar, M., 354
Alachkar, F., 391
Alberman, E., 146
Albers, J.J., 188
Albert, M.L., 37
Albert, P., 297
Aldrich, E.F., 322
Alexander, M.P., 40
Al-Mefty, O., 218, 241
Al-Rajeh, S.M., 142
Altenburger, H., 172
Altschuler, E.M., 236
Aminoff, M.J., 21
Andersen, A.R., 105
Andersen, L.B., 143
Anderson, D.E., 284
Anderson, G., 155
Ando, T., 297
Andoh, T., 287
Andrewes, D.G., 131
Angelini, C., 189
Anscher, M., 365
Anson, J.A., 277
Antti-Poika, I., 327
Aparisi, R., 175
Appel, S., 161
Apuzzo, M.L.J., 368
Ariyasu, L., 192
Armstrong, D., 374
Arnaudo, E., 189
Arnon, R., 161
Arrótegui, J., 329
Asada, M., 274
Asano, Y., 297
Asari, S., 289
Asfora, W.T., 305
Asner, N.G., 370
Assouline, E., 340
Aubourg, P., 190
Aurelius, E., 164
Ausman, J.I., 271
Autret, E., 96
Avery, D., 109
Avril, M.-F., 256
Awad, I.A., 302
Aymard, A., 225, 230
Aymard, G.A., 223

B

Baba, H., 339
Babikian, V.K., 37
Backhovens, H., 45
Bailes, J.E., 208
Bamford, J., 38
Banzet, P., 256
Barnes, R.W., 312
Barnett, G.H., 234
Barnett, H.J.M., 57, 387
Barnwell, S.L., 226, 233, 301
Barrios, C., 329
Barrow, D.L., 290
Barry, M.E., 215
Barta, P.E., 32
Basham, J.K., 137
Batjer, H.H., 228, 282
Batzdorf, U., 328
Baumann, S.B., 376
Baykut, L., 354
Beaglehole, R., 53
Beauvois, M.F., 35
Becker, D., 202
Becker, G.M., 205
Becker, L.E., 359
Beckman, C.S., 183
Beierwaltes, W.H., 235
Bell, R., 115
Bell, W.H., III, 314
Belles, A., 352
Belman, A.L., 87
Benech, F., 73
Benedetti, A., 239
Benedetti, T.J., 366
Bentson, J., 202
Berenstein, A., 342
Berger, M.L., 164
Berglund, G., 75
Bergman, H., 136
Berney, J., 248
Bernstein, L., 87
Bernstein, M., 235, 253
Bertrand, P., 96
Biary, N., 172
Bichard, W., 208
Bien, S., 225
Billard, C., 96
Biller, J., 56
Binda, A., 189
Bird, T.D., 49
Bisson, B.D., 188
Bissonette, D.J., 240
Bizzari, J.P., 256
Björnsson, A., 329
Black, K., 202
Black, K.L., 250
Bladin, P.F., 131
Blair, S.J., 343
Blanchard, P., 379
Blanche, S., 190
Blau, J.N., 114
Blisard, K.S., 164
Blumbergs, P., 246
Bogdahn, U., 205
Bohner, D., 154
Bonerandi, J.J., 256
Bonita, R., 53
Bonneterre, J., 256

Bornstein, M.B., 161
Borovich, B., 349, 350
Bose, A., 25
Bougnères, P.-F., 190
Bouvard, G., 391
Bowers, J., 113
Brann, B.S., IV, 85
Brass, L.M., 64
Brasswell, R., 235
Braun, J., 349, 350
Brega, K., 255
Breger, R.K., 8
Brem, H., 250
Brenton, D., 181
Brereton, A., 143
Bresolin, N., 189
Brody, B.A., 79
Brook, R.H., 71
Brooke, M.H., 149
Brown, G., 188
Brown, J., 46
Brown, L.M., 376
Brown, R.H., Jr., 150
Brown, S., 161
Brownstein, B.H., 143
Bruner, B.W., 325
Bruni, A.C., 45
Bruns, G.A.P., 150
Brzustowicz, L.M., 142
Bucholz, R.D., 210
Bucknall, R.C., 139
Buehler, B.A., 83
Bugat, R., 256
Bullock, R., 356
Bulstrode, C., 332
Burchiel, K.J., 381
Burger, P.C., 17, 250, 365
Burkhart, L.E., 258
Burton, L.E., 135
Busto, R., 318
Byl, F.M., 192

C

Camaert, J.J., 357
Camfield, C.S., 97
Camfield, P.R., 97
Campbell, J.N., 333
Cantu, J.-M., 45
Carenzi, A., 189
Carlson, A.M., 98
Carr, L.A., 137
Carter, L.P., 208, 300
Casasco, A., 230
Cascino, G.D., 17
Casentini, L., 239
Cassady, J.R., 250
Castellano, G., 73
Castelli, E., 189
Cech, T., 334
Cendra, E., 58
Cetas, T.C., 250
Chabal, S., 125

413

A Simple, Once-a-Year Dose!

Review the partial list of titles below. And then request your own FREE 30-day preview. When you purchase a Year Book, we'll also send you an automatic notice of future volumes about two months before they publish.

This system was designed for your convenience and to take up as little of your time as possible. If you do not want the Year Book, the advance notice makes it easy for you to let us know. And if you elect to receive the new Year Book, you need do nothing. We will send it on publication.

No worry. No wasted motion. And, of course, every Year Book is yours to examine FREE of charge for thirty days.

Year Book of **Anesthesia**® (22137)
Year Book of **Cardiology**® (22114)
Year Book of **Critical Care Medicine**® (22091)
Year Book of **Dermatology**® (22108)
Year Book of **Diagnostic Radiology**® (22132)
Year Book of **Digestive Diseases**® (22081)
Year Book of **Drug Therapy**® (22139)
Year Book of **Emergency Medicine**® (22085)
Year Book of **Endocrinology**® (22107)
Year Book of **Family Practice**® (20801)
Year Book of **Geriatrics and Gerontology** (22121)
Year Book of **Hand Surgery**® (22096)
Year Book of **Hematology**® (22604)
Year Book of **Health Care Management**® (21145)
Year Book of **Infectious Diseases**® (22606)
Year Book of **Infertility** (22093)
Year Book of **Medicine**® (22087)
Year Book of **Neonatal-Perinatal Medicine** (22117)
Year Book of **Neurology and Neurosurgery**® (22120)
Year Book of **Nuclear Medicine**® (22140)
Year Book of **Obstetrics and Gynecology**® (22118)
Year Book of **Occupational and Environmental Medicine** (22092)
Year Book of **Oncology** (22128)
Year Book of **Ophthalmology**® (22135)
Year Book of **Orthopedics**® (22116)
Year Book of **Otolaryngology – Head and Neck Surgery**® (22086)
Year Book of **Pathology and Clinical Pathology**® (22104)
Year Book of **Pediatrics**® (22088)
Year Book of **Plastic and Reconstructive Surgery**® (22112)
Year Book of **Psychiatry and Applied Mental Health**® (22110)
Year Book of **Pulmonary Disease**® (22109)
Year Book of **Sports Medicine**® (22115)
Year Book of **Surgery**® (22084)
Year Book of **Ultrasound** (21170)
Year Book of **Urology**® (22094)
Year Book of **Vascular Surgery**® (22105)

Mosby-Year Book, Inc. • 11830 Westline Industrial Drive • St. Louis, MO 63146